PSYCHOPHARMACOLOGY

PSYCHOPHARMACOLOGY
A Concise Overview

THIRD EDITION

ARASH ANSARI, MD

Assistant Professor of Psychiatry
Harvard Medical School
Cambridge, MA

DAVID N. OSSER, MD

Associate Professor of Psychiatry
Harvard Medical School
VA Boston Healthcare System
Brockton, MA

OXFORD
UNIVERSITY PRESS

Oxford University Press is a department of the University of Oxford. It furthers
the University's objective of excellence in research, scholarship, and education
by publishing worldwide. Oxford is a registered trade mark of Oxford University
Press in the UK and certain other countries.

Published in the United States of America by Oxford University Press
198 Madison Avenue, New York, NY 10016, United States of America.

Library of Congress Cataloging-in-Publication Data
Names: Ansari, Arash, author. | Osser, David N. (David Neal), author.
Title: Psychopharmacology : a concise overview / Arash Ansari, MD,
Assistant Professor of Psychiatry, Harvard Medical School
David N. Osser, MD, Associate Professor of Psychiatry, Harvard Medical School.
Description: 3rd edition. | New York : Oxford University Press, [2020] |
Includes bibliographical references and index.
Identifiers: LCCN 2020012365 (print) | LCCN 2020012366 (ebook) |
ISBN 9780197537046 (paperback) | ISBN 9780197537060 (epub) |
ISBN 9780197537077
Subjects: LCSH: Psychopharmacology. | Psychotropic drugs.
Classification: LCC RM315 .A63 2020 (print) |
LCC RM315 (ebook) | DDC 615.7/8—dc23
LC record available at https://lccn.loc.gov/2020012365
LC ebook record available at https://lccn.loc.gov/2020012366

9 8 7 6 5 4 3 2
Printed by Marquis, Canada

Contents

List of Tables

About the Authors

Arash Ansari, MD, is an Assistant Professor of Psychiatry at Harvard Medical School. Over the past 20 years, he has taught psychopharmacology to Harvard Medical School students and psychiatric residents. Dr. Ansari practiced inpatient and outpatient psychiatry at the Brigham and Women's Faulkner Hospital, where he received the 2008 Arthur R. Kravitz, MD Award for Excellence in Psychiatric Teaching and Education. He has subsequently practiced psychiatry in private practice and at the Harvard University Health Services in Cambridge, MA.

David N. Osser, MD, is an Associate Professor of Psychiatry at Harvard Medical School and attending psychiatrist at the VA Boston Healthcare System, Brockton Division, where he organizes the psychopharmacology curriculum for residents at the Harvard South Shore Psychiatry Residency Training Program. He is general editor of the website www.psychopharm.mobi. Dr. Osser was the recipient of the 2012 Mentorship Award from the American Psychiatric Association "in recognition of substantial and formative contributions to the mentoring of students and residents throughout a distinguished career in psychiatric research" and the 2015 Stuart T. Hauser Mentorship Award in Psychiatry from the Harvard Medical School Psychiatry Executive Committee.

Dr. Ansari and Dr. Osser do not have any affiliations with the pharmaceutical industry.

Author Disclaimer

The information presented in this manuscript is meant to be an overview of some of the major topics in psychopharmacology and an introduction to the field, but not a handbook for the administration of available psychotropics. Specifics regarding clinical use of medications including doses are presented for educational purposes only. Although every effort has been made to present the material accurately, we cannot rule out typographical or other errors. As always, the package insert of each medication should be reviewed prior to prescription and administration, and treatment should be customized to the needs and characteristics of the individual patient after a thorough psychiatric evaluation.

Preface

This book is an updated and expanded edition of the authors' previous editions of the books titled *Psychopharmacology: A Concise Overview for Students and Clinicians, 2nd Edition*, published in 2015, and *Psychopharmacology for Medical Students*, published in 2009.

Information about newly available and emerging medications has been included. Although much of what was known about psychopharmacology and included in the previous editions is still current, this new text addresses recent areas of controversy and further changes in emphasis that have developed over the past few years. Sections related to the clinical use of psychotropics for the treatment of relevant psychiatric (and some nonpsychiatric) disorders have been expanded significantly in this edition. New sections on recently emerging pharmacotherapies, as well as sections on the use of psychiatric medications in women of childbearing potential (including implications in pregnancy and breastfeeding) have been added. As before, the authors' goal in this edition has been to help practicing clinicians as well as students gain access to information that may help them provide optimum patient care.

Introduction

The use of psychotropic medicines to treat psychiatric illness has increased dramatically in recent times. Although the biological etiologies of most psychiatric disorders are still unclear, effective pharmacological treatments have been developed over the past 60 to 70 years that have become part of the standard of care.

Psychiatric medications are part of the armamentarium of most practicing physicians and prescribers, regardless of medical specialty. Although more severe types of mental illness are likely to be treated by psychiatrists, most prescriptions for psychotropics (e.g., anxiolytics and newer antidepressants) are written by non-psychiatrists (Stagnitti 2008). Psychiatric medications remain consistently prominent in the list of the top 200 most prescribed medications and in the top 20 pharmaceuticals in terms of sales in the United States (ClinCalc 2019). From 2008 to 2012, medications for "mental health" were ranked as the third top therapeutic class (after antihypertensives and pain medications) in the number of dispensed prescriptions (IMS Health 2014).

As in the treatment of all medical disorders, a thorough evaluation must precede psychiatric diagnosis and subsequent psychopharmacological treatment. A complete history should be obtained, and the patient should be examined. Medical or neurological etiologies that may contribute to the presentation of psychiatric illness should be identified and addressed. Nearly 10% of patients presenting with a psychiatric complaint will turn out to have a medical problem as the primary cause (Hall, Popkin et al. 1978). Active substance abuse, if present, should be treated before or at the same time that pharmacological therapies are initiated. Obtaining collateral information from other treating clinicians and patients' significant others may also be needed in many cases.

Once a clear diagnosis is made, one should consider whether the condition requires medication treatment. Mild to moderate anxiety and depression, for example, often respond equally well to supportive interventions or psychotherapy (King, Sibbald et al. 2000; Barkham and Hardy 2001; American Psychiatric Association [APA] 2010; Farah, Alsawas et al. 2016), and the addition of pharmacological treatments may provide only minor benefit (Cuijpers, van Straten et al. 2010; Tolin 2017). Antidepressants may be less efficacious than previously thought for the treatment of milder forms of depression (see chapter on antidepressants).

On the other hand, if the psychiatric disorder or symptoms are severe, or if psychosis, mania, or dangerousness is present, then psychopharmacological treatments (and referral to a psychiatrist) are usually indicated. Although many primary care physicians may be quite comfortable with their ability to manage psychiatric illness, the amount of monitoring that is required to provide adequate follow-up should be taken into account before initiating treatment. When treating moderate to severe psychiatric illness, optimum therapy often includes the use of concomitant psychotherapy in addition to pharmacotherapeutic measures (Keller, McCullough et al. 2007; Banerjee, Shamash et al. 1996; Reynolds, Frank et al. 1999; Katon, Von Korff et al. 1999; Miklowitz 2008; APA 2010; Oestergaard and Moldrup 2011).

***

The following chapters review the major categories of psychiatric medications, including antidepressants, anxiolytics, antipsychotics, mood stabilizers, and medicines for attention-deficit/

hyperactivity disorder and substance use disorders. The most commonly used medications in each category are discussed. For each medication, its mechanism of action and specific properties and characteristics are reviewed. Potential adverse effects are thoroughly discussed given that medication tolerability is a significant determinant of appropriate therapy. The primary injunction for physicians is to "first, do no harm."

Of note, the focus of this book is psychopharmacology as it pertains to adults only. Children and adolescents may tolerate or respond to these medications differently—and the use of psychopharmacological therapies in these younger age groups is outside the scope of this book. Observations about medication responses in adolescents are included here only where they are relevant to discussions about adult pharmacotherapy.

For some disorders, there are new and emerging pharmacotherapies that are being studied. Some remain investigational in the United States. Others have been recently approved by the Food and Drug Administration (FDA) but have not yet become part of routine treatment. Their safety has not yet been established in clinical practice—they are works in progress.

After a thorough discussion of prescription psychiatric medications, the most commonly studied alternative and complementary medicines (e.g., compounds that are considered "dietary" or "herbal" supplements) are also briefly discussed. Over-the-counter supplements are often considered by patients as a way to avoid the use of conventional (but evidence-based) antidepressants and their real (or imagined) potential adverse effects. However, these supplements are often not as well studied as available prescription drugs. Furthermore, the lack of regulation by the FDA allows for significant variability in available formulations, and there are concerns that what is ostensibly sold might not be what is actually in the bottle. Although many herbal and nutritional supplements are well tolerated, it should not be assumed that they have no risks. Systemic risks cannot be ruled out, and risks relevant to a particular agent should be investigated before a supplement is considered. The main focus of this book, however, is a review of available prescription drugs, which have benefited from being more stringently regulated.

***

Appropriate clinical use of evidence-supported prescription medications depends on findings from pre- and post-marketing studies as well as from available treatment algorithms and consensus guidelines.

Randomized placebo-controlled trials, using strict exclusionary criteria when selecting subjects, have traditionally been used to study a psychiatric medication's *efficacy* (i.e., the ability of the medication to treat the condition better than placebo under controlled conditions). For example, studies comparing an antidepressant to placebo may use an eight-week double-blind parallel design and include subjects with major depression but without any other medical or psychiatric comorbidities. Response may be defined as a 50% improvement in a chosen outcome rating scale. These efficacy studies provide the response data that pharmaceutical companies must submit to the FDA to obtain approvals and specific indications for developed drugs. However, in these studies, the use of exclusionary criteria and varying definitions of response limit their applicability to the general patient population, which often presents with more complex comorbid problems.

Post-marketing *effectiveness* studies, on the other hand, are often larger, naturalistic studies that attempt to approximate real-world conditions by studying patients who may have psychiatric and medical comorbidities and by relying on broader outcome measures for assessing response. These studies may compare outcomes of treatment with multiple medications. As such, effectiveness studies add to our understanding of how well the drugs work (Summerfelt and Meltzer 1998). National Institute of Mental

Health–sponsored effectiveness studies have the added benefit of funding from a neutral (non-pharmaceutical industry) source, thereby avoiding possible study design shortcomings or evaluator biases that may influence study results (Heres, Davis et al. 2006; Osser 2008). These studies include (a) the Clinical Antipsychotic Trials of Intervention Effectiveness (CATIE; Keefe, Bilder et al. 2007; Lieberman, Stroup et al. 2005; Fervaha, Agid et al. 2014; Jakubovski, Carlson et al. 2015), (b) the Sequenced Treatment Alternatives to Relieve Depression Study (STAR*D; Rush, Trivedi et al. 2006; McGrath, Stewart et al. 2006; Nierenberg, Fava et al. 2006; Trivedi, Fava et al. 2006; Fava, Rush et al. 2006; Pigott 2015; Mojtabai 2017; Steiner, Boulos et al. 2017), (c) the Systematic Treatment Enhancement Program for Bipolar Disorder (STEP-BD; Sachs, Nierenberg et al. 2007; Goldberg, Perlis et al. 2007; Miklowitz, Otto et al. 2007; Tada, Uchida et al. 2015; Mousavi, Johnson et al. 2018), (d) the Clinical Antipsychotic Trials of Intervention Effectiveness–Alzheimer's Disease (CATIE-AD; Schneider, Tariot et al. 2006; Sultzer, Davis et al. 2008; Vigen, Mack et al. 2011; Yoshida, Roberts et al. 2017), and (e) the National Institute of Alcohol Abuse and Alcoholism (NIAAA) sponsored Combined Pharmacotherapies and Behavioral Interventions study (COMBINE; Anton, O'Malley et al. 2006; Anton, Oroszi et al. 2008; Leggio, Ray et al. 2009). Findings from these studies continue to influence clinical psychiatric practice.

Students and clinicians can access available treatment guidelines and algorithms to help guide the choice of treatment for each disorder. Numerous international guidelines—for example, those from the APA, the UK-based National Institute for Health and Clinical Excellence, and the World Federation of Societies of Biological Psychiatry—exist to help clinicians.

Evidence-based algorithms, such as those of the Psychopharmacology Algorithm Project of the Harvard South Shore Program (of which one of this book's authors [D.O.] is the general editor; Ansari and Osser 2010; Osser and Dunlop 2010;

Bajor, Ticlea et al. 2011; Tang and Osser 2012; Osser, Roudsari et al. 2013; Mohammad and Osser 2014; Hamoda and Osser 2008; Stein, Baldwin et al. 2010; Stein, Koen et al. 2012; Abejuela and Osser 2016; Giakoumatos and Osser 2019; Beaulieu, Tabasky et al. 2019; Wang and Osser 2019) can be helpful in guiding and prioritizing treatments when multiple agents are available for the same condition.

Even after the characteristics, efficacy, effectiveness, and risk profiles of individual medications have been understood, the student or clinician should still consider multiple clinical variables prior to selecting a specific agent. The prescriber should take the following into account: (a) patient acuity and the need to address the most dangerous presenting symptoms (e.g., behavioral agitation, suicidality, catatonia, etc.) first, (b) the patient's past treatment history, (c) pre-existing medical conditions to minimize any increase in medical risk, (d) possible medication interactions, (e) the time required for amelioration of symptoms, (f) a medication's known side effects and how these may subsequently affect presenting symptoms, (g) the desirability of minimizing the use of unnecessary polytherapy, (h) possible pharmacogenetic factors and hereditary patterns of drug response and tolerance, and (i) financial cost–benefit considerations (Ansari, Osser et al. 2009). Regardless of which disorder is being treated, these factors play a significant role in arriving at the appropriate pharmacotherapy. This is a time-consuming process, but only by evaluating the patient thoroughly, including gaining understanding of psychosocial and developmental circumstances that may be contributing to the current symptoms, can proper psychopharmacology be administered. Unfortunately, in the current healthcare environment, time is the resource that may be the least available to the prescriber. Healthcare professionals need to insist on being allowed the necessary time with their patients to minimize errors and optimize outcomes.

In addition to the indication for which a psychiatric medication is initially FDA-approved (e.g., an antidepressant for major depressive disorder), other indications may be established at later dates. Furthermore, medicines are frequently used for non-approved ("off-label") psychiatric indications (e.g., an antidepressant for insomnia) or for the treatment of other medical or neurological disorders. Where applicable, these other uses are also discussed in the following chapters.

***

The use of psychotropics in pregnant women and during lactation is also discussed in each chapter. It has been estimated that up to 50% of all pregnancies in the United States may be unplanned (Mosher and Bachrach 1996). If so, it behooves the clinician to consider the specific risks and benefits of medications during pregnancy for all women of childbearing potential.

The use of psychotropics during pregnancy has been widely studied and broad conclusions have been drawn from retrospective and prospective observational studies of registries of pregnant women taking psychotropic medications. The observed rates of congenital anomalies have been compared to the baseline rate of 2% to 4% (Holmes 1976; Centers for Disease Control and Prevention 2008). It is important to note that due to obvious ethical considerations, prospective double-blind placebo-controlled studies can never be used to arrive at more definitive conclusions about the tolerability and safety of medicines used during pregnancy. There is even less known about any long-term neurodevelopmental effects of these medicines on the fetus. Data about adverse effects of psychiatric medications can be accessed through the Developmental and Toxicology Reproductive Database (DART): http://toxnet.nlm.nih.gov/newtonxnet/dart.htm.

The risks and benefits of taking medications during pregnancy should be balanced against the risks and benefits of not taking medications (i.e., leaving the untreated pregnant mother vulnerable to psychiatric illness). Often there are relevant studies available showing the impact of untreated illness on the mother and fetus. The severity of the untreated illness, along with the availability of alternative non-psychopharmacological therapies are also factors that should be considered. Ultimately, the decision to accept or decline a psychiatric medication is a very personal one for the mother, although access to information and consultation with other psychiatric and non-psychiatric healthcare providers are often helpful as the mother is supported through the decision-making process.

The clinician should also have some familiarity with the risks and benefits of medications during breastfeeding. The National Institute of Health's Toxicology Data Network (TOXNET): LactMed database, https://toxnet.nlm.nih.gov/newtoxnet/lactmed.htm, is an online database that summarizes current evidence about medications and breastfeeding and serves as an excellent updated reference for both patients and prescribers.

***

Finally, each chapter includes a table of relevant psychiatric medications that are most commonly encountered in clinical practice. Adult dosing, additional characteristics, "black box" warnings, and FDA-approved indications for each medication are listed. The information provided is for educational purposes only; the package insert should be consulted and specific patient characteristics should be reviewed before any treatment is initiated.

***

As in other areas of medical practice, the appropriate use of psychiatric medications is an art as well as a science. Art and science are combined when a clinician is able to support a patient in the acceptance of evidence-supported treatments with reasonable safety. However, sometimes the patient will have a strong preference for a treatment other than the one that is recommended by the clinician, who will need then to be prepared to work with those preferences. Still, safety concerns may need to override patient preferences.

The prescriber's relationship with his or her patient is of paramount importance. The patient's distress needs to be understood holistically within the person's overall life context. When the patient's distress is understood and the patient is respected, subjective distress is often diminished and therapeutic alliance and treatment adherence are more likely to be improved (Salzman, Glick et al. 2010; Stahl 2000). Treatment is then more likely to be successful.

Pharmacotherapy may be associated with complicated biological consequences (e.g., adverse side effects) and psychosocial implications (e.g., stigmatizing consequences of having a psychiatric illness and taking medication), and the clinician needs to remain attentive to his or her patients' needs during treatment. The psychopharmacological treatment of psychiatric disorders can be a complex endeavor.

References

Abejuela HR, Osser DN (2016). The Psychopharmacology Algorithm Project at the Harvard South Shore Program: an algorithm for generalized anxiety disorder. Harv Rev Psychiatry 24(4): 243–256.

American Psychiatric Association (2010). Practice guideline for the treatment of patients with major depressive disorder, third edition. Am J Psychiatry, 167(10, Suppl): 1–118.

Ansari A, Osser DN (2010). The Psychopharmacology Algorithm Project at the Harvard South Shore Program: an update on bipolar depression. Harv Rev Psychiatry 18(1): 36–55.

Ansari A, Osser DN, Lai LS, Schoenfeld PM, Potts KC (2009). Pharmacological approach to the psychiatric inpatient, in Ovsiew F, Munich RL (eds),

Principles of inpatient psychiatry. Philadelphia, PA: Lippincott Williams & Wilkins. Pages 43–69.

Anton RF, O'Malley SS, et al. (2006). Combined pharmacotherapies and behavioral interventions for alcohol dependence: the COMBINE study: a randomized controlled trial. JAMA 295: 2003–2017.

Anton RF, Oroszi G, et al. (2008). An evaluation of mu-opioid receptor (OPRM1) as a predictor of naltrexone response in the treatment of alcohol dependence: results from the Combined Pharmacotherapies and Behavioral Interventions for Alcohol Dependence (COMBINE) study. Arch Gen Psychiatry 65: 135–144.

Bajor LA, Ticlea AN, et al. (2011). The Psychopharmacology Algorithm Project at the Harvard South Shore Program: an update on posttraumatic stress disorder. Harv Rev Psychiatry 19(5): 240–258.

Banerjee S, Shamash K, et al. (1996). Randomized controlled trial of effect of intervention by psychogeriatric team on depression in frail elderly people at home. Brit Med J 313: 1058–1061.

Barkham M, Hardy GE (2001). Counseling and interpersonal therapies for depression: towards securing an evidence-base. Brit Med Bull 57: 115–132.

Beaulieu AM, Tabasky E, Osser DN (2019). The psychopharmacology algorithm project at the Harvard South Shore Program: an algorithm for adults with obsessive-compulsive disorder. Psychiatry Res 281: 112583.

Centers for Disease Control and Prevention (2008). Update on overall prevalence of major birth defects—Atlanta, Georgia, 1978–2005. MMWR 57(1): 1–5.

ClinCalc (2019). The top 200 drugs of 2018. http://clincalc.com/DrugStats

Cuijpers P, Van Straten A, et al. (2010). The contribution of active medication to combined treatments of psychotherapy and pharmacotherapy for adult depression: a meta-analysis. Acta Psychiatr Scand 121(6): 415–423.

Farah WH, Alsawas M, Mainou M, et al. (2016). Non-pharmacological treatment of depression: a systematic review and evidence map. Evid Based Med 21(6): 214–221.

Fava M, Rush AJ, et al. (2006). A comparison of mirtazapine and nortriptyline following two consecutive failed medication treatments for depressed outpatients: a STAR*D report. Am J Psychiatry 163: 1161–1172.

Fervaha G, Agid O, et al. (2014). Effect of antipsychotic medication on overall life satisfaction among individuals with chronic schizophrenia: findings from the NIMH CATIE study. Eur Neuropsychopharmacol 24(7): 1078–1085.

Giakoumatos CI, Osser D (2019). The Psychopharmacology Algorithm Project at the Harvard South Shore Program: an update on unipolar nonpsychotic depression. *Harv Rev Psychiatry* 27(1): 33–52.

Goldberg JF, Perlis RH, et al. (2007). Adjunctive antidepressant use and symptomatic recovery among bipolar depressed patients with concomitant manic symptoms: findings from the STEP-BD. Am J Psychiatry 164: 1348–1355.

Hall RC, Popkin MK, et al. (1978). Physical illness presenting as psychiatric disease. Arch Gen Psychiatry 35: 1315–1320.

Hamoda HM, Osser DN (2008). The Psychopharmacology Algorithm Project at the Harvard South Shore Program: an update on psychotic depression. Harv Rev Psychiatry 16(4): 235–247.

Heres S, Davis J, et al. (2006). Why olanzapine beats risperidone, risperidone beats quetiapine, and quetiapine beats olanzapine: an exploratory analysis of head-to-head comparison studies of second-generation antipsychotics. Am J Psychiatry 163: 185–194.

Holmes LB (1976). Current concepts in genetics: congenital malformations. N Engl J Med 295(4): 204–207.

IMS (2014). IMS Health. Top therapeutic classes by dispensed prescriptions (U.S.). http://www.imshealth.com/deployedfiles/imshealth/Global/Content/Corporate/Press Room/2012_U.S/Top_Therapeutic_Classes_Dispensed_Prescriptions_2012.pdf

Jakubovski E, Carlson JP, Bloch MH (2015). Prognostic subgroups for remission, response, and treatment continuation in the Clinical Antipsychotic Trials of Intervention Effectiveness (CATIE) trial. J Clin Psychiatry 76(11): 1535–1545.

Katon W, Von Korff M, et al. (1999). Stepped collaborative care for primary care patients with persistent symptoms of depression: a randomized trial. Arch Gen Psychiatry 56: 1109–1115.

Keefe RS, Bilder RM, et al. (2007). Neurocognitive effects of antipsychotic medications in patients with chronic schizophrenia in the CATIE trial. Arch Gen Psychiatry 64: 633–647.

Keller MB, McCullough JP, et al. (2007). A comparison of nefazodone, the cognitive behavioral-analysis system of psychotherapy, and their combination for the treatment of chronic depression. N Engl J Med 342: 1462–1470.

King M, Sibbald B, et al. (2000). Randomized controlled trial of non-directive counseling, cognitive-behavior therapy and usual general practitioner care in the management of depression as well as mixed anxiety and depression in primary care. Health Technol Assess 4: 1–83.

Leggio L, Ray LA, et al. (2009). Blood glucose level, alcohol heavy drinking, and alcohol craving during treatment for alcohol dependence: results from the Combined Pharmacotherapies and Behavioral Interventions for Alcohol Dependence (COMBINE) study. Alcohol Clin Exp Res 33(9): 1539–1544.

Lieberman JA, Stroup TS, et al. (2005). Effectiveness of antipsychotic drugs in patients with chronic schizophrenia. N Engl J Med 353: 1209–1223.

McGrath PJ, Stewart JW, et al. (2006). Tranylcypromine versus venlafaxine plus mirtazapine following three failed antidepressant medication trials for depression: a STAR*D report. Am J Psychiatry 163: 1531–1541.

Miklowitz, D. J. (2008). Adjunctive psychotherapy for bipolar disorder: state of the evidence. Am J Psychiatry 165: 1408–1419.

Miklowitz DJ, Otto MW, et al. (2007). Psychosocial treatments for bipolar depression: a 1-year randomized trial from the Systematic Treatment Enhancement Program. Arch Gen Psychiatry 64: 419–426.

Mohammad OM, Osser DN (2014). The Psychopharmacology Algorithm Project at the Harvard South Shore Program: an algorithm for acute mania. Harv Rev Psychiatry 22(5): 274–294.

Mojtabai R (2017). Nonremission and time to remission among remitters in major depressive disorder: revisiting STAR*D. Depress Anxiety 34(12): 1123–1133.

Mosher WD, Bachrach CA (1996). Understanding U.S. fertility: continuity and change in the National Survey of Family Growth, 1988–1995. Fam Plann Perspect 28(1): 4–12.

Mousavi Z, Johnson S, Li D (2018). Does recent mania affect response to antidepressants in bipolar disorder? A re-analysis of STEP-BD data. J Affect Disord 236: 136–139.

Nierenberg AA, Fava M, et al. (2006). A comparison of lithium and T(3) augmentation following two failed medication treatments for depression: a STAR*D report. Am J Psychiatry 163: 1519–1530.

Oestergaard S, Moldrup C (2011). Optimal duration of combined psychotherapy and pharmacotherapy for patients with moderate and severe depression: a meta-analysis. J Affect Disord 131(1–3): 24–36.

Osser DN (2008). Cleaning up evidence-based psychopharmacology. Psychopharm Review 43: 19–25.

Osser DN, Dunlop LR (2010). The Psychopharmacology Algorithm Project at the Harvard South Shore Program: an update on generalized social anxiety disorder. Psychopharm Review 45: 91–98.

Osser DN, Roudsari MJ, et al. (2013). The Psychopharmacology Algorithm Project at the Harvard South Shore Program: an update on schizophrenia. Harv Rev Psychiatry 21(1): 18–40.

Pigott HE (2015). The STAR*D trial: it is time to reexamine the clinical beliefs that guide the treatment of major depression. Can J Psychiatry 60(1): 9–13.

Reynolds CF, Frank E, et al. (1999). Nortriptyline and interpersonal psychotherapy as maintenance therapies for recurrent major depression: a randomized controlled trial in patients older than 59 years. JAMA 281: 39–45.

Rush AJ, Trivedi MH, et al. (2006). Acute and longer-term outcomes in depressed outpatients requiring one or several treatment steps: A STAR*D report. Am J Psychiatry 163: 1905–1917.

Sachs GS, Nierenberg AA, et al. (2007). Effectiveness of adjunctive antidepressant treatment for bipolar depression. N Engl J Med 356: 1711–1722.

Salzman C, Glick I, et al. (2010). The 7 sins of psychopharmacology. J Clin Psychopharmacol 30(6): 653–655.

Schneider LS, Tariot PN, et al. (2006). Effectiveness of atypical antipsychotic drugs in patients with Alzheimer's disease. N Engl J Med 355: 1525–1538.

Stagnitti MN (2008). Antidepressants prescribed by medical doctors in office based and outpatient settings by specialty for the U.S. civilian non-institutionalized population, 2002 and 2005. Statistical Brief #206. Medical Expenditure Panel Survey. Agency for Healthcare Research and Quality.

Stahl SM (2000). The 7 habits of highly effective psychopharmacologists: overview. J Clin Psychiatry 61(4): 242–243.

Stein, DJ, Baldwin DS, et al. (2010). A 2010 evidence-based algorithm for the pharmacotherapy of social anxiety disorder. Curr Psychiatry Rep 12(5): 471–477.

Stein, DJ, Koen N, et al. (2012). A 2012 evidence-based algorithm for the pharmacotherapy for obsessive-compulsive disorder. Curr Psychiatry Rep 14(3): 211–219.

Steiner AJ, Boulos N, et al. (2017). Major depressive disorder in patients with doctoral degrees: patient-reported depressive symptom severity, functioning, and quality of life before and after initial treatment in the STAR*D study. J Psychiatr Pract 23(5): 328–341.

Sultzer DL, Davis SM, et al. (2008). Clinical symptom responses to atypical antipsychotic medications in Alzheimer's disease: phase 1 outcomes from the CATIE-AD effectiveness trial. Am J Psychiatry 165: 844–854.

Summerfelt WT, Meltzer HY (1998). Efficacy vs. effectiveness in psychiatric research. Psychiatr Serv 49: 834–835.

Tada M, Uchida H, et al. (2015). Antidepressant dose and treatment response in bipolar depression: reanalysis of the Systematic Treatment Enhancement Program for Bipolar Disorder (STEP-BD) data. J Psychiatr Res 68: 151–156.

Tang, M, Osser DN (2012). The Psychopharmacology Algorithm Project at the Harvard South Shore program: 2012 update on psychotic depression. J Mood Dis 2(4): 168–179.

Tolin DF (2017). Can cognitive behavioral therapy for anxiety and depression be improved with pharmacotherapy? A meta-analysis. Psychiatr Clin North Am 40(4): 715–738.

Trivedi MH, Fava M, et al. (2006). Medication augmentation after the failure of SSRIs for depression. N Engl J Med 354: 1243–1252.

Vigen CL, Mack WJ, et al. (2011). Cognitive effects of atypical antipsychotic medications in patients with Alzheimer's disease: Outcomes from CATIE-AD. Am J Psychiatry 168(8): 831–839.

Wang D, Osser DN (2019). The psychopharmacology algorithm project at the Harvard South Shore Program: an update on bipolar depression. Bipolar Disord. doi:10.1111/bdi.12860

Yoshida K, Roberts R, et al. (2017). Lack of early improvement with antipsychotics is a marker for subsequent nonresponse in behavioral and psychological symptoms of dementia: analysis of CATIE-AD data. Am J Geriatr Psychiatry 25(7): 708–716.

1

Antidepressants

Antidepressants are medications that have been found to be effective for the treatment of depressive syndromes, including (acute and chronic) major depression and persistent depressive disorder (dysthymia). These syndromal states are characterized by the presence of depressed mood or loss of interest for most of the day (nearly every day for at least two weeks in the case of major depression and for more days than not for most of two years in the case of dysthymia) plus associated clinical symptoms (i.e., neurovegetative changes such as loss of energy, disturbed sleep and appetite, and cognitive symptoms). Depressive syndromes are sometimes described as "clinical depression" to distinguish them from unhappiness or sadness that occurs in reaction to distressing life events. Antidepressants are not generally better than placebo or general supportive measures for treating "depressed mood" alone when no other associated symptoms are present. However, lay misconceptions that antidepressants act as "happy pills" are unfortunately still common.

Theories about the pathophysiology of depression are plentiful, but none are proven. The inexact term "chemical imbalance," ubiquitously used or implied in the pharmaceutical industry marketing of antidepressant products, can be helpful in reducing the stigma of mental disorders by characterizing them as a biological (i.e., medical) illnesses. However, this term, which is best avoided in scientific as well as doctor–patient discourse, is a gross misrepresentation of the complexities in the pathophysiological mechanism of depression. It also tends to obfuscate the psychosocial factors that may have contributed to the development of the depressive state. Antidepressants are only one aspect of the treatment of patients with depression, and they should be used along with psychosocial treatment modalities when indicated (Cuijpers 2014).

Most available antidepressants primarily affect the serotonin (i.e., 5-hydroxytryptamine [5-HT]) and norepinephrine neurotransmitter systems. Serotonin and norepinephrine (along with dopamine and histamine) are monoamines (Nestler, Hyman et al. 2015). Norepinephrine secreting neurons originate primarily from the locus ceruleus (and lateral tegmental areas) and project widely to almost all areas of the brain and spinal cord. Serotonergic neurons reside in the dorsal and median raphé nuclei in the brainstem and diffusely make contact with most areas of the brain. Most antidepressants increase the available amount of norepinephrine and/or serotonin at the neuronal synapse by decreasing the reuptake of these neurotransmitters into the presynaptic cell. They do so by inhibiting the norepinephrine transporter and/or the serotonin transporter or by delaying the metabolism of these neurotransmitters. Other antidepressants have direct effects on monoamine receptors.

Genetic polymorphisms of the norepinephrine and serotonin reuptake transporters (Kim, Lim et al. 2006; Porcelli, Fabbri et al. 2012) as well as polymorphisms of post-synaptic serotonin receptors (McMahon, Buervenich et al. 2006) have been associated with differences in responses to different antidepressants. Once synaptic changes have taken place with treatment, long-term adaptations in post-synaptic neurons, which include changes in intracellular mediators and resultant changes in gene expression, may be responsible for alleviating depression (Nestler, Hyman et al. 2015; Niciu, Ionescu et al. 2013; Hodgson, Tansey et al. 2016).

Other mechanisms of action have also been proposed for the therapeutic effects of currently available antidepressants. Antidepressants may increase brain-derived neurotrophic factor, which may serve to undo the downregulation of hippocampal neurogenesis that may occur secondary to stress (Masi and Brovedani 2011). Hippocampal neurogenesis, and/or the formation of new synapses, and re-organization of new neurons may also explain the therapeutic effects of antidepressants (Tang, Helmeste et al. 2012). Anti-inflammatory effects have also been proposed as antidepressants' mechanisms of action (Nazimek, Strobel et al. 2017; Galecki, Mossakowska-Wojcik et al. 2018). Anti-inflammatory agents have not been found to be particularly effective, but there are some promising data showing that markers for inflammation such as C-reactive protein might help predict response to certain antidepressants (Jha, Minhajuddin et al. 2017).

Tricyclic Antidepressants

Beginning with the introduction of imipramine in the late 1950s (Kuhn 1958), tricyclic antidepressants were among the first classes of antidepressants developed. They share a tricyclic structure (two benzene rings on either side of a seven-member ring), exhibit variable degrees of norepinephrine and serotonin reuptake inhibition, and are antagonists at several other neurotransmitter receptors (Yildiz, Gonul & Tamam 2002). Examples of tricyclic antidepressants (TCAs) that were commonly used include the tertiary amines **imipramine, amitriptyline, clomipramine,** and **doxepin,** and the secondary amines **desipramine** (metabolite of imipramine) and **nortriptyline** (metabolite of amitriptyline). Use of TCAs has dramatically declined since the development of newer antidepressants with fewer side effects starting in the 1980s. TCAs are difficult to tolerate: in a recent study of augmentation strategies after unsatisfactory response to a TCA, it took 14 years for a clinic in Barcelona, Spain to recruit 100 subjects (Navarro, Boulahfa et al. 2019).

All TCAs can cause the following adverse effects: (a) slowing of intracardiac conduction by inhibiting sodium channels as measured by QRS and QT prolongation, (b) anticholinergic effects such as dry mouth, urinary retention, and constipation due to muscarinic acetylcholine receptor antagonism, (c) orthostatic hypotension due to peripheral alpha-1-adrenergic antagonism, and (d) sedation and weight gain (except perhaps for desipramine) due to histamine (H1) receptor antagonism. For these reasons, TCAs need to be started at low doses and increased gradually, giving the patient time to accommodate to some of these effects. Individual differences in both severity of side effects and therapeutic effects (along with differences in therapeutic serum levels; Perry, Zeilmann et al. 1994) do exist among individual TCAs. There is some evidence to suggest that TCAs may have efficacy in the treatment of psychotic depression (Hamoda and Osser 2008; Tang and Osser 2012).

The cardiac effects of TCAs have contributed to a reduction in their use over the past 30 years. Prolonged QT interval (designated as the QTc when corrected for heart rate) may be associated with torsades de pointes, a potentially fatal ventricular arrhythmia. QT prolongation is also an issue with the use of other antidepressants like citalopram and some antipsychotic agents like ziprasidone, quetiapine, and risperidone (see antipsychotic chapter). All patients should have an electrocardiogram (ECG) to rule out any existing conduction abnormalities (such as bundle branch block) prior to considering TCAs. Patients with recent myocardial infarctions should not initiate treatment with these antidepressants. In addition, TCAs (more so than other antidepressants) may be associated with an increase in cardiovascular disease even in those not known to have a cardiac history prior to treatment (Hamer, David Batty et al. 2011). They may be associated with lower heart rate variability and increased mortality (Zimmermann-Viehoff, Kuehl et al. 2014; Noordam, van den Berg et al. 2016).

Most important, depressed patients who are at risk for suicide and overdose may not be appropriate for treatment with TCAs. It should be noted that a 1- to 2-week supply of these medications could be fatal in overdose due to the risk of cardiac arrhythmias. Therefore, depending on the patient's risk of suicide, clinicians may need to limit the number of tablets prescribed with each refill. This concern is significantly lessened with the use of many of the newer antidepressants that are safer in overdose.

TCAs are often used for their mild to moderate analgesic effects in the treatment of chronic pain syndromes including migraine headaches (Magni 1991). Analgesic effects are thought to be due to effects at the locus coeruleus as well as to noradrenergic changes in descending pathways in the spinal cord and inhibitory effects on peripheral dorsal ganglia (Kremer, Salvat et al. 2016; Obata 2017). These modest analgesic effects are independent of any effect on mood, with efficacy starting at lower doses and with response seen earlier than when used for depression (Magni 1991; Max, Culnane et al. 1987; Onghena and Van Houdenhove 1992). Analgesic effects may be independent of antidepressant serum concentrations (Sindrup, Holbech et al. 2017). TCAs may be more effective for chronic pain than primarily serotonergic antidepressants (selective serotonin reuptake inhibitors [SSRIs]; see later discussion; Ansari 2000; Fishbain 2000; Saarto and Wiffen 2007; Jackson, Mancuso et al. 2017).

Monoamine Oxidase Inhibitors

Monoamine oxidase is an enzyme that acts to metabolize monoamines, both intracellularly and extracellularly. Its inhibition increases the amount of the monoamines serotonin, norepinephrine, and dopamine available for neurotransmission. Monoamine oxidase inhibitors (MAOIs) can act on two isomers of monoamine oxidase enzymes: MAO-A (found in the brain as well as intestines—it metabolizes all the previously discussed neurotransmitters) and MAO-B (found in the brain and platelets and primarily metabolizes dopamine). If an MAOI acts on both isomers, it is termed "nonselective"; it is "selective" if only acting on one or the other isomer. Generally MAO-A inhibition is thought to be necessary for antidepressant effect (Thase 2012; Goldberg & Thase 2013).

The first MAOI, iproniazid, an antituberculosis drug, was discovered in the 1950s. The nonselective MAOIs **tranylcypromine, phenelzine, isocarboxazid**, and the more recently available **transdermal selegiline** (an anti-parkinsonian MAO-B selective agent that is nonselective at higher doses) are MAOIs that are currently available in the United States for the treatment of depression. These antidepressants may be particularly effective for patients with depressive syndromes also meeting criteria for the atypical features specifier (in DSM-5; i.e., two of the following four symptoms: hyperphagia, hypersomnia, a heavy leaden feeling in the limbs, and severe sensitivity to criticism or rejection as a personality trait; Quitkin, Stewart et al. 1993). Atypical depression is not rare. A recent large study found the prevalence of atypical depression was about 15% among depressed patients in China (Xin, Chen et al. 2019).

Although mild serotonergic side effects (see later discussion on SSRIs) and orthostatic hypotension can occur with routine MAOI use, there are two other primary areas of concern that limit the use of these agents (Lippman and Nash 1990). First, dangerous interactions can occur with certain foods containing tyramine, such as aged cheeses and red wines. MAOIs inhibit the metabolism of tyramine in the intestine, increasing its general circulation and ultimately leading to an increase in sympathetic outflow. This can produce an adrenergic ("hypertensive") crisis characterized by severe hypertension, headache, and increased risk of stroke and cerebral hemorrhage. Patients need to be advised regarding dietary restrictions before treatment. Also, to prevent a hypertensive crisis, MAOIs cannot be combined with medications that have sympathomimetic properties such as some over-the-counter decongestant cold remedies, amphetamines, and epinephrine (which is often added to local anesthetics as a vasoconstrictor).

Second, MAOIs, if used concomitantly with serotonergic agents, such as SSRIs (see following discussion), may lead to "serotonin syndrome," a potentially fatal condition that is characterized by hyperreflexia, hyperthermia, and tachycardia and may lead to delirium, seizures, coma, and death. The triad of (a) mental status changes, (b) alterations in neuromuscular tone, and (c) autonomic hyperactivity (not all of which may occur simultaneously) must be recognized promptly and managed carefully with hospitalization and the use of serotonin antagonists (Iqbal, Basil et al. 2012). To reduce the risk of developing serotonin syndrome, a 2-week washout period is required when switching from SSRIs (or any other agents with serotonergic effects) to MAOIs, or vice versa. An exception is when the SSRI fluoxetine is being discontinued: a 5-week washout period is needed before starting an MAOI because of the long half-life of its metabolite norfluoxetine (Boyer and Shannon 2005). Another exception is the new antidepressant vortioxetine (see following discussion), which requires a 3-week washout period before starting an MAOI (PDR 2019). The prescribing clinician can and should access online drug interaction databases when considering the use of an MAOI. In addition to SSRIs, other serotonergic drugs that should not be combined with MAOIs include serotonin-norepinephrine reuptake inhibitors (SNRIs; see following discussion), TCAs, buspirone, triptans, cyclobenzaprine, dextromethorphan, and opioids with serotonergic activity such as meperidine, tramadol, and methadone (Goldberg and Thase 2013). Similarly, linezolid, an antibiotic with mild MAOI activity, should not be combined with serotonergic antidepressants (Frykberg, Gordon et al. 2015). Trazodone (discussed later) has been reported to be safe and effective as a sleep aid in patients on MAOIs (Zimmer, Daly & Benjamin 1984).

Selective Serotonin Reuptake Inhibitors

SSRIs are antidepressants with a more favorable side effect profile than TCAs and MAOIs and, as such, are among the first-line antidepressants. SSRI efficacy is comparable to that of TCAs (Qin, Zhang et al. 2014; Undurraga and Baldessarini 2017). As their name implies, SSRIs inhibit the serotonin transporter from taking up serotonin at the neuronal synapse. Interestingly, polymorphisms at the promoter region of the serotonin transporter gene (SLC6A4) may influence response to SSRIs: the presence of the "short" form of the serotonin transporter gene may be associated with poor response to SSRIs and more adverse effects, whereas the presence of the "long" allele may be associated with positive drug response (Malhotra, Murphy et al. 2004) and better tolerability (Murphy, Hollander et al. 2004; Zhu, Klein-Fedyshin et al. 2017). Data from the large National Institute of Mental Health Sequenced Treatment Alternatives to Relieve Depression (STAR*D) study, however, failed to support the association between this polymorphism and drug response (Kraft, Peters et al. 2007; Lekman, Paddock et al. 2008). The association may be stronger in some groups than in others (i.e., stronger in Whites than in Asians; Porcelli, Fabbri et al. 2012) and therefore may be less apparent in studies with mixed populations. More recently, the European Genome–Based Therapeutic Drugs for Depression (GENDEP) project looked for associations between multiple other genetic polymorphisms involved in serotonin signaling and antidepressant response, but their results have been mixed (Uher, Huezo-Diaz et al. 2009; Garcia-Gonzalez, Tansey et al. 2017; Fabbri, Tansey et al. 2018).

Currently available SSRIs include **fluoxetine, paroxetine, sertraline, fluvoxamine**, and **citalopram** and its S-enantiomer **escitalopram**. Possible mild early side effects (that can be minimized by starting the SSRI at a low dose and increasing the dose gradually) include gastrointestinal (GI) upset, sweating, dizziness, headaches, jitteriness, or sedation. These mild side effects are often transient and do not indicate a need for SSRI discontinuation. Continuation of these agents may be associated with usually (but not always) reversible (Ben-Sheetrit, Aizenberg et al. 2015) sexual side effects (e.g., decreased libido, erectile dysfunction, delayed ejaculation, or inability to climax) in 2% to 73% of treated patients (depending on how questions regarding sexual side effects are asked; Montejo, Llorca et al. 2001). A later meta-analysis showed that adverse sexual effects may occur in up to 80% of treated patients (Serretti and Chiesa 2009). If sexual side effects persist (as they can in up to 80% of patients; Montejo, Llorca et al. 2001), SSRI dose reduction, addition of a phosphodiesterase inhibitor (e.g., sildenafil), or switching to another antidepressant may need to be considered (Keltner, McAfee et al. 2002; Rizvi and Kennedy 2013; Taylor, Rudkin et al. 2013).

SSRIs differ in their propensities to inhibit hepatic cytochrome P450 enzymes (e.g., CYP1A2, CYP2C9, CYP2C19, CYP2D6, CYP3A4; Ereshefsky, Jhee et al. 2005). Inhibition of hepatic enzymes may lead to decreased metabolism of substrate medications such as warfarin, metoprolol, tricyclic antidepressants, and antipsychotics. This may increase serum levels of these drugs and lead to increased risk of dangerous adverse effects such as bleeding, hypotension, cardiac arrhythmias, and parkinsonian effects, respectively. Among the SSRIs, fluoxetine, fluvoxamine, and paroxetine are the most likely to inhibit CYP450 enzymes. Citalopram and escitalopram, followed by sertraline, are the least likely to inhibit the metabolism of other drugs and are therefore preferred in patients concomitantly treated with multiple other medications. However, citalopram should not be used with other medications that can prolong the QT interval (see following discussion).

Other drug-drug interactions may also occur with SSRIs. As previously noted, the combination of SSRIs (or other serotonergic agents) and MAOIs can lead to serotonin syndrome. Serotonin syndrome can also occur, however, if SSRIs are added to other serotonergic medications. These include but are not limited to SNRIs (and other serotonergic medication discussed later), TCAs (especially clomipramine), triptans (although risks are low; Orlova, Rizzoli et al. 2018), tramadol, opioids with serotonergic activity, dextromethorphan, and drugs of abuse such as 3,4-methylenedioxymethamphetamine. One cannot rule out the possibility that SSRI monotherapy can lead to serotonin syndrome (Abadie, Rousseau et al. 2015), but this is rare in clinical practice unless the patient has overdosed on the medication.

Despite the relatively benign side effect profiles of the SSRIs as a class, they do have significant medical risks:

1. SSRIs have anticoagulant effects and are associated with a greater risk of bleeding syndromes and operative bleeding risk (Quinn, Singer et al. 2014; Roose and Rutherford 2016; Renoux, Vahey et al. 2017) especially if the treated patient is already taking nonsteroidal anti-inflammatory drugs, warfarin, or corticosteroids. Gastrointestinal bleeding risk, for example, may increase ninefold when an SSRI and nonsteroidal anti-inflammatory drugs are combined. This risk is markedly reduced with the use of protein pump inhibitors or H2 blockers (de Abajo and Garcia-Rodriguez 2008).

2. SSRIs are associated with worsening osteoporosis, increased risk of falls in the elderly and a twofold risk of increased factures. There may also be some "confounding by indication" in that decreased bone density may be associated with underlying depression (Bolton, Metge et al. 2008; Ziere, Dieleman et al. 2008; Verdel, Souverein et al. 2010; Sterke, Ziere et al. 2012; Diem, Harrison et al. 2013). A prospective cohort study controlling for various confounders found no increased bone loss compared to untreated controls (Diem, Ruppert et al. 2013). However, a more recent larger study found that there is a higher risk of major osteoporotic fractures and hip fractures in patients over 40 years old who take SSRIs (or antipsychotics) and that this risk may be even slightly higher than for those who take benzodiazepines (Bolton, Morin et al. 2017). Perimenopausal women taking SSRIs may also be at higher risk of fractures (Sheu, Lanteigne et al. 2015).

3. SSRIs may lead to hyponatremia, and may be more likely to do so than other antidepressants such as TCAs or mirtazapine (see following discussion; Farmand, Lindh et al. 2018). The elderly and those already taking diuretics may be at higher risk (Movig, Leufkens et al. 2002).

4. SSRIs have been generally considered to be weight neutral. However, recent studies suggest a possible association between weight gain and SSRI treatment (Uguz, Sahingoz et al. 2015), especially if treatment is coupled with a sedentary life style (Shi, Atlantis et al. 2017). Only fluoxetine was associated with no significant weight gain in the Uguz et al. study. Paroxetine has been associated with significant weight gain (Serretti and Mandelli 2010), but in Uguz et al., the gain was just as great with escitalopram. Also, an observational study of patients treated with SSRIs for obsessive-compulsive disorder found that both paroxetine and citalopram were associated with >14% of patients gaining more than 7% of their body weight versus <5% with sertraline (Maina, Albert et al. 2004).

5. As previously mentioned, citalopram has been found to produce dose-related QT prolongation. The maximum allowed dose has been lowered to 40 mg per day or 20 mg per day in the elderly. It should not be used in patients who are otherwise at risk for QT prolongation or who are taking other medications (e.g., some antipsychotics, methadone as discussed later) that may also prolong QT. Citalopram, which is a substrate of the CYP2C19 enzyme, also should be used at lower doses or avoided in patients taking inhibitors of this enzyme, such as cimetidine, proton pump inhibitors, modafinil, and (possibly) oral contraceptives (Sheeler, Ackerman et al. 2012). Bupropion (discussed later) may also potentially increase citalopram serum levels by 30% or 40% (depending on the metric used), although the mechanism for this interaction is not known (PDR 2019).

QT prolongation seemed to be much less with escitalopram, the active enantiomer (Castro, Clements et al. 2013; Food and Drug Administration [FDA] 2012). Although one large observational study did not detect any adverse effects from 60 mg of citalopram (Zivin, Pfeiffer et al. 2013), another did confirm significant arrhythmia risk for citalopram as well as escitalopram (Girardin, Gex-Fabry et al. 2013). More recent data suggest that increases in escitalopram plasma levels do not appear to be associated with increases in QT prolongation (Carceller-Sindreu, de Diego-Adelino et al. 2017). However, 30 mg/day doses of escitalopram (which exceeds the package insert maximum of 20 mg/day) can significantly prolong the QT interval (FDA 2012). Other SSRIs have a much lower risk of prolonging QT (for which the effect is primarily noted in the setting of antidepressant overdose; Funk and Bostwick 2013).

6. SSRIs may contribute to cataract formation (Etminan, Mikelberg et al. 2010), but more recent results have been mixed (Becker, Jick et al. 2017).

The relatively benign side effect profiles of SSRIs and their ease of use have contributed to widespread use by clinicians who might not have been comfortable using earlier antidepressants such as TCAs and MAOIs. In cases of atypical presentations of depression, or depression in the context of recent substance abuse, SSRIs are more readily used even before there is absolute clarity in diagnosis. Under these circumstances, many clinicians believe that the benefits of treatment may outweigh the risks. However, evidence suggests that SSRIs are less effective, and possibly even ineffective, when compared to placebo in the treatment of depressed patients with concomitant alcohol abuse or dependence (Iovieno, Tedeschini et al. 2011; Atigari, Kelly et al. 2013).

Although empirical "trials" of an SSRI (as an antidepressant with a *relatively* benign side effect profile) in situations where there is less than optimum diagnostic clarity may be appropriate for some patients, the physician should still be aware of at least two other major areas of risk. First, all antidepressants can induce mania in the short-term and overall mood instability in the long-term in patients with a vulnerability to bipolar disorder. A clear family history should be obtained to investigate whether there is a genetic predisposition to bipolar disorder. Also, clinicians should be aware that younger depressed patients, who may go on later to exhibit manic symptoms, may be incorrectly diagnosed with unipolar depression when in fact they may have a bipolar diathesis. A "pre-bipolar" presentation of depression (Rihmer, Dome et al. 2013; O'Donovan, Garnham et al. 2008) should be suspected in patients with (a) a family history of bipolar depression; (b) a younger age of onset; (c) a family history of completed suicide; (d) past poor response to antidepressants; (e) a history of treatment-emergent agitation, irritability, or suicidality; and (f) a history of postpartum psychosis (Chaudron and Pies 2003). Depressed patients with these characteristics may have bipolar rather than unipolar depression and therefore should not be reflexively started on an antidepressant (Ghaemi, Ko et al. 2002; O'Donovan, Garnham et al. 2008; Phelps 2008). Also, patients frequently deny symptoms of hypomania, thinking that they are part of their normal temperament and not recognizing that they occur in discreet episodes. The bipolar diagnosis can be missed for years because of this. Family members and significant others may recognize the discreet episodes well before the patient becomes aware of them.

Second, antidepressant use has been associated with an increased risk of treatment-emergent suicidality—this occurs in about 4% of treated patients versus 2% on placebo—especially in children, adolescents, and young adults as noted in the current package inserts of all antidepressants. It is still unclear if this risk is significant in adults over the age of 25. The reasons for this increase in suicidality are not clear, although increased agitation (e.g., akathisia) or activation as a side effect (Harada, Sakamoto et al. 2008) or the possible emergence of "mixed" manic symptoms (mania combined with dysphoric mood) in depressed bipolar patients as previously noted may be responsible.

Despite the concern and subsequent FDA "black box" warnings that antidepressants may infrequently increase suicide risk, it should be noted that the overall rates of suicide in the United States had actually decreased over a prior 15-year span probably due to the increasingly widespread use of SSRI antidepressants (Grunebaum, Ellis et al. 2004). Except for a more recent uptick in suicides, earlier longitudinal data suggested that overall antidepressant use has been associated with a significant reduction in suicidal behavior (Leon, Solomon et al. 2011). Nevertheless, the concern about treatment-emergent suicidality argues for a need for careful evaluation and diagnosis, increased discussion of risks and benefits of treatment with patients (and family when appropriate), and close monitoring of all patients beginning antidepressant therapy. Prescribing antide-pressants when indicated, coupled with these steps, is more appropri-ate than withholding antidepressants in unipolar depressed patients who are much more likely to benefit rather than come to harm from these treatments (Bridge, Iyengar et al. 2007). Unfortunately, sur-veys found that after the black box warning about suicide risk was publicized, instead of the hoped for increase in the monitoring of patients undergoing antidepressant therapy (Morrato, Libby et al. 2008), there was an overall decrease in the use of antidepressants and an increase in the overall rates of suicide (Gibbons, Brown et al. 2007). Since the possible reluctance to prescribe antidepressant prescriptions, especially by primary care providers, may deprive many depressed patients of needed treatment, some have called for removal of these black box warnings (Friedman 2014).

Serotonin-Norepinephrine Reuptake Inhibitors

The SNRIs **venlafaxine**, **desvenlafaxine** (the major active metab-olite of venlafaxine), and **duloxetine** are dual-action serotoner-gic and noradrenergic antidepressants that might be expected to have efficacy similar to TCAs though without their anticholiner-gic, antihistaminic, hypotensive, or significant cardiac side effects. Milnacipran is an SNRI which is FDA labeled in the United States for the treatment of fibromyalgia but not for depression. Its enan-tiomer **levomilnacipran**, however, was released in 2013 and FDA-approved for the treatment of depression.

Venlafaxine is primarily serotonergic at lower doses and has a dual action only at higher doses (Feighner 1999; Richelson 2003). Using venlafaxine at lower doses (i.e., less than 150 mg per day), therefore, should be presumed to be similar to using an SSRI. At higher doses, it can have a mild to moderate dose-related hypertensive effect (Johnson, Whyte et al. 2006; Mbaya, Alam et al. 2007), although patients with effectively treated hypertension can tolerate venlafaxine without an increase in blood pressure (Feighner 1999). Desvenlafaxine is the major active metabolite of venlafaxine and has similar properties to the parent compound. However, the once-daily starting dose for desvenlafaxine is equivalent to the target dose, and no titration is usually needed. Also, its metabolism is independent of the cytochrome enzymes of the liver, and therefore no dose adjustments are needed in patients with hepatic illness (Reddy, Kane et al. 2010). Duloxetine, which exerts a dual action effect throughout its dose range (i.e., not only at higher doses as with venlafaxine; Stahl and Grady 2003; Chappell, Eisenhofer et al. 2014) can also increase blood pressure, although the effect may be less pronounced and clinically insignificant (Raskin, Goldstein et al. 2003; Wohlreich, Mallinckrodt et al. 2007). Notably, there has been no correlation of duloxetine's consistent dual-action effect with any evidence of improved efficacy. Indeed, it remains unclear whether there is any advantage of dual-action agents over SSRIs, except perhaps in severely depressed inpatients with melancholia (Giakoumatos and Osser 2019). However, SNRIs, like TCAs, are more likely to induce mania in bipolar patients than SSRIs (Leverich, Altshuler et al. 2006).

Because low-dose TCAs have been shown to be modestly effective in the treatment of chronic pain syndromes, and SNRIs have a similar dual action, they have been proposed for the treatment of chronic pain symptoms as well. However, there is insufficient clinical evidence to support the use of venlafaxine for pain, particularly at low doses where it has no noradrenergic effect (Gallagher, Gallagher et al. 2015). In the case of duloxetine, despite considerable advertising to the contrary, it may not have a clinically significant effect on pain symptoms in most depressed patients (Spielmans 2008; Gebhardt, Heinzel-Gutenbrunner & Konig 2016). It has been found to be effective, and has FDA approval, for pain associated with diabetic neuropathy and fibromyalgia (although in the latter, its effects may be more modest and partially due to improvements in psychiatric symptoms; Lunn, Hughes et al. 2014; Welsch, Uceyler et al. 2018). Milnacipran, as previously noted, has an indication for fibromyalgia but not for depression in the United States. Although the more benign side effect profile of duloxetine may make it the preferred agent in a patient for whom the risks associated with a TCA are unacceptable, there is no evidence to suggest it would be more efficacious for the treatment of pain than low dose TCAs. Additionally, when used as an antidepressant, duloxetine has been found to be less tolerable overall than venlafaxine and the SSRIs, without providing any advantages in efficacy (Schueler, Koesters et al. 2011; Cipriani, Koesters et al. 2012).

Levomilnacipran, the newest available SNRI, is reported to have greater potency for norepinephrine reuptake inhibition relative to its inhibition of serotonin reuptake (Auclair, Martel et al. 2013). It also shows significantly greater selectivity for norepinephrine reuptake inhibition when compared to venlafaxine and duloxetine. There has been no suggestion that these properties confer any clinical advantages over other antidepressants (Wagner, Schultes et al. 2018).

Antidepressants With Other Mechanisms of Action

Bupropion is an antidepressant with a poorly understood mechanism of action. It is believed to exert its effect through dopamine reuptake inhibition although it is unclear why this mechanism alone should provide it with an antidepressant effect. It may also exhibit norepinephrine reuptake inhibition (Richelson 2003; Rosenbaum, Arana et al. 2005). Bupropion has a different side effect profile from serotonergic antidepressants and can have mild stimulant-like properties. It can decrease appetite and is nonsedating, but constipation is fairly common. It is unlikely to cause sexual side effects or weight gain—two of the most common reasons for medication nonadherence in patients—and is reasonably safe in cardiac patients. However, bupropion can lower seizure threshold and is therefore contraindicated in patients who have a history of seizures or conditions that increase seizure risk such as eating disorders or active withdrawal from alcohol or benzodiazepines. The risk of seizure is dose dependent: this should be kept in mind when combining bupropion with CYP2D6 inhibitors such as paroxetine or fluoxetine that may increase bupropion serum levels. Among antidepressants, bupropion is least likely to cause mania in bipolar patients (Leverich, Altshuler et al. 2006; Post, Altshuler et al. 2006). Recent preliminary data suggest that bupropion, in contrast to TCAs and citalopram, may be associated with a shortening of the QT interval (Castro, Clements et al. 2013). Bupropion has comparable benefit to SSRIs for anxiety symptoms in depressed patients (Trivedi, Rush et al. 2001). It is a very reasonble first-line treatment for a wide range of depressed patients.

Mirtazapine increases both serotonin and norepinephrine at the neuronal synapse (and therefore like SNRIs has "dual actions") through mechanisms distinct from reuptake inhibition. It is an antagonist at alpha-2-adrenergic autoreceptors thereby increasing norepinephrine and serotonin release, and it blocks postsynaptic 5-HT2A, 5-HT2C, and 5-HT3 serotonin receptors (Feighner 1999). (Mianserin, an earlier analog of mirtazapine marketed in Europe, has a similar mechanism of action.) Mirtazapine can improve appetite (likely through 5-HT3 and H1 antagonism) and sleep (through histamine antagonism). As expected, these immediate effects can be very beneficial in the treatment of the acutely depressed patient with poor oral intake and insomnia. Weight gain over the long term, however, can be a concern that might outweigh these advantages.

Nefazodone is a postsynaptic 5-HT2 antagonist with weak serotonin and norepinephrine reuptake inhibition (DeVane, Grothe et al. 2002). Although nefazodone can improve sleep, is neutral in regard to weight gain, and less likely than SSRIs to cause sexual side effects, it is used much less often since it was found to produce rare (1 in 250,000–300,000 patient-years) but severe hepatotoxicity (Gelenberg 2002). This product was withdrawn by its original manufacturer, but it is available as a generic.

Trazodone, an antidepressant structurally similar to nefazodone, is used primarily as a hypnotic (as it proved to be too sedating for most patients at doses necessary for antidepressant effect). Trazodone can commonly cause orthostasis and should be used cautiously in the elderly. Priapism is a rare side effect that should be discussed with male patients before treatment. Recently, a new extended release formulation of trazodone with once-daily dosing has been introduced for the treatment of depression, although it is still unclear if this newer formulation would have any advantages over the generic compound. Both formulations do not appear to cause weight gain or significant sexual side effects (Sheehan, Croft et al. 2009).

Vilazodone, a relatively new antidepressant, is both a selective serotonin reuptake inhibitor and a partial agonist at the 5-HT1A receptor (Dawson and Watson 2009; Khan 2009). The 5-HT1A receptor is a presynaptic receptor in raphe nuclei that is thought to be autoinhibited by increased serotonin in the synapse, so lowering this inhibition with partial agonism is meant to augment the serotonin reuptake inhibition effect. Also, 5-HT1A is a postsynaptic receptor in limbic areas and in the neocortex, and partial agonism there is thought to possibly decrease sexual side effects. Therefore, vilazodone is claimed to have a quicker antidepressant effect as well as fewer sexual side effects than SSRIs. However, it is not clear if either of these aspirations is true as comparative studies are nonexistent. The side effect profile generally appears to be similar to SSRIs, with GI symptoms limiting rapid dose titration (de Paulis 2007; Rickels, Athanasiou et al. 2009; Khan, Cutler et al. 2011; Laughren, Gobburu et al. 2011). Other common side effects may include sleep changes, dry mouth, and dizziness (Shi, Wang et al. 2016). There is still insufficient evidence to recommend this newer drug over less expensive alternatives (Wagner, Schultes et al. 2018).

Vortioxetine was FDA-approved in 2013. It is referred to as a "multimodal" antidepressant with a wide range of neurotransmitter and receptor effects (Mork, Montezinho et al. 2013). In addition to inhibiting the serotonin transporter, it is an antagonist at 5-HT1D, 5-HT3, and 5-HT7 receptors; a partial agonist at the 5-HT1B receptor; and a full agonist at the 5-HT1A receptor. Based on animal studies, it is postulated to have a positive effect on memory and attention due to its antagonism at the 5-HT7 receptor. In humans, improvements in a subset of cognitive measures have been noted (Frampton 2016), but their overall degree of clinical relevance is unclear. The FDA did not approve the manufacturer's application for a special indication for cognitively impaired depressed patients. Results of controlled trials for efficacy in depression are mixed (Jain, Mahableshwarkar et al. 2013; Citrome 2014; Koesters, Ostuzzi et al. 2017). Nausea may be a common adverse effect. As with vilazodone, there is insufficient evidence at this time to recommend its use over already available and less costly antidepressants (Wagner, Schultes et al. 2018).

Emerging Pharmacotherapies

Most available antidepressants have been "me too drugs," seeming to offer the same results through fairly similar mechanisms of action. There are some novel agents, however, but limitations due to cost and the settings needed to administer some of these medications may slow the process by which they enter routine clinical practice.

Ketamine, a rapid-acting *N*-methyl-D-aspartate glutamate receptor antagonist, appears to have short-term antidepressant effects (Fond, Loundou et al. 2014). Most notably, it has been observed that ketamine can produce a rapid response within 2 hours after a single intravenous infusion, and the effect can last up to a week (Zarate, Singh et al. 2006; Covvey, Crawford et al. 2012; Mathew, Shah et al. 2012; McGirr, Berlim et al. 2015). It is not yet clear if the response can be sustained over the longer term. Reviews also suggest a possible role for ketamine in decreasing suicidal ideation (Wilkinson, Ballard et al. 2018) and for treatment-resistant depression (Medeiros da Frota Ribeiro and Riva-Posse 2017). Inhaled preparations of ketamine may be a more practical method for sustained administration (Lapidus, Levitch et al. 2014; Andrade 2015). The newly studied intranasal **esketamine** (s-enantiomer of ketamine) appears to have some efficacy for the treatment of depessive symptoms and suicidality (Canuso, Singh et al. 2018) and has recently received FDA approval for treatment-resistant depression and suicidality. The drug is extremely costly and must be administered in a healthcare setting.

The proposed mechanism of action of ketamine (and esketamine) as a glutamate receptor antagonist had been considered to be through a disinhibition of glutamergic transmission leading to an increase in synaptogenesis in the medial prefrontal cortex (Duman and Li 2012). However, a review of other glutamate receptor modulators (e.g., memantine, riluzole) did not find similar antidepressants effects (Caddy, Amit et al. 2015). Recently, a small randomized controlled study found that ketamine had no antidepressant effect if administered to patients who were pretreated with the opioid antagonist naltrexone, suggesting that the observed mood altering effects of ketamine may be opioid mediated (Williams, Heifets et al. 2018). As such, opioid receptor stimulation would seem unlikely to be a major advance for the treatment of long-term problems like treatment-resistant depression. There has been a flurry of editorials pro and con about this study and about what other mechanisms could be involved. Until there is more clarity on this, it seems that ketamine use should be restricted to short term use in severely ill patients such as inpatients with melancholic depression.

Rapastinel, another glutamatergic modulator, may also show some promise for treatment-resistant depression (Ragguett, Rong et al. 2019).

Opioids have been studied for the treatment of depression, treatment-resistant depression and suicidality (Stanciu, Glass et al. 2017). **Buprenorphine**, a mu-opioid receptor partial agonist (discussed later), has shown some promise for these indications, but it is not clear if its use would provide any benefit over currently available treatments for depression. Buprenorphine may have antidepressant effects through kappa-opioid receptor antagonism, even when mu-receptors are blocked by naltrexone (Almatroudi, Husbands et al. 2015).

Brexanolone, a synthetic version of the steroid allopregnanolone (a metabolite of progesterone), is a gamma-aminobutyric-acid receptor modulator. It has been postulated that the rapid fall of allopregnanolone after delivery may contribute to the emergence of postpartum depression. Brexanolone has been shown to have efficacy for the treatment of postpartum depression (Meltzer-Brody, Colquhoun et al. 2018). It recently obtained FDA approval for the treatment of postpartum depression. Each treatment is extremely costly, and it must be administered as an intravenous infusion over 60 hours in a healthcare facility and under medical supervision; severe sedation and loss of consciousness may occur during treatment. The response to brexanolone is often rapid. It has not been studied for other types of depression.

Complementary, Alternative, and Other Pharmacotherapies

Evidence available for the use of over-the-counter supplements is often either lacking or of very poor quality. There is a dearth of large randomized controlled clinical trials for most of the available agents. Although some evidence suggests that **S-adenosyl** methionine, omega-3 fatty acids, L-methylfolate, St. John's wort, **tryptophan**, and **vitamin D** have mild antidepressant effects (for some as adjuncts to conventional antidepressants), the evidence is of limited utility given the poor quality of the data supporting their use (Appleton, Sallis et al. 2015; Galizia, Oldani et al. 2016; Sarris, Murphy et al. 2016; Asher, Gartlehner et al. 2017; Asher, Gerkin et al. 2017; Schefft, Kilarski et al. 2017). Of these, the best evidence for acute antidepressant effects as monotherapy is associated with S-adenosyl methionine and St. John's wort (Sharma, Gerbarg et al. 2017; Linde, Berner & Kriston 2008). Recent evidence suggests that **curcumin**, found in turmeric, may help alleviate depressive symptoms (Ng, Koh et al. 2017), but there is very little clinical experience with this agent.

Adverse drug reactions may occur as they do with prescribed antidepressants (Hoban, Byard et al. 2015). Psychiatric risks, such as the risk of treatment-emergent mania or suicidality with the use of these "natural antidepressants," have not been investigated and cannot be ruled out.

The addition of over-the-counter complementary agents to a patient's existing drug regimen or the initiation of a prescribed antidepressant for a patient who is in the habit of taking multiple herbal medicines greatly increases the risk of drug–drug interactions (Schefft, Kilarski et al. 2017). Of note, the combination of tryptophan or St. Johns wart and a serotonergic antidepressant or an MAOI may increase the risk of serotonin syndrome. Also, St. John's wort can induce the CYP3A4 hepatic enzyme, thereby increasing the metabolism of several medications, including some psychiatric medications and oral contraceptives (Lynch and Price 2007).

Testosterone has been studied for the treatment of depressed men but may be primarily beneficial to men with low baseline testosterone (Zarrouf, Artz et al. 2009). A new meta-analysis concluded that testosterone may reduce depressive symptoms, especially at higher dose ranges (Walther, Breidenstein et al. 2018). However, risks of exogenously administered testosterone (e.g., cardiovascular risks, potential risk of testosterone-dependent prostate cancer, and worsened sleep apnea) preclude the routine or high-dose use of this hormone for the treatment of depression.

Further Notes on the Clinical Use of Antidepressants for Unipolar Depression

Do Antidepressants Work?

Although numerous published randomized controlled trials comparing individual antidepressants with placebo have historically shown antidepressants to be superior to placebo (50% to ~60% over 30% to ~40%), concerns have been raised about the overall clinical effectiveness of these medications. First, there is the concern that data are selectively published, so that many studies unfavorable to the studied antidepressants may have never been publicly reported, thus biasing the evidence base. A review of antidepressant effect size including data from published and unpublished studies (available to the FDA) showed a lower antidepressant effect size than that derived from reviews of published literature only (Turner, Matthews et al. 2008). This lower effect size has been described as "clinically insignificant" (Kirsch, Deacon et al. 2008; Turner and Rosenthal 2008). One of the reasons for this marginal net efficacy is an increasing placebo response rate in the more recent antidepressant efficacy studies (Walsh, Seidman et al. 2002). These rates may be a result of the recruitment of more mildly ill subjects in clinical trials, leading to a greater likelihood of a placebo response in less ill patients, although this has been disputed by some (Furukawa, Cipriani et al. 2018). The Hamilton Depression Rating Scale as an outcome measure, used in almost all studies, has been shown to be deeply flawed and contributing strongly to the lack of differences between SSRIs and placebo (Hieronymus, Emilsson et al.

2016). Some analyses have found that patients who are only mildly to moderately ill do not respond better to antidepressants than to placebo, but as severity increases, the benefits become significant (Kirsch, Deacon et al. 2008; Khin, Chen et al. 2011). However, a review of data on fluoxetine and venlafaxine found benefit at all levels of severity (Gibbons, Hur et al. 2012). In summary, antidepressants may still be efficacious, but perhaps not as often as previously thought, and they may be more likely to be clinically effective in the severely depressed. However, some would assert that problems with research conduct and design, rather than problems with the medications, account for most of the disappointing outcomes.

Starting, Continuing, and Terminating Antidepressant Therapy

Once the decision has been made to start an antidepressant, the starting dose should be a low dose to minimize adverse effects. It is then titrated as tolerated to a therapeutic dose. Response may begin by the end of the first week, but generally 2 to 6 weeks of treatment are needed for a more substantial response (Taylor, Freemantle et al. 2006). Significant response in the first 1 to 2 weeks is possible, but it could be a placebo response or the sign of a possible manic switch, the latter suggesting the advisability of discontinuing the antidepressant. Patients (especially teenagers and young adults) should also be monitored early on for treatment-emergent suicidality. New suicidality may be accompanied with restlessness, impulsivity, and ego-dystonic thoughts of self-harm (Stubner, Grohmann et al. 2018) and may occur when initiating or increasing the dose of the antidepressant. If treatment-emergent suicidality occurs, the antidepressant must be discontinued.

Other more common and typical physical side effects of antidepressants can occur in the first days of treatment; some may even target and alleviate certain depression symptoms. For example, the sleep- and appetite-enhancing effects of mirtazapine, which can be seen early in treatment, are likely to be helpful to a patient who has been suffering from insomnia and poor oral intake because of his or her depression. Such an antidepressant could help a patient symptomatically feel better within the first few days. However, the onset of effects on the core symptoms of depression may still require several weeks. Still, early improvement in depressive symptoms by the second week may be a predictor of later response and remission (Vermeiden, Kamperman et al. 2015; Wagner, Engel et al. 2017). If no improvement, no matter how small, is seen by 2 to 4 weeks (or 1–2 weeks in the inpatient setting), then an increase in dose (if appropriate) or a change of antidepressant is likely to be warranted. Once improvement begins, however, gradual subtle changes in mood, affect, and cognition may then continue for the duration of the medication trial, which may take up to 12 weeks.

Patients who respond to treatment and have had only one depressive episode are often recommended to remain on the antidepressant for 9 to 12 months before considering discontinuation. However, if there have been repeated depressive episodes or a history of suicidality, psychotic features, or other dangerous symptoms, a longer period of many years of continuation treatment is usually recommended. Although questions have been raised about the effectiveness of antidepressants in treating acute depression (see previous discussion), there is less question about the benefits of antidepressants in relapse prevention (Geddes, Carney et al. 2003; Glue, Donovan et al. 2010).

If a decision is made to discontinue antidepressant treatment, the medication should be tapered off slowly, particularly to avoid the occurrence of an SSRI or SNRI "discontinuation syndrome." This is particularly true when tapering off paroxetine, venlafaxine, or duloxetine but is less frequently seen with fluoxetine given the long half-life of its active metabolite norfluoxetine. The discontinuation syndrome is characterized by vague neurological symptoms ("brain zaps"), dizziness, GI symptoms, headache, and flu-like symptoms. Although variability in onset and persistence have been reported, the syndrome is generally mild, lasting a few days to a few weeks and can be reversed by reintroducing the withdrawn agent (Haddad 1998; Fava, Gatti et al. 2015; Papp and Onton 2018). Generally, the syndrome is not known to be life threatening, but in some individuals, it can be extremely distressing. Often patients assume that the symptoms indicate that their depression is returning: they should be reassured that these immediate symptoms are probably withdrawal-related, and they may wait to see if an actual mood syndrome redevelops over the coming months. Tapering over 4 weeks is usually adequate except with paroxetine and venlafaxine/duloxetine; 8 or more weeks may be required for them.

First-Line Treatments

Clinical practice today emphasizes the use of newer ("second-generation") antidepressants including SSRIs, SNRIs, bupropion, and mirtazapine. As discussed previously, the older tricyclics and MAOIs are not first-line because of their greater toxicity and risk of harm from overdose. In a meta-analysis of 203 studies comparing the efficacy and side effects of these newer antidepressants, no substantial differences in effectiveness were found (Gartlehner, Gaynes et al. 2008). The authors recommended that antidepressants be selected on the basis of differences in expected side effects and cost (i.e., use generic products over brand items). A subsequent review of 117 trials concluded that sertraline had the most favorable balance among benefits, side effects, and acquisition cost (Cipriani, Furukawa et al. 2009). Escitalopram also had slightly better efficacy, but was still an expensive brand product at the time of that study. A subsequent review supported sertraline's overall better efficacy and acceptability compared to a broad range of other antidepressants (Cipriani, La Ferla et al. 2010). The most recent "network meta-analysis" of 21 antidepressants found that they were all more efficacious than placebo for the treatment of major depressive disorder and confirmed that escitalopram was among the more effective and sertraline was among the more tolerable antidepressants (Cipriani, Furukawa et al. 2018). Escitalopram and sertraline, therefore, appear to be reasonable first-line SSRIs, especially if one also considers their low propensities for CYP450 drug interactions and low cost.

Antidepressants may have similar efficacy in dysthymic disorder as well, with an even larger separation from placebo (due to a smaller placebo response) than found in studies for major depressive disorder (Levkovitz, Tedeschini et al. 2011).

Another option for first-line use is bupropion. As noted, its effectiveness overall and on anxiety symptoms accompanying major depression is the same as with SSRIs (Zimmerman, Posternak et al. 2005). The risk of seizures with the sustained release formulation was 0.1%, comparable to SSRIs and other antidepressants, at least at doses up to 300 mg daily (Dunner, Zisook et al. 1998; Tripp 2010). Bupropion rarely causes weight gain or sexual side effects. This is a significant benefit, given that sexual dysfunction is one of the major causes of disability and treatment dropout in the outpatient treatment of depression in primary care (Gandhi, Weingart et al. 2003). Patients should be informed that there are choices for initial treatment of their depression because of side effect differences.

Outcome Studies

The STAR*D study, sponsored by the National Institute of Mental Health was a study of medications for the treatment of major depression. It produced important insights into the optimum use of pharmacotherapy for this disorder (Wisniewski, Rush et al. 2009). STAR*D started with almost 4,000 heterogeneous "real-world" patients with major depression, who were treated by a mixture of psychiatrists and primary care physicians. Patients agreed to have up to four sequential medication trials with the goal of achieving remission from their depression. Each trial lasted up to 14 weeks. Patients started with citalopram for the first trial. If response was unsatisfactory, they could have a switch to one of three antidepressants, or an augmentation with one of two augmenting agents. For the third trial, there were other switches or augmentations available, and finally for those still depressed and still willing to undergo the fourth trial, there was the choice of an MAOI or a combination of venlafaxine and mirtazapine. The latter combination has been referred to informally as "rocket fuel" because of the four different neurotransmitter alterations that it is thought to induce (McGrath, Stewart et al. 2006). Key findings from STAR*D include the following:

- Citalopram did not work well if patients met the DSM-IV criteria for melancholic features (McGrath, Khan et al. 2008).
- The switches in the second trial (to another SSRI: sertraline to bupropion or venlafaxine) had equal efficacy although there was a nonsignificant numerical advantage to the switch to venlafaxine.
- The augmentations in the second trial (buspirone— discussed in the anxiolytic chapter—or bupropion) worked equally well.
- Nothing worked well in the first two trials if patients had significant anxiety symptoms along with their depression (Fava, Rush et al. 2008). However, a recent study with adjunctive aripiprazole (an antipsychotic discussed later) added to an SSRI found good results in patients with depression mixed with anxiety, in a post-hoc analysis (Trivedi, Thase et al. 2008). This needs replication in a prospectively designed study with comparison to other augmentations.
- In the third trial, switching to a TCA worked fairly well. It might have worked better if clinicians had dosed the TCA properly and used plasma levels to monitor adequacy of dosage.

- Adding lithium (discussed in the later section on mood stabilizers) did not work as well as adding triiodothyronine in the third trial, but lithium might have done better if clinicians had dosed it properly.
- In the fourth trial, the MAOI did not do well compared to the venlafaxine/mirtazapine combination, but clinicians underdosed the MAOI. Unfortunately, for the few patients who remitted from either treatment, early relapse occurred in 75% (Rush, Trivedi et al. 2006).

As a group, STAR*D subjects were not particularly interested in psychotherapeutic treatment for their depression. Psychotherapy was available as an option in the second treatment trial, but patients could elect to drop it from the randomization option list, and most did so (Wisniewski, Fava et al. 2007). The modest remission rates seen in STAR*D may reflect that a major component of the improvement in depression seen in research and clinical settings comes from the nonspecific, interpersonal supportive aspects of care including the therapeutic alliance. STAR*D patients might have been less susceptible to these benefits than other patients who are more invested in psychosocial treatments of their disorder. It is hoped that future studies will improve our ability to select the best treatments for each patient, psychopharmacological and psychotherapeutic, depending on their needs and preferences.

Monotherapy Versus Combination Antidepressants

There had been interest in the possibility that a combination of two or more antidepressants might benefit a wider spectrum of patients or work more rapidly than a single agent like an SSRI or bupropion (Blier, Ward et al. 2010). However, the Combining Medications to Enhance Depression Outcomes (CO-MED) study seemed to settle the issue in favor of monotherapy (Rush, Trivedi et al. 2011; Sung,

Haley et al. 2012). Six hundred sixty-five outpatients were treated in psychiatric and primary care sites. They were randomized to either escitalopram 10 to 20 mg daily, escitalopram plus bupropion, or mirtazapine plus venlafaxine. At 12 weeks, remission rates were 39% for the first two options and 38% for the "rocket fuel" combination, which had worse adverse effects. The study added to the evidence that escitalopram may be a particularly good monotherapy to select initially. However, given escitalopram's sexual side effects, many patients may still prefer to start with bupropion monotherapy (not an option in CO-MED).

Treatment-Resistant Depression

Treatment-resistant depression, or depression that is refractory to 2 or more adequately dosed antidepressant trials, requires further evaluation. A review of the initial diagnosis of unipolar depression, along with a consideration of other possible alternative diagnoses such as bipolar depression, comorbid disorders such as anxiety or posttraumatic disorders, personality disorders, and substance use disorders, as well as the presence of overwhelming psychosocial stressors and/or poor patient adherence to provided treatment should be taken into account before rushing to the next pharmacological treatment. If further pharmacotherapy is indicated, options include increasing the dose to the maximum tolerable dose, switching to an antidepressant with a different mechanism of action, or the addition of an augmenting agent if there is any indication that the current treatment has been partially helpful. There is insufficient evidence to guide the clinician as to which action has a greater chance of success (Connolly and Thase 2011). In clinical practice, switching to another antidepressant including a TCA, or augmenting treatment with lithium, thyroid hormone, a second-generation antipsychotic (e.g., aripiprazole, quetiapine, olanzapine—although olanzapine is not recommended due to severe metabolic side effects—or risperidone; Zhou, Keitner et al. 2015), or a second antidepressant with a different mechanism of action (e.g., the addition of bupropion or mirtazapine to an SSRI) may all be tried. Electroconvulsive therapy is an option to consider (see following discussion). If not already in place, psychotherapy should be considered whenever response to available antidepressants is suboptimal (Li, Zhang et al. 2018). Poor antidepressant response may be associated with a history of trauma in early childhood (Williams, Debattista et al. 2016), and "dyadic discord" or significant ongoing conflict in important relationships (Denton, Carmody et al. 2010).

Electroconvulsive therapy (ECT), which has been found to be effective for treatment-resistant depression, may need to be considered early on (Kellner, Greenberg et al. 2012; Ross, Zivin et al. 2018). In the setting of severe depression, ECT may be more appropriate than subjecting a patient to numerous medication trials with decreasing chances of success. Ketamine (or esketamine) may also be considered. Lastly, repetitive transcranial magnetic stimulation (rTMS) is an FDA-approved treatment for major depression that has failed one pharmacotherapy trial. It is not approved for treatment-resistant depression defined as two or more failed trials (despite its frequent use in this population), and the lack of efficacy was recently confirmed in a randomized sham-controlled trial in 164 veterans (Yesavage, Fairchild et al. 2018). Thirty-nine percent remitted in this trial, but there was no difference between active and sham treatments. rTMS, like pharmacotherapy, has a high placebo-response rate, and clinicians who rely on their "clinical experience" for determining what is effective can be misled by the placebo effect.

Clinical Use of Antidepressants in Other Psychiatric Disorders

The clinical use of antidepressants in anxiety disorders, obsessive-compulsive disorder and posttraumatic stress disorder is reviewed in the chapter on anxiolytics.

Post-Myocardial Infarction Depression

SSRIs are often the treatment of choice in depressed patients with severe cardiovascular disease (Mavrides and Nemeroff 2013). Among the SSRIs, sertraline, followed by escitalopram, are favored due to their overall tolerability (especially in the elderly) and their low risk of drug–drug interactions. However, it should be noted that sertraline was only effective in patients with a prior history of depressive episodes before their coronary artery disease became a problem (Glassman, O'Connor et al. 2002). It was not different from placebo in patients who had their first depression in that context. Those patients might have an adjustment disorder. In the escitalopram study, they did not evaluate the relationship with prior histories of depression (Kang, Bae et al. 2016). Citalopram and TCAs are avoided given their potential effects on cardiac conduction and increased risk of QT prolongation. Venlafaxine is not considered a first-line treatment given its potential to increase blood pressure and heart rate (Diaper, Rich et al. 2013). Similar adrenergic effects on blood pressure are possible with duloxetine.

Post-Stroke Depression

Due to their tolerability, SSRIs are considered the treatment of choice for post-stroke depression; however, it is unclear whether antidepressant therapy improves functional outcomes such as activities of daily living (Xu, Zou et al. 2016; Paolucci 2017).

Depression in Parkinson's Disease

Moderate to severe depression associated with Parkinson's disease (PD), which is often characterized by anhedonia and/or low mood, requires treatment. Although both TCAs and SSRIs have been found to be helpful for depression in PD, TCA side effects such as orthostatic hypotension and anticholinergic effects suggest that SSRIs (despite their rare potential to worsen PD motor symptoms; Gerber and Lynd 1998) would be more appropriate first-line treatments, especially in the elderly (Costa, Rosso et al.

2012). Bupropion, despite a lack of randomized control trials supporting its use in PD, may be beneficial to patients given its inhibition of dopamine reuptake at the synapse (Zaluska and Dyduch 2011). Pramipexole (a D3 dopamine receptor agonist) may also have efficacy for depression in PD (Barone, Scarzella et al. 2006; Harada, Ishizaki et al. 2011). Consideration of pramipexole or an MAOI (e.g., transdermal selegiline) for depression in patients with PD would necessitate consultation with the patient's neurologist, given that these medications are often used to directly affect the core motor symptoms of PD. Finally, potential medication interactions should be taken into account (e.g., if an SSRI is being considered for a patient who is already taking an MAOI for PD).

Eating Disorders

Antidepressants (and psychiatric medications in general) appear ineffective for patients with anorexia nervosa, unless the patient has concurrent depression (Frank and Shott 2016). Mirtazapine, which is often considered due to its potential for weight gain, did not appear to have a significant effect in one small study (Hrdlicka, Beranova et al. 2008). Although antidepressants may have minimal efficacy for acute treatment of anorexia, they may have a role in relapse prevention once the patient's weight has been restored (Marvanova and Gramith 2018).

Fluoxetine (primarily effective at higher doses) is the only SSRI that is FDA-approved for the treatment of bulimia, and its effectiveness is independent of its effect on mood (Fluoxetine Bulimia Nervosa Collaborative Study Group 1992; Goldstein, Wilson et al. 1999). However, other SSRIs, such as sertraline and citalopram, have also been noted to reduce the frequency of binging and purging episodes (Leombruni, Amianto et al. 2006; Milano, Petrella et al. 2004).

Fluoxetine, sertraline, and citalopram may be modestly effective in the treatment of binge eating disorder (McElroy, Casuto et al. 2000; Arnold, McElroy et al. 2002; McElroy, Hudson et al. 2003; Leombruni, Piero et al. 2008). Bupropion is often considered for its appetite suppressant properties in patients with binge-eating disorder, and its use may result in modest short-term weight loss (White and Grilo 2013). The combination of bupropion and naltrexone has been recently approved by the FDA for weight loss, but its role in the treatment of eating disorders per se is not clear (despite a possible effect in binge eating behaviors; Guerdjikova, Walsh et al. 2017)). Finally, as previously noted, bupropion is contraindicated in patients with anorexia nervosa or bulimia given the increased risk of seizures in these patients.

Premenstrual Dysphoric Disorder

Premenstrual dysphoric disorder is characterized by mood and anxiety symptoms that occur during the second half (luteal phase) of the menstrual cycle. Serotonergic antidepressants (e.g., SSRIs and SNRIs) appear to improve premenstrual dysphoric disorder symptoms and are considered to be first-line treatments (Maharaj and Trevino 2015; Reid and Soares 2018).

Perimenopausal Depression

Depressive symptoms during the perimenopausal period are often associated with vasomotor symptoms (de Kruif et al. 2016). Aside from hormonal treatments that are often used when physical symptoms are predominant, SSRIs and SNRIs can be treatments of choice for perimenopausal depression. Of note, paroxetine has an FDA indication for vasomotor symptoms associated with menopause, although its side effect profile makes it generally less desirable compared to other SSRIs.

Clinical Use of Antidepressants in Nonpsychiatric Disorders

The use of antidepressants for pain syndromes has been discussed earlier in this chapter.

Irritable Bowel Syndrome

Although the evidence is mixed, there is some evidence that SSRIs and TCAs may improve global well-being in patients with irritable bowel syndrome (IBS; Tack, Broekaert et al. 2006; Ford, Talley et al. 2009; Ruepert, Quartero et al. 2011; Bundeff and Woodis 2014). More recent reviews, however, have found SSRIs to be not as effective as previously thought (Xie, Tang et al. 2015) and less effective than TCAs (Kulak-Bejda, Bejda et al. 2017) for IBS. TCAs and SNRIs may be considered for their modest effects on IBS-related pain (Chen, Ilham et al. 2017).

Functional Dyspepsia and Gastroparesis

Persistent dyspepsia without organic pathology is termed "functional dyspepsia" (FD). There is some evidence to suggest that TCAs and mirtazapine may improve FD (Jiang, Jia et al. 2016; Lu, Chen et al. 2016; Moayyedi, Lacy et al. 2017), but venlafaxine may not (although the doses of venlafaxine may have been too low to have had any noradrenergic effects). SSRIs do not appear to improve FD (Lu, Chen et al. 2016). Mirtazapine appears also to be helpful for nausea and vomiting associated with refractory gastroparesis (Malamood, Roberts et al. 2017).

Use in Women of Childbearing Potential, Pregnancy, and Breastfeeding

Pregnancy

Untreated depression is associated with low birth weight, higher preterm birth rates, poor adherence with prenatal care, postpartum depression, and an overall worsened health status in pregnant women (Orr, Blazer et al. 2007; Yonkers, Wisner et al. 2009). Antidepressant discontinuation during pregnancy increases the risk of relapse (Cohen, Altshuler et al. 2006). These factors suggest that the potential risks and benefits of using antidepressants during pregnancy should be weighed against the known risks of untreated depression.

TCAs (with the exception of clomipramine) do not appear to increase the rate of congenital anomalies, although they may be associated with poor neonatal adaptation syndrome (see following discussion; Reis and Kallen 2010; Gentile 2014; Ornoy, Weinstein-Fudim et al. 2017; Vasilakis-Scaramozza et al. 2013). There is insufficient evidence to support the use of MAOIs in pregnancy.

Most SSRIs do not appear to increase the risk of congenital malformations (Addis and Koren 2000; Einarson and Einarson 2005; Rahimi, Nikfar et al. 2006; Kjaersgaard, Parner et al. 2013; Payne 2017), but they may slightly increase the risk of spontaneous abortions (Almeida, Basso et al. 2016). Paroxetine should be avoided given a potential risk of atrial septal defects (Reefhuis, Devine et al. 2015; Berard, Iessa et al. 2016). Apparent associations between SSRIs and persistent pulmonary hypertension in the newborn (PPHN; a rare but potentially lethal complication; Alwan, Bandoli et al. 2016), preterm birth, low birth weight, and autism may be the result of confounding by the mother's underlying psychiatric illness (Koren and Nordeng 2013; Jimenez-Solem 2014; Andrade 2017; Payne 2017). To address concerns about PPHN, an updated FDA (2011) advisory noted that "given the conflicting results from different studies, it is premature to reach any conclusion about a possible link between SSRI use and PPHN." The clinician should be aware, however, that despite the overall evidence-based consensus that SSRIs do not seem to increase the risk of malformations and seem to only minimally increase the risk of perinatal and postnatal complications, recent studies and reviews continue to suggest inconsistencies and areas of concern (Berard, Zhao et al. 2015; Berard, Zhao et al. 2017; Gao, Wu et al. 2017; Shen, Gao et al. 2017; Tak, Job et al. 2017).

Exposure to antidepressants (TCAs, SSRIs, mirtazapine) during late pregnancy may lead to poor neonatal adaptation syndrome, which may occur in up to a third of exposed newborns and is usually characterized by mild and transient irritability, jitteriness, feeding problems, and respiratory distress (Moses-Kolko, Bogen et al. 2005). Poor neonatal adaptation syndrome may be dose dependent and in a quarter of infants may last for 3 days or longer (Galbally, Spigset et al. 2017; Hogue, Temple-Cooper et al. 2017). Again, confounding by indication could explain these associations.

Although bupropion is considered to have low teratogenicity and to be comparable to other commonly used antidepressants in this regard (Cole, Modell et al. 2007), it has been associated with a small increased risk in cardiovascular malformations (Alwan, Reefhuis et al. 2010; Hendrick, Suri et al. 2017). It may also increase the risk of miscarriage (Chun-Fai-Chan, Koren et al. 2005).

A few studies suggest that mirtazapine, venlafaxine, duloxetine, nefazodone, and trazodone do not increase the risk of congenital malformations (Einarson, Bonari et al. 2003; Furu, Kieler et al. 2015; Smit, Wennink et al. 2015; Lassen, Ennis et al. 2016; Smit, Dolman et al. 2016), but more data would be needed to support these findings. Given the propensity of venlafaxine and duloxetine to increase blood pressure, they are often avoided during pregnancy due to the concern that they would increase the risk of preeclampsia (Palmsten, Huybrechts et al. 2013).

The newest antidepressants (e.g., vilazodone and vortioxetine) are underrepresented in large studies of antidepressant exposure in pregnant women. There are insufficient data to support their use during pregnancy.

Long-term neurobehavioral risks to children as a result of maternal antidepressant treatment are not known. Both untreated maternal depression and maternal antidepressant therapy may contribute to long-term risks of speech, motor, and learning disorders in children, although these are difficult to quantify and causal relationships are difficult to establish (Suri, Lin et al. 2014; Brown, Gyllenberg et al. 2016).

In reviewing pregnancy and conception it should also be noted that exposure to newer antidepressants, specifically SSRIs, may have deleterious effects on male spermatozoa and reduced sperm count and motility (Anonymous 2015). Whether SSRIs clinically reduce fertility in male patients who are trying to conceive is not known. The evidence as to whether SSRI therapy in women affects fertility is mixed (Sylvester, Menke et al. 2019).

Breastfeeding

Antidepressants that have been effective and tolerated during pregnancy are often continued during the postpartum period (Payne 2017). The amount of antidepressant transferred from the mother to the infant via breast milk is generally very low or undetectable, and the drug's effects on the newborn are thought to be generally mild (Berle and Spigset 2011).

Among TCAs, amitriptyline appears to be compatible with breastfeeding, while insufficient data for clomipramine, doxepin, and nortriptyline and the long half-life of imipramine argue against the use of these latter agents (Kronenfeld, Berlin et al. 2017).

Among SSRIs, higher concentrations in breast milk have been found for fluoxetine and citalopram. The other SSRIs are considered to have very low or undetectable levels in breast milk (Weissman, Levy et al. 2004). Duloxetine, bupropion, mirtazapine, and trazodone levels are often low in breast milk; however, the potential risk of seizures with bupropion is of some concern (Kronenfeld, Berlin et al. 2017).

Table of Antidepressants

Table 1.1 summarizes characteristics of commonly discussed antidepressants (Ansari and Osser 2015; WHO 2019; Lexicomp 2019; PDR 2019).

TABLE 1.1 Antidepressants

Medication[a]	Adult Dosing[b]	Comments/FDA *Indication*
Imipramine (TCA) (Tofranil®)	See nortriptyline, except increase gradually to 100–200 mg po qhs. Max 300 mg/day in hospitalized adults. Use with caution in patients with hepatic or renal impairments.	Check baseline ECG; therapeutic serum level of imipramine + its metabolite desipramine: 175–350 ng/mL; TCA most commonly used in comparative anxiety studies; CYP1A2, CYP2D6 substrate. Black Box Warning: Suicidality *Major Depression/Temporary adjunct in childhood enuresis in patients greater or equal to 6 years of age*
Amitriptyline (TCA) (Elavil®)	See nortriptyline, except increase gradually to 100–200 mg po qhs. Max 300 mg/day in hospitalized patients. Reduce initial dose for patients with hepatic impairment. Use with caution in patients with hepatic or renal impairments.	Check baseline ECG; possible therapeutic serum level of amitriptyline + its metabolite nortriptyline: 93–140 ng/mL; frequently used in low doses for chronic pain; most anticholinergic TCA; TCA with most overall adverse effects; CYP1A2, CYP2D6 substrate. On WHO Essential Medicines List for depressive disorders. Black Box Warning: Suicidality *Major Depression*
Clomipramine (TCA) (Anafranil®)	See nortriptyline, except increase gradually to 100–200 mg po qhs. Max 250 mg/day. Reduce initial dose for patients with hepatic impairment. Use with caution in patients with hepatic or renal impairments.	Check baseline ECG; most serotonergic TCA; CYP1A2, CYP2D6 substrate. Effective in low doses for chronic pain. On WHO Essential Medicines List for OCD. Black Box Warning: Suicidality *OCD*

(continued)

TABLE 1.1 Continued

Medication[a]	Adult Dosing[b]	Comments/FDA Indication
Doxepin (TCA) (Sinequan®, Adapin®, Silenor®)	See nortriptyline, except increase gradually to 100–200 mg po qhs. Max 300 mg/day. Newly marketed as a hypnotic in doses of 3 or 6 mg max nightly (Silenor®). Reduce initial dose and use with caution in patients with hepatic impairment.	Check baseline ECG; very sedating TCA, usually used as adjunct for insomnia; CYP2D6 substrate. Black Box Warning: Suicidality *Depression/Anxiety* For Silenor®: *Insomnia characterized by difficulties with sleep maintenance*
Desipramine (TCA) (Norpramin®)	See nortriptyline, except give in am and/ or in divided doses, gradually increase to 100–200 mg/day. Max 300 mg/day in severely depressed or hospitalized patients. Reduce initial dose and use with caution in patients with hepatic impairment.	Check baseline ECG; serum therapeutic level of desipramine: greater than 115 ng/mL; least sedating (possibly activating) TCA; most noradrenergic TCA; CYP2D6 substrate. Black Box Warning: Suicidality *Major Depression*
Nortriptyline (TCA) (Aventyl®, Pamelor®)	Start: 10–25 mg po qhs and increase by 10–25 mg every 2 days until 50–150 mg/ day in divided doses then check serum level after 4–5 days. Max 150 mg/day. Use with caution in patients with hepatic or renal impairments	Check baseline ECG; therapeutic serum level of nortriptyline: 58–148 ng/mL (TCA with most defined therapeutic serum level—inverted U dose-response curve); TCA with least postural hypotension so best for use in elderly; CYP2D6 substrate. Black Box Warning: Suicidality *Major Depression*

TABLE 1.1 Continued

Medication[a]	Adult Dosing[b]	Comments/FDA *Indication*
Phenelzine (MAOI) (Nardil®)	Start: 15 mg po bid and increase weekly by 15 mg/day to 45–60 mg/day. Max 90 mg/day. Contraindicated in patients with hepatic impairment or severe renal impairment.	Nonselective MAOI; dangerous medication and food interactions (see package insert). Black Box Warning: Suicidality *Treatment of atypical, nonendogenous, or neurotic depression*
Tranylcypromine (MAOI) (Parnate®)	Start: 10 mg po bid and increase weekly by 10 mg/day to 30–60 mg/day. Max 60 mg/day. Contraindicated in patients with hepatic impairment or severe renal impairment.	Nonselective MAOI; dangerous food and drug interactions (see package insert). Black Box Warning: Suicidality; Hypertensive Crisis *Treatment-resistant depression*
Transdermal Selegiline (MAOI) (Emsam®)	Start: 6 mg transdermal q day then increase by 3 mg patches as needed to max of 12 mg/day.	Selective MAO-B inhibitor; at 6 mg dose may not need diet restrictions (but perhaps with less antidepressant effect), but at higher doses a nonselective MAOI and needs diet restrictions; dangerous food and drug interactions (see package insert). Black Box Warning: Suicidality; Hypertensive Crisis *MDD*

(continued)

TABLE 1.1 Continued

Medication[a]	Adult Dosing[b]	Comments/FDA *Indication*
Fluoxetine (SSRI) (Prozac®, Prozac Weekly®, Sarafem®)	For daily fluoxetine, Prozac®: Start: 5–20 mg po q am then hold at 20 mg for 4 weeks then if needed increase by 10–20 mg every 4 weeks as tolerated, stop if no improvement after 4 weeks at 60 mg/day. Max 80 mg/day. Use lower doses in patients with hepatic impairment.	SSRI with longest ½ life, metabolite norfluoxetine with even longer ½ life; possibly works a little slower than other antidepressants; inhibits CYP2C9, CYP2D6, CYP3A4. On WHO Essential Medicines List for depressive disorders. Black Box Warning: Suicidality *MDD/OCD/PMDD/Bulimia Nervosa/Panic Disorder*
Paroxetine (SSRI) (Paxil®, Paxil CR®, Brisdelle®)	For paroxetine, Paxil®: Start: 10–20 mg po qhs and if needed increase by 10 mg increments in 2–4 weeks to 30–40 mg/day as tolerated. Max 60 mg/day. Reduce initial dose to 10 mg/day, and use caution in adjusting dose, with a max of 40 mg/day in patients with hepatic or renal impairment.	SSRI most likely to cause discontinuation symptoms; SSRI most associated with treatment-emergent suicidality; produces weight gain; may have most sexual side effects; inhibits CYP2D6. Black Box Warning: Suicidality *MDD/OCD/Panic Disorder/ Social anxiety disorder PTSD/ GAD/PMDD* For Brisdelle®: *Severe Vasomotor Symptoms associated with Menopause*

TABLE 1.1 Continued

Medication[a]	Adult Dosing[b]	Comments/FDA *Indication*
Sertraline (SSRI) (Zoloft®)	Start: 25–50 mg po q day and maintain for 2–4 weeks, increase by 25–50 mg/day every 4 weeks if needed. Max 200 mg/day but unclear if more helpful than 100 mg/day. Doses should be halved in patients with mild hepatic impairment; sertraline should not be used in patients with severe hepatic impairment.	Less enzymatic inhibition than fluoxetine, paroxetine, and fluvoxamine (although may increase lamotrigine levels); well-tolerated SSRI; may have the most favorable balance among benefits, side effects, and cost; a substrate of multiple CYP450 enzymes, primarily of CYP2B6; modest inhibitor of CYP2D6. Black Box Warning: Suicidality *MDD/PMDD/Panic disorder PTSD/Social anxiety disorder OCD*
Fluvoxamine (SSRI) (Luvox®, Luvox CR®)	For fluvoxamine, Luvox®: Start: 25 mg po bid and increase in 4 days to 100 mg/day in single or divided doses, if needed may increase to 200 mg/day in divided doses, max of 300 mg daily in divided doses. Reduced doses may be needed in patients with hepatic impairment.	Primarily used for OCD in U.S. due to initial application to FDA for this indication, but may not be more effective than other SSRIs for OCD; inhibits CYP1A2, CYP2C9, CYP2C19, CYP3A4. Black Box Warning: Suicidality *OCD*

(continued)

TABLE 1.1 Continued

Medication[a]	Adult Dosing[b]	Comments/FDA *Indication*
Citalopram (SSRI) (Celexa®)	Start: 10–20 mg po q day and increase to 40 mg/day in 7 days, (20 mg/day may equal placebo in some studies), do not increase beyond 40 mg/day given risk of QT prolongation at higher doses. Max dose of 20 mg po q day in those over 60 years old. Max dose of 20 mg in those with hepatic impairment. Use with caution in patients with severe renal impairment.	Least likely SSRI (along with escitalopram and sertraline) to cause CYP450 medication interactions; well tolerated overall, except that it can prolong QT on doses higher than 40 mg/day. Avoid in patients who are already at higher risk of QT prolongation, with an underlying heart condition, or if QTc ≥500 milliseconds. Avoid use with other medications that can prolong QT. CYP2C19 substrate (avoid with other medications that may inhibit this enzyme). Black Box Warning: Suicidality *Major Depression*
Escitalopram (SSRI) (Lexapro®)	Start: 10 mg po q day; higher doses not shown to be better but dose may be increased to 20 mg po q day after a minimum of 1 week. Max 20 mg/day. Reduce dose to 10 mg daily for patients with hepatic impairment; use with caution in patients with severe renal impairment.	S-citalopram; well tolerated; low risk of medication interactions; comparison with citalopram showed about 15% better efficacy with escitalopram but this may have been an artifact of doses used; modest inhibitory effect on CYP2D6. Black Box Warning: Suicidality *MDD/GAD*

TABLE 1.1 Continued

Medication[a]	Adult Dosing[b]	Comments/FDA Indication
Venlafaxine (SNRI) (Effexor®, Effexor XR®)	For venlafaxine, Effexor®: Start: 37.5 mg po q day for 4 days then increase to 75 mg daily, then add 75mg/day every week until 225 mg/day (which is max for XR). Maximum is 375 mg/day for regular release venlafaxine. Doses should be decreased by 50% or more for patients with hepatic or renal impairment.	Check baseline blood pressure, then every 3–6 months; an SSRI at low doses; >150 mg needed for norepinephrine effect—but increases blood pressure at these higher doses; significant discontinuation syndrome; low risk of enzyme inhibition; substrate of CYP2D6 Black Box Warning: Suicidality *MDD/GAD/Social anxiety disorder/Panic disorder*
Desvenlafaxine (SNRI) (Pristiq®; Khedezla®)	Start: 50 mg po daily and continue; may go up to usual max of 100 mg daily but no clear benefit from doses higher than 50 mg/day. Max dose is 50 mg every other day in patients with severe renal impairment.	Active metabolite of venlafaxine. Check baseline blood pressure, then every 3–6 months; significant discontinuation syndrome; low risk of enzyme inhibition; nausea may be early adverse effect; still an expensive brand SNRI. CYP3A4 substrate. Black Box Warning: Suicidality *MDD*

(continued)

TABLE 1.1 Continued

Medication[a]	Adult Dosing[b]	Comments/FDA Indication
Duloxetine (SNRI) (Cymbalta®)	Start: 20–40 mg/day in single or divided doses, increase to 60 mg/day in divided doses after 7 days. Max 120 mg/day but no evidence that increasing to maximum is more helpful. Avoid in patients with liver disease or severe renal impairment.	Check baseline blood pressure, then every 3–6 months; serotonergic and noradrenergic effects at all doses; no clinically significant benefit on physical pain that often accompanies depression; avoid if substantial alcohol use; significant discontinuation syndrome; modest inhibition of CYP2D6, CYP1A2. Black Box Warning: Suicidality *MDD/GAD/Diabetic neuropathy/Fibromyalgia/ Chronic musculoskeletal pain*
Bupropion (Wellbutrin®, Wellbutrin SR®, Wellbutrin XL®, ForFivo®, Zyban®)	For Wellbutrin XL®: Start: 150 mg po q am and increase to 300 mg q am after 4–7 days, max of 450 mg q am; different dosing for different formulations. Reduce doses in patients with hepatic or renal impairments.	Contraindicated in patients with history of seizure, eating disorder or if otherwise at high seizure risk; least likely to cause sexual side effects or weight gain; moderate inhibition of CYP2D6. Black Box Warning: Suicidality *MDD/Prevention of MDE in patients with seasonal affective disorder/Aid to smoking cessation treatment*

TABLE 1.1 Continued

Medication[a]	Adult Dosing[b]	Comments/FDA *Indication*
Mirtazapine (Remeron®)	Start: 7.5–15 mg po qhs and increase to 30 mg qhs after 1–2 weeks, max 45 mg po qhs. Clearance may be decreased therefore, use with caution in patients with hepatic or renal impairments	Improves appetite and sleep as early side effects; can cause weight gain; low risk of medication interactions; less sexual side effects than SSRIs; may be more sedating at lower doses; may work faster than other antidepressants. Rare agranulocytosis may occur; substrate of CYP2D6, CYP1A2, CYP3A4 Black Box Warning: Suicidality *MDD*
Trazodone (Desyrel®, Oleptro®)	For trazodone, Desyrel®, for insomnia only: Start: 25 mg po qhs, if needed increase to 50 mg, then can increase by 25–50 mg increments every 3–4 days up to 200 mg at bedtime. Extended release trazodone (Oleptro®): Start: 150 mg po qhs, increase by 75 mg every 4th day, maximum 375 mg po qhs. Use with caution in patients with hepatic or renal impairments.	Used primarily for insomnia; may cause orthostasis, priapism; generally not used as an antidepressant but when it was used as an antidepressant the dose was 400 mg daily; extended release formulation is recently marketed for depression; CYP3A4 substrate. Prolongs QT interval. Black Box Warning: Suicidality *MDD*

(continued)

TABLE 1.1 Continued

Medication[a]	Adult Dosing[b]	Comments/FDA *Indication*
OTHER NEWER ANTIDEPRESSANTS:		
Vilazodone (Viibryd®)	Start: 10 mg per day for first week then 20 mg per day for 2nd week, then 30 mg daily for 3rd week, then 40 mg per day; lower than 40 mg daily dose may not be effective. Take with food. Titration limited by GI symptoms. Mildly sedating. Max 40 mg/day.	Expensive. Unclear if it has any benefits over cost-effective SSRIs and SNRIs. Inhibits CYP2C8; CYP3A4 substrate, expected to have low drug-drug interactions. Black Box Warning: Suicidality *MDD*
Isocarboxazid (MAOI) (Marplan®)	Start 10 mg po bid, if tolerated increase by 10 mg increments every 2–4 days to 40 mg po/daily total, bid to qid dosing. Max is 60 mg/day in divided doses. Contraindicated in patients with hepatic impairment or severe renal impairment.	Nonselective MAOI. Available for decades so not actually a "new" MAOI but generic is now unavailable. New brand name drug is very expensive. Dangerous food and drug interactions (see package insert) Black Box Warning: Suicidality *Depression*
Levomilnacipran ER (SNRI) (Fetzima®)	Start: 20 mg po daily for 2 days then increase to 40 mg po daily, then may increase in 40 mg daily increments every 2 or more days as tolerated, max is 120 mg per day. Reduced dose is needed in patients with hepatic impairment. Do not use in patients with severe renal impairment.	Check baseline blood pressure, then every 3–6 months; potent norepinephrine reuptake inhibition; CYP3A4 substrate Black Box Warning: Suicidality *MDD*

TABLE 1.1 Continued

Medication[a]	Adult Dosing[b]	Comments/FDA *Indication*
Vortioxetine (Trintellix®)	Start: 10 mg po daily, reduce to 5 mg daily if higher doses are not tolerated. May increase to 20 mg po daily if tolerated, max is 20 mg per day.	Multiple serotonin receptor effects; nausea most common adverse effect. May displace other highly protein bound drugs; CYP2D6 substrate Black Box Warning: Suicidality *MDD*
EMERGING PHARMACOTHERAPIES:		
Esketamine Nasal Spray (Spravato®)	Avoid food for 2 hours, and liquids for 30 minutes, before administration. Start: 28 mg spray to each nostril for a total of 56 mg twice weekly. If needed and tolerated, subsequent doses may be increased to 84 mg twice weekly (max dose). Assess at 4 weeks if needed to continue. For maintenance: beginning on week 5 may administer once weekly. At week 9 and afterwards adjust frequency for lowest interval needed to maintain remission (e.g., once a week or once every 2 weeks). Patients with moderate hepatic impairments may need longer monitoring period, and not recommended in those with severe impairment.	New antidepressant with minimal clinical experience, therefore risks may not be fully known. Administration requires certified healthcare setting and direct observation and is very expensive. Depersonalization, derealization, dissociation, dizziness, nausea may be frequent. Increased blood pressure may be seen. Contraindicated in patients with aneurysmal vascular disease or arteriovenous malformations or history of intracerebral hemorrhage. Not recommended during pregnancy or breastfeeding. Should not be combined with other CNS depressants. Metabolized by CYP2B6 and CYP3A4. Black Box Warning: Sedation, dissociation, needing monitoring for 2 hours or more after each treatment; abuse and misuse potential. Risk Evaluation and Mitigation Strategy (REMS); suicidality *Treatment-resistant depression in adults, in conjunction with an oral antidepressant*

(continued)

TABLE 1.1 Continued

Medication[a]	Adult Dosing[b]	Comments/FDA *Indication*
Brexanolone (Zulresso®)	Administered intravenously over 60-hour continuous infusion. See package insert for IV dose titration. Infusion must be stopped if "excessive" sedation or hypoxia occurs. Not recommended in patients with moderate to severe renal impairment.	New antidepressant with minimal clinical experience, therefore risks may not be fully known. Extremely expensive. Administration requires certified healthcare setting and direct observation. Risks of excessive sedation, syncope and hypoxia. Should not be combined with other CNS depressants. Black Box Warning: Monitoring needed with continuous pulse oximetry given risk of excessive sedation, sudden loss of consciousness; Risk Evaluations and Mitigation Strategy *Postpartum depression in adults*

SEE PACKAGE INSERT FOR DOSING AND OTHER INFORMATION BEFORE PRESCRIBING MEDICATIONS. Dosing should be adjusted downward ("start low, go slow" strategy) for the elderly and/or the medically compromised. Abbreviations: bid (bis in die), twice a day; CYP, Cytochrome P450 enzyme; FDA, Food and Drug Administration; GAD, generalized anxiety disorder; MAOI, monoamine oxidase inhibitor; MAO, B-monoamine oxidase inhibitor, B subtype; MDD, major depressive disorder; MDE, major depressive episode; mg, milligram; ng/mL, nanogram per milliliter; OCD, obsessive compulsive disorder; PMDD, pre-menstrual dysphoric disorder; po (per os), orally; PTSD, posttraumatic stress disorder; q (quaque), every; qhs, (quaque hora somni) at bedtime; SNRI, serotonin norepinephrine reuptake inhibitor; SSRI, selective serotonin reuptake inhibitor; TCA, tricyclic antidepressant; WHO, World Health Organization.

[a]Generic and U.S. brand name(s).

[b]Doses are provided for educational purposes only.

References

Abadie D, Rousseau V, et al. (2015). Serotonin syndrome: analysis of cases registered in the French Pharmacovigilance Database. J Clin Psychopharmacol 35(4): 382–388.

Addis A, Koren G (2000). Safety of fluoxetine during the first trimester of pregnancy: a meta-analytical review of epidemiological studies. Psychol Med 30(1): 89–94.

Almatroudi A, Husbands SM, et al. (2015). Combined administration of buprenorphine and naltrexone produces antidepressant-like effects in mice. J Psychopharmacol 29(7): 812–821.

Almeida NDO, Basso O, et al. (2016). Risk of miscarriage in women receiving antidepressants in early pregnancy, correcting for induced abortions. Epidemiology 27(4): 538–546.

Alwan S, Bandoli G, et al. (2016). Maternal use of selective serotonin-reuptake inhibitors and risk of persistent pulmonary hypertension of the newborn. Clin Pharmacol Ther 100(1): 34–41.

Alwan S, Reefhuis J, et al. (2010). Maternal use of bupropion and risk for congenital heart defects. Am J Obstet Gynecol 203(1): 52 e51–56.

Andrade C (2015). Intranasal drug delivery in neuropsychiatry: focus on intranasal ketamine for refractory depression. J Clin Psychiatry 76(5): e628–631.

Andrade C (2017). Antidepressant exposure during pregnancy and risk of autism in the offspring, 1: meta-review of meta-analyses. J Clin Psychiatry 78(8): e1047–e1051.

Anonymous (2015). Semen abnormalities with SSRI antidepressants. Prescrire Int 24(156): 16–17.

Ansari A (2000). The efficacy of newer antidepressants in the treatment of chronic pain: a review of current literature. Harvard Rev Psychiatry 7: 257–277.

Ansari A, Osser DN (2015). *Psychopharmacology, A Concise Overview for Students and Clinicians, 2nd Edition*. North Charleston, SC: CreateSpace.

Appleton KM, Sallis HM, et al. (2015). Omega-3 fatty acids for depression in adults. Cochrane Database Syst Rev 11: CD004692.

Arnold LM, McElroy SL, et al. (2002). A placebo-controlled, randomized trial of fluoxetine in the treatment of binge-eating disorder. J Clin Psychiatry 63(11): 1028–1033.

Asher GN, Gartlehner G, et al. (2017). Comparative benefits and harms of complementary and alternative medicine therapies for initial treatment of major depressive disorder: systematic review and meta-analysis. J Altern Complement Med 23(12): 907–919.

Asher GN, Gerkin J, et al. (2017). Complementary therapies for mental health disorders. Med Clin North Am 101(5): 847–864.

Atigari OV, Kelly AM, et al. (2013). New onset alcohol dependence linked to treatment with selective serotonin reuptake inhibitors. Int J Risk Saf Med 25(2): 105–109.

Auclair AL, Martel JC, et al. (2013). Levomilnacipran (F2695), a norepinephrine-preferring SNRI: profile in vitro and in models of depression and anxiety. Neuropharmacology 70: 338–347.

Barone P, Scarzella L, et al. (2006). Pramipexole versus sertraline in the treatment of depression in Parkinson's disease: a national multicenter parallel-group randomized study. J Neurol 253(5): 601–607.

Becker C, Jick SS, et al. (2017). Selective serotonin reuptake inhibitors and cataract risk: a case-control analysis. Ophthalmology 124(11): 1635–1639.

Ben-Sheetrit J, Aizenberg D, et al. (2015). Post-SSRI sexual dysfunction: clinical characterization and preliminary assessment of contributory factors and dose–response relationship. J Clin Psychopharmacol 35(3): 273–278.

Berard A, Iessa N, et al. (2016). The risk of major cardiac malformations associated with paroxetine use during the first trimester of pregnancy: a systematic review and meta-analysis. Br J Clin Pharmacol 81(4): 589–604.

Berard A, Zhao JP, et al. (2015). Sertraline use during pregnancy and the risk of major malformations. Am J Obstet Gynecol 212(6): 795 e791–795 e712.

Berard A, Zhao JP, et al. (2017). Antidepressant use during pregnancy and the risk of major congenital malformations in a cohort of depressed pregnant women: an updated analysis of the Quebec Pregnancy Cohort. BMJ Open 7(1): e013372.

Berle JO and Spigset O (2011). Antidepressant use during breastfeeding. Curr Womens Health Rev 7(1): 28–34.

Blier P, Ward HE, et al. (2010). Combination of antidepressant medications from treatment initiation for major depressive disorder: a double-blind randomized study. Am J Psychiatry 167(3): 281–288.

Bolton JM, Metge C, et al. (2008). Fracture risk from psychotropic medications: a population-based analysis. J Clin Psychopharmacol 28(4): 384–391.

Bolton JM, Morin SN, et al. (2017). Association of mental disorders and related medication use with risk for major osteoporotic fractures. JAMA Psychiatry 74(6): 641–648.

Boyer EW, Shannon M (2005). The serotonin syndrome. New Engl J Med 352: 1112–1120.

Bridge JA, Iyengar S, et al. (2007). Clinical response and risk for reported suicidal ideation and suicide attempts in pediatric antidepressant treatment: a meta-analysis of randomized controlled trials. JAMA 297: 1683–1696.

Brown AS, Gyllenberg D, et al. (2016). Association of selective serotonin reuptake inhibitor exposure during pregnancy with speech, scholastic, and motor disorders in offspring. JAMA Psychiatry 73(11): 1163–1170.

Bundeff AW and Woodis CB (2014). Selective serotonin reuptake inhibitors for the treatment of irritable bowel syndrome. Ann Pharmacother 48(6): 777–784.

Caddy C, Amit BH, et al. (2015). Ketamine and other glutamate receptor modulators for depression in adults. Cochrane Database Syst Rev 9: CD011612.

Canuso CM, Singh JB, et al. (2018). Efficacy and safety of intranasal esketamine for the rapid reduction of symptoms of depression and suicidality in patients at imminent risk for suicide: results of a double-blind, randomized, placebo-controlled study. Am J Psychiatry 175(7): 620–630.

Carceller-Sindreu M, de Diego-Adelino J, et al. (2017). Lack of relationship between plasma levels of escitalopram and QTc-interval length. Eur Arch Psychiatr Clin Neurosci 267(8): 815–822.

Castro VM, Clements CC, et al. (2013). QT interval and antidepressant use: a cross sectional study of electronic health records. BMJ 346: f288.

Chappell JC, Eisenhofer G, et al. (2014). Effects of duloxetine on norepinephrine and serotonin transporter activity in healthy subjects. J Clin Psychopharmacol 34(1): 9–16.

Chaudron LH and Pies RW (2003). The relationship between postpartum psychosis and bipolar disorder: a review. J Clin Psychiatry 64: 1284–1292.

Chen L, Ilham SJ, et al. (2017). Pharmacological approach for managing pain in irritable bowel syndrome: a review article. Anesth Pain Med 7(2): e42747.

Chun-Fai-Chan B, Koren G, et al. (2005). Pregnancy outcome of women exposed to bupropion during pregnancy: a prospective comparative study. Am J Obstet Gynecol 192(3): 932–936.

Cipriani A, Furukawa TA, et al. (2009). Comparative efficacy and acceptability of 12 new-generation antidepressants: a multiple-treatments meta-analysis. Lancet 373(9665): 746–758.

Cipriani A, Furukawa TA, et al. (2018). Comparative efficacy and acceptability of 21 antidepressant drugs for the acute treatment of adults with major depressive disorder: a systematic review and network meta-analysis. Lancet 391(10128): 1357–1366.

Cipriani A, Koesters M, et al. (2012). Duloxetine versus other anti-depressive agents for depression. Cochrane Database Syst Rev 10: CD006533.

Cipriani A, La Ferla T, et al. (2010). Sertraline versus other antidepressive agents for depression. Cochrane Database Syst Rev 4: CD006117.

Citrome L (2014). Vortioxetine for major depressive disorder: a systematic review of the efficacy and safety profile for this newly approved antidepressant—what is the number needed to treat, number needed to harm and likelihood to be helped or harmed? Int J Clin Pract 68(1): 60–82.

Cohen LS, Altshuler LL, et al. (2006). Relapse of major depression during pregnancy in women who maintain or discontinue antidepressant treatment. JAMA 295(5): 499–507.

Cole JA, Modell JG, et al. (2007). Bupropion in pregnancy and the prevalence of congenital malformations. Pharmacoepidemiol Drug Saf 16(5): 474–484.

Connolly KR, Thase ME (2011). If at first you don't succeed: a review of the evidence for antidepressant augmentation, combination and switching strategies. Drugs 71(1): 43–64.

Costa FH, Rosso AL, et al. (2012). Depression in Parkinson's disease: diagnosis and treatment. Arq Neuropsiquiatr 70(8): 617–620.

Covvey JR, Crawford AN, et al. (2012). Intravenous ketamine for treatment-resistant major depressive disorder. Ann Pharmacother 46(1): 117–123.

Cuijpers P (2014). Combined pharmacotherapy and psychotherapy in the treatment of mild to moderate major depression? JAMA Psychiatry 71(7): 747–748.

Dawson LA, Watson JM (2009). Vilazodone: a 5-HT1A receptor agonist/serotonin transporter inhibitor for the treatment of affective disorders. CNS Neurosci Ther 15(2): 107–117.

de Abajo FJ, Garcia-Rodriguez LA (2008). Risk of upper gastrointestinal tract bleeding associated with selective serotonin reuptake inhibitors and venlafaxine therapy: interaction with nonsteroidal anti-inflammatory drugs and effect of acid-suppressing agents. Arch Gen Psychiatry 65(7): 795–803.

de Kruif M, Spijker AT, et al. (2016). Depression during the perimenopause: a meta-analysis. J Affect Disord 206: 174–180.

Denton WH, Carmody TJ, et al. (2010). Dyadic discord at baseline is associated with lack of remission in the acute treatment of chronic depression. Psychol Med 40(3): 415–424.

de Paulis T (2007). Drug evaluation: vilazodone—a combined SSRI and 5-HT1A partial agonist for the treatment of depression. IDrugs 10(3): 193–201.

DeVane CL, Grothe DR, et al. (2002). Pharmacology of antidepressants: focus on nefazodone. J Clin Psychiatry 63(Suppl 1): 10–17.

Diaper A, Rich AS, et al. (2013). Changes in cardiovascular function after venlafaxine but not pregabalin in healthy volunteers: a double-blind, placebo-controlled study of orthostatic challenge, blood pressure and heart rate. Hum Psychopharmacol 28(6): 562–575.

Diem SJ, Harrison SL, et al. (2013). Depressive symptoms and rates of bone loss at the hip in older men. Osteoporosis Int 24(1): 111–119.

Diem SJ, Ruppert K, et al. (2013). Rates of bone loss among women initiating antidepressant medication use in midlife. J Clin Endocrinol Metab 98(11): 4355–4363.

Duman RS, Li N (2012). A neurotrophic hypothesis of depression: role of synaptogenesis in the actions of NMDA receptor antagonists. Philos Trans R Soc Lond B Biol Sci 367(1601): 2475–2484.

Dunner DL, Zisook S, et al. (1998). A prospective safety surveillance study for bupropion sustained-release in the treatment of depression. J Clin Psychiatry 59(7): 366–373.

Einarson AL, Bonari S, et al. (2003). A multicentre prospective controlled study to determine the safety of trazodone and nefazodone use during pregnancy. Can J Psychiatry 48(2): 106–110.

Einarson TR, Einarson A (2005). Newer antidepressants in pregnancy and rates of major malformations: a meta-analysis of prospective comparative studies. Pharmacoepidemiol Drug Saf 14(12): 823–827.

Ereshefsky L, Jhee S, et al. (2005). Antidepressant drug-drug interaction profile update. Drugs R & D 6: 323–336.

Etminan M, Mikelberg FS, et al. (2010). Selective serotonin reuptake inhibitors and the risk of cataracts: a nested case-control study. Ophthalmology 117(6): 1251–1255.

Fabbri, C, Tansey KE, et al. (2018). New insights into the pharmacogenomics of antidepressant response from the GENDEP and STAR*D studies: rare variant analysis and high-density imputation. Pharmacogenomics J 18(3): 413–421.

Farmand S, Lindh JD, et al. (2018). Differences in associations of antidepressants and hospitalization due to hyponatremia. Am J Med 131(1): 56–63.

Fava GA, Gatti A, et al. (2015). Withdrawal symptoms after selective serotonin reuptake inhibitor discontinuation: a systematic review. Psychother Psychosom 84(2): 72–81.

Fava M, Rush AJ, et al. (2008). Difference in treatment outcome in outpatients with anxious versus nonanxious depression: a STAR*D report. Am J Psychiatry 165: 342–351.

Feighner JP (1999). Mechanism of action of antidepressant medications. J Clin Psychiatry 60(Suppl 4): 4–11.

Fishbain D (2000). Evidence-based data on pain relief with antidepressants. Anna Med 32: 305–316.

Fluoxetine Bulimia Nervosa Collaborative Study Group (1992). Fluoxetine in the treatment of bulimia nervosa. A multicenter, placebo-controlled, double-blind trial. Arch Gen Psychiatry 49(2): 139–147.

Fond G, Loundou A, et al. (2014). Ketamine administration in depressive disorders: a systematic review and meta-analysis. Psychopharmacology (Berl) 231(18): 3663–3676.

Food and Drug Administration (2011). FDA drug safety communication: selective serotonin reuptake inhibitor (SSRI) antidepressant use during pregnancy and reports of a rare heart and lung condition in newborn babies. https://www.fda.gov/Drugs/DrugSafety/ucm283375.htm

Food and Drug Administration (2012). FDA drug safety communication: revised recommendations for Celexa (citalopram hydrobromide)

related to a potential risk of abnormal heart rhythms with high doses. http://www.fda.gov/drugs/drugsafety/ucm297391.htm

Ford AC, Talley NJ, et al. (2009). Efficacy of antidepressants and psychological therapies in irritable bowel syndrome: systematic review and meta-analysis. Gut 58(3): 367–378.

Frampton JE (2016). Vortioxetine: a review in cognitive dysfunction in depression. Drugs 76(17): 1675–1682.

Frank GK, Shott ME (2016). The role of psychotropic medications in the management of anorexia nervosa: rationale, evidence and future prospects. CNS Drugs 30(5): 419–442.

Friedman RA (2014). Antidepressants' black-box warning—10 years later. N Engl J Med 371(18): 1666–1668.

Frykberg RG, Gordon S, et al. (2015). Linezolid-associated serotonin syndrome: a report of two cases. J Am Podiatr Med Assoc 105(3): 244–248.

Funk KA, Bostwick JR (2013). A comparison of the risk of QT prolongation among SSRIs. Ann Pharmacother 47(10): 1330–1341.

Furu K, Kieler H, et al. (2015). Selective serotonin reuptake inhibitors and venlafaxine in early pregnancy and risk of birth defects: population based cohort study and sibling design. BMJ 350: h1798.

Furukawa TA, Cipriani A, et al. (2018). Is placebo response in antidepressant trials rising or not? A reanalysis of datasets to conclude this long-lasting controversy. Evid Based Ment Health 21(1): 1–3.

Galbally M, Spigset O, et al. (2017). Neonatal adaptation following intrauterine antidepressant exposure: assessment, drug assay levels, and infant development outcomes. Pediatr Res 82(5): 806–813.

Galecki P, Mossakowska-Wojcik J, et al. (2018). The anti-inflammatory mechanism of antidepressants—SSRIs, SNRIs. Prog Neuropsychopharmacol Biol Psychiatry 80(Pt C): 291–294.

Galizia I, Oldani L, et al. (2016). S-adenosyl methionine (SAMe) for depression in adults. Cochrane Database Syst Rev 10: CD011286.

Gallagher HC, Gallagher RM, et al. (2015). Venlafaxine for neuropathic pain in adults. Cochrane Database Syst Rev 8: CD011091.

Gandhi TK, Weingart SN, et al. (2003). Adverse drug events in ambulatory care. N Engl J Med 348(16): 1556–1564.

Gao SY, Wu QJ, et al. (2017). Fluoxetine and congenital malformations: a systematic review and meta-analysis of cohort studies. Br J Clin Pharmacol 83(10): 2134–2147.

Garcia-Gonzalez, J, Tansey KE, et al. (2017). Pharmacogenetics of antidepressant response: a polygenic approach. Prog Neuropsychopharmacol Biol Psychiatry 75: 128–134.

Gartlehner G, Gaynes BN, et al. (2008). Comparative benefits and harms of second-generation antidepressants: background paper for the American College of Physicians. Anna Intern Med 149: 734–750.

Gebhardt S, Heinzel-Gutenbrunner M, Konig U (2016). Pain relief in depressive disorders: a meta-analysis of the effects of antidepressants. J Clin Psychopharmacol 36(6): 658–668.

Geddes JR, Carney SM, et al. (2003). Relapse prevention with antidepressant drug treatment in depressive disorders: a systematic review. Lancet 361(9358): 653–661.

Gelenberg AJ (2002). Nefazodone hepatotoxicity: Black Box Warning. Biol Therap Psychiatr Newsl 25.

Gentile, S. (2014). Tricyclic antidepressants in pregnancy and puerperium. Expert Opin Drug Saf 13(2): 207–225.

Gerber PE, Lynd LD (1998). Selective serotonin-reuptake inhibitor-induced movement disorders. Ann Pharmacother 32(6): 692–698.

Ghaemi SN, Ko JY, et al. (2002). "Cade's disease" and beyond: misdiagnosis, antidepressant use, and a proposed definition for bipolar spectrum disorder. Can J Psychiatry 47: 125–134.

Giakoumatos CI, Osser DN (2019). The Psychopharmacology Algorithm Project at the Harvard South Shore Program: an update on unipolar nonpsychotic depression. Harv Rev Psychiatry 27(1): 33–52.

Gibbons RD, Brown CH, et al. (2007). Early evidence on the effects of regulators' suicidality warnings on SSRI prescriptions and suicide in children and adolescents. Am J Psychiatry 164: 1356–1363.

Gibbons RD, Hur K, et al. (2012). Benefits from antidepressants: synthesis of 6-week patient-level outcomes from double-blind placebo-controlled randomized trials of fluoxetine and venlafaxine. Arch Gen Psychiatry 69(6): 572–579.

Girardin FR, Gex-Fabry M, et al. (2013). Drug-induced long QT in adult psychiatric inpatients: the 5-year cross-sectional ECG Screening Outcome in Psychiatry study. Am J Psychiatry 179(12): 1468–1476.

Glassman AH, O'Connor CM, et al. (2002). Sertraline treatment of major depression in patients with acute MI or unstable angina. JAMA 288(6): 701–709.

Glue P, Donovan MR, et al. (2010). Meta-analysis of relapse prevention antidepressant trials in depressive disorders. Aust N Z J Psychiatry 44(8): 697–705.

Goldberg JF, Thase ME (2013). Monoamine oxidase inhibitors revisited: what you should know. J Clin Psychiatry 74(2): 189–191.

Goldstein DJ, Wilson MG, et al. (1999). Effectiveness of fluoxetine therapy in bulimia nervosa regardless of comorbid depression. Int J Eat Disord 25(1): 19–27.

Grunebaum MF, Ellis SP, et al. (2004). Antidepressants and suicide risk in the United States, 1985–1999. J Clin Psychiatry 65: 1456–1462.

Guerdjikova AI, Walsh B, et al. (2017). Concurrent improvement in both binge eating and depressive symptoms with naltrexone/bupropion therapy in overweight or obese subjects with major depressive disorder in an open-label, uncontrolled study. Adv Ther 34(10): 2307–2315.

Haddad P (1998). The SSRI discontinuation syndrome. J Psychopharmacol 12(3): 305–313.

Hamer M, David Batty G, et al. (2011). Antidepressant medication use and future risk of cardiovascular disease: the Scottish Health Survey. Eur Heart J 32(4): 437–442.

Hamoda HM, Osser DN (2008). The Psychopharmacology Algorithm Project at the Harvard South Shore Program: an update on psychotic depression. Harv Rev Psychiatry 16(4): 235–247.

Harada T, Ishizaki F, et al. (2011). New dopamine agonist pramipexole improves parkinsonism and depression in Parkinson's disease. Hiroshima J Med Sci 60(4): 79–82.

Harada T, Sakamoto K, et al. (2008). Incidence and predictors of activation syndrome induced by antidepressants. Depression Anxiety 25: 1014–1019.

Hendrick V, Suri R, et al. (2017). Bupropion use during pregnancy: a systematic review. Prim Care Companion CNS Disord 19(5): 17r02160.

Hieronymous F, Emilsson JF, et al. (2016). Consistent superiority of selective serotonin reuptake inhibitors over placebo in reducing depressed mood in patients with major depression. Mol Psychiatry 21(4): 523–530.

Hoban CL, Byard RW, et al. (2015). A comparison of patterns of spontaneous adverse drug reaction reporting with St. John's wort and fluoxetine during the period 2000–2013. Clin Exp Pharmacol Physiol 42(7): 747–751.

Hodgson K, K. Tansey KE, et al. (2016). Transcriptomics and the mechanisms of antidepressant efficacy. Eur Neuropsychopharmacol 26(1): 105–112.

Hogue AN, Temple-Cooper ME, et al. (2017). Effects of in-utero exposure to selective serotonin reuptake inhibitors and venlafaxine on term and preterm infants. J Neonatal Perinatal Med 10(4): 371–380.

Hrdlicka M, Beranova I, et al. (2008). Mirtazapine in the treatment of adolescent anorexia nervosa: case-control study. Eur Child Adolesc Psychiatry 17(3): 187–189.

Iovieno N, Tedeschini E, et al. (2011). Antidepressants for major depressive disorder and dysthymic disorder in patients with comorbid alcohol use disorders: a meta-analysis of placebo-controlled randomized trials. J Clin Psychiatry 72(8): 1144–1151.

Iqbal MM, Basil MJ, et al. (2012). Overview of serotonin syndrome. Ann Clin Psychiatry 24(4): 310–318.

Jackson JL, Mancuso JM, et al. Kay (2017). Tricyclic and tetracyclic antidepressants for the prevention of frequent episodic or chronic tension-type headache in adults: a systematic review and meta-analysis. J Gen Intern Med 32(12): 1351–1358.

Jain R, Mahableshwarkar AR, et al. (2013). A randomized, double-blind, placebo-controlled 6-wk trial of the efficacy and tolerability of 5 mg vortioxetine in adults with major depressive disorder. Int J Neuropsychopharmacol 16(2): 313–321.

Jha MK, Minhajuddin A, et al. (2017). Can C-reactive protein inform antidepressant medication selection in depressed outpatients? Findings from the CO-MED trial. Psychoneuroendocrinology 78: 105–113.

Jiang SM, Jia L, et al. (2016). Beneficial effects of antidepressant mirtazapine in functional dyspepsia patients with weight loss. World J Gastroenterol 22(22): 5260–5266.

Jimenez-Solem E. (2014). Exposure to antidepressants during pregnancy—prevalences and outcomes. Dan Med J 61(9): B4916.

Johnson EM, Whyte E, et al. (2006). Cardiovascular changes associated with venlafaxine in the treatment of late-life depression. Am J Geriatr Psychiatry 14: 796–802.

Kang HJ, Bae KY, et al. (2016). Associations between serotonergic genes and escitalopram treatment responses in patients with depressive disorder and acute coronary syndrome: the EsDEPACS study. Psychiatry Investig 13(1): 157–160.

Kellner CH, Greenberg RM, et al. (2012). ECT in treatment-resistant depression. Am J Psychiatry 169(12): 1238–1244.

Keltner NL, McAfee KM, et al. (2002). Mechanisms and treatments of SSRI-induced sexual dysfunction. Perspect Psychiatr Care 38(3): 111–116.

Khan A (2009). Vilazodone, a novel dual-acting serotonergic antidepressant for managing major depression. Expert Opin Investig Drugs 18(11): 1753–1764.

Khan A, Cutler AJ, et al. (2011). A randomized, double-blind, placebo-controlled, 8-week study of vilazodone, a serotonergic agent for the treatment of major depressive disorder. J Clin Psychiatry 72(4): 441–447.

Khin NA, Chen YF, et al. (2011). Exploratory analyses of efficacy data from major depressive disorder trials submitted to the US Food and Drug Administration in support of new drug applications. J Clin Psychiatry 72(4): 464–472.

Kim H, Lim SW, et al. (2006). Monoamine transporter gene polymorphisms and antidepressant response in Koreans with late-life depression. JAMA 296: 1609–1618.

Kirsch I, Deacon BJ, et al. (2008). Initial severity and antidepressant benefits: a meta-analysis of data submitted to the Food and Drug Administration. PLoS Med 5(2): e45.

Kjaersgaard MI, Parner ET, et al. (2013). Prenatal antidepressant exposure and risk of spontaneous abortion—a population-based study. PLoS One 8(8): e72095.

Koesters M, Ostuzzi G, et al. (2017). Vortioxetine for depression in adults. Cochrane Database Syst Rev 7: CD011520.

Koren G, Nordeng HM (2013). Selective serotonin reuptake inhibitors and malformations: case closed? Semin Fetal Neonatal Med 18(1): 19–22.

Kraft JB, Peters EJ, et al. (2007). Analysis of association between the serotonin transporter and antidepressant response in a large clinical sample. Biol Psychiatry 61: 734–742.

Kremer M, Salvat E, et al. (2016). Antidepressants and gabapentinoids in neuropathic pain: mechanistic insights. Neuroscience 338: 183–206.

Kronenfeld N, Berlin M, et al. (2017). Use of Psychotropic Medications in Breastfeeding Women. Birth Defects Res 109(12): 957–997.

Kuhn R (1958). The treatment of depressive states with G 22355 (imipramine hydrochloride). Am J Psychiatry 115: 459–464.

Kulak-Bejda A, Bejda G, et al. (2017). Antidepressants for irritable bowel syndrome-A systematic review. Pharmacol Rep 69(6): 1366–1379.

Lapidus KA, Levitch CF, et al. (2014). A randomized controlled trial of intranasal ketamine in major depressive disorder. Biol Psychiatry 76(12): 970–976.

Lassen D, Ennis ZN, et al. (2016). First-trimester pregnancy exposure to venlafaxine or duloxetine and risk of major congenital malformations: a systematic review. Basic Clin Pharmacol Toxicol 118(1): 32–36.

Laughren TP, Gobburu J, et al. (2011). Vilazodone: clinical basis for the US Food and Drug Administration's approval of a new antidepressant. J Clin Psychiatry 72(9): 1166–1173.

Lekman M, Paddock S, et al. (2008). Pharmacogenetics of major depression: insights from level 1 of the Sequenced Treatment Alternatives to Relieve Depression (STAR*D) trial. Molec Diag Ther 12: 321–330.

Leombruni P, Amianto F, et al. (2006). Citalopram versus fluoxetine for the treatment of patients with bulimia nervosa: a single-blind randomized controlled trial. Adv Ther 23(3): 481–494.

Leombruni P, Piero A, et al. (2008). A randomized, double-blind trial comparing sertraline and fluoxetine 6-month treatment in obese patients with Binge Eating Disorder. Prog Neuropsychopharmacol Biol Psychiatry 32(6): 1599–1605.

Leon AC, Solomon DA, et al. (2011). Antidepressants and risks of suicide and suicide attempts: a 27-year observational study. J Clin Psychiatry 72(5): 580–586.

Leverich GS, Altshuler LL, et al. (2006). Risk of switch in mood polarity to hypomania or mania in patients with bipolar depression during acute and continuation trials of venlafaxine, sertraline, and bupropion as adjuncts to mood stabilizers. Am J Psychiatry 163: 232–239.

Levkovitz Y, Tedeschini E, et al. (2011). Efficacy of antidepressants for dysthymia: a meta-analysis of placebo-controlled randomized trials. J Clin Psychiatry 72(4): 509–514.

Lexicomp (2019). https://www.wolterskluwercdi.com/lexicomp-online/

Li JM, Zhang Y, et al. (2018). Cognitive behavioral therapy for treatment-resistant depression: a systematic review and meta-analysis. Psychiatry Res 268: 243–250.

Linde K, Berner MM, Kriston L (2008). St John's wort for major depression. Cochrane Database Syst Rev 8(4): CD000448.

Lippman SB, Nash K (1990). Monoamine oxidase inhibitor update. Potential adverse food and drug interactions. Drug Safety 5: 195–204.

Lu Y, Chen M, et al. (2016). Antidepressants in the Treatment of Functional Dyspepsia: a Systematic Review and Meta-Analysis. PLoS One 11(6): e0157798.

Lunn MP, Hughes RA, et al. (2014). Duloxetine for treating painful neuropathy, chronic pain or fibromyalgia. Cochrane Database Syst Rev 1: CD007115.

Lynch T, Price A (2007). The effect of cytochrome P450 metabolism on drug response, interactions, and adverse effects. Am Fam Physician 76(3): 391–396.

Magni G (1991). The use of antidepressants in the treatment of chronic pain. A review of the current evidence. Drugs 42: 730–748.

Maharaj S, Trevino K (2015). A comprehensive review of treatment options for premenstrual syndrome and premenstrual dysphoric disorder. J Psychiatr Pract 21(5): 334–350.

Maina G, Albert U, et al. (2004). Weight gain during long-term treatment of obsessive-compulsive disorder: a prospective comparison between serotonin reputake inhibitors. J Clin Psychiatry 65(10): 1365–1371.

Malamood M, Roberts A, et al. (2017). Mirtazapine for symptom control in refractory gastroparesis. Drug Des Devel Ther 11: 1035–1041.

Malhotra AK, Murphy GM Jr., et al. (2004). Pharmacogenetics of psychotropic drug response. Am J Psychiatry 161: 780–796.

Marvanova M, Gramith K (2018). Role of antidepressants in the treatment of adults with anorexia nervosa. Ment Health Clin 8(3): 127–137.

Masi G, Brovedani P (2011). The hippocampus, neurotrophic factors and depression: possible implications for the pharmacotherapy of depression. CNS Drugs 25(11): 913–931.

Mathew SJ, Shah A, et al. (2012). Ketamine for treatment-resistant unipolar depression: current evidence. CNS Drugs 26(3): 189–204.

Mavrides N, Nemeroff C (2013). Treatment of depression in cardiovascular disease. Depress Anxiety 30(4): 328–341.

Max MB, Culnane M, et al. (1987). Amitriptyline relieves diabetic neuropathy pain in patients with normal or depressed mood. Neurology 37: 589–596.

Mbaya P, Alam F, et al. (2007). Cardiovascular effects of high dose venlafaxine XL in patients with major depressive disorder. Hum Psychopharmacol 22: 129–133.

McElroy SL, Casuto LS, et al. (2000). Placebo-controlled trial of sertraline in the treatment of binge eating disorder. Am J Psychiatry 157(6): 1004–1006.

McElroy SL, Hudson JL, et al. (2003). Citalopram in the treatment of binge-eating disorder: a placebo-controlled trial. J Clin Psychiatry 64(7): 807–813.

McGirr A, Berlim MT, et al. (2015). A systematic review and meta-analysis of randomized, double-blind, placebo-controlled trials of ketamine in the rapid treatment of major depressive episodes. Psychol Med 45(4): 693–704.

McGrath PJ, Khan AY, et al. (2008). Response to a selective serotonin reuptake inhibitor (citalopram) in major depressive disorder with melancholic features: a STAR*D report. J Clin Psychiatry 69: 1847–1855.

McGrath PJ, Stewart JW, et al. (2006). Tranylcypromine versus venlafaxine plus mirtazapine following three failed antidepressant medication trials for depression: a STAR*D report. Am J Psychiatry 163: 1531–1541.

McMahon FJ, Buervenich S, et al. (2006). Variation in the gene encoding the serotonin 2A receptor is associated with outcome of antidepressant treatment. Am J Hum Genet 78: 804–814.

Medeiros da Frota Ribeiro C, Riva-Posse P (2017). Use of ketamine in elderly patients with treatment-resistant depression. Curr Psychiatry Rep 19(12): 107.

Meltzer-Brody S, Colquhoun H, et al. (2018). Brexanolone injection in post-partum depression: two multicentre, double-blind, randomised, placebo-controlled, phase 3 trials. Lancet 392(10152): 1058–1070.

Milano W, Petrella C, et al. (2004). Treatment of bulimia nervosa with sertraline: a randomized controlled trial. Adv Ther 21(4): 232–237.

Moayyedi PM, Lacy BE, et al. (2017). ACG and CAG clinical guideline: management of dyspepsia. Am J Gastroenterol 112(7): 988–1013.

Montejo AL, Llorca G, et al. (2001). Incidence of sexual dysfunction associated with antidepressant agents: a prospective multicenter study of 1022 outpatients. Spanish Working Group for the Study of Psychotropic-Related Sexual Dysfunction. J Clin Psychiatry 62(Suppl 3): 10–21.

Mork A, Montezinho LP, et al. (2013). Vortioxetine (Lu AA21004), a novel multimodal antidepressant, enhances memory in rats. Pharmacol Biochem Behav 105: 41–50.

Morrato EH, Libby AM, et al. (2008). Frequency of provider contact after FDA advisory on risk of pediatric suicidality with SSRIs. Am J Psychiatry 165: 42–50.

Moses-Kolko EL, Bogen D, et al. (2005). Neonatal signs after late in utero exposure to serotonin reuptake inhibitors: literature review and implications for clinical applications. JAMA 293(19): 2372–2383.

Movig KL, Leufkens HG, et al. (2002). Association between antidepressant drug use and hyponatraemia: a case-control study. Br J Clin Pharmacol 53(4): 363–369.

Murphy GM Jr, Hollander SB, et al. (2004). Effects of the serotonin transporter gene promoter polymorphism on mirtazapine and paroxetine efficacy and adverse events in geriatric major depression. Arch Gen Psychiatry 61: 1163–1169.

Navarro V, Boulahfa I, et al. (2019). Lithium agumentation versus citalopram combination in imipramine-resistant major depression: a 10-week randomized open-label study. J Clin Psychopharmacol 39(3): 254–257.

Nazimek K, Strobel S, et al. (2017). The role of macrophages in anti-inflammatory activity of antidepressant drugs. Immunobiology 222(6): 823–830.

Nestler EJ, Hyman SE, et al. (2015). *Molecular Neuropharmacology, A Foundation for Clinical Neuroscience, 3rd Edition*. New York, NY: McGraw-Hill.

Ng QX, Koh SSH, et al. (2017). Clinical Use of Curcumin in Depression: a Meta-Analysis. J Am Med Dir Assoc 18(6): 503–508.

Niciu MJ, Ionescu DF, et al. (2013). Second messenger/signal transduction pathways in major mood disorders: moving from membrane to mechanism of action, part I: major depressive disorder. CNS Spectr 18(5): 231–241.

Noordam R, van den Berg ME, et al. (2016). Antidepressants and heart-rate variability in older adults: a population-based study. Psychol Med 46(6): 1239–1247.

O'Donovan C, Garnham JS, et al. (2008). Antidepressant monotherapy in pre-bipolar depression; predictive value and inherent risk. J Affect Dis 107: 293–298.

Obata H (2017). Analgesic mechanisms of antidepressants for neuropathic pain. Int J Mol Sci 18(11): E2483.

Ornoy A, Weinstein-Fudim L, et al. (2017). Antidepressants, antipsychotics, and mood stabilizers in pregnancy: what do we know and how should we treat pregnant women with depression. Birth Defects Res 109(12): 933–956.

Onghena P, Van Houdenhove B (1992). Antidepressant-induced analgesia in chronic non-malignant pain: a meta-analysis of 39 placebo-controlled studies. Pain 49: 205–219.

Orlova Y, Rizzoli P, et al. (2018). Association of coprescription of triptan antimigraine drugs and selective serotonin reuptake inhibitor or selective norepinephrine reuptake inhibitor antidepressants with serotonin syndrome. JAMA Neurol 75(5): 566–572.

Orr ST, Blazer DG, et al. (2007). Depressive symptoms and indicators of maternal health status during pregnancy. J Womens Health (Larchmt) 16(4): 535–542.

Palmsten K, Huybrechts KF, et al. (2013). Antidepressant use and risk for preeclampsia. Epidemiology 24(5): 682–691.

Paolucci S (2017). Advances in antidepressants for treating post-stroke depression. Expert Opin Pharmacother 18(10): 1011–1017.

Papp A, Onton JA (2018). Brain zaps: an underappreciated symptom of antidepressant discontinuation. Prim Care Companion CNS Disord 20(6): 18m02311.

Payne JL (2017). Psychopharmacology in pregnancy and breastfeeding. Psychiatr Clin North Am 40(2): 217–238.

PDR (2019). Prescriber's digital reference. http://www.pdr.net

Perry PJ, Zeilmann C, et al. (1994). Tricyclic antidepressant concentrations in plasma: an estimate of their sensitivity and specificity as a predictor of response. J Clin Psychopharmacol 14: 230–240.

Phelps J (2008). The bipolar spectrum, in Parker G, Ed., *Bipolar II Disorder. Modeling, Measuring, and Managing.* Cambridge, UK: Cambridge University Press. Pages 15–45.

Porcelli S, Fabbri C, et al. (2012). Meta-analysis of serotonin transporter gene promoter polymorphism (5-HTTLPR) association with antidepressant efficacy. Eur Neuropsychopharmacol 22(4): 239–258.

Post RM, Altshuler LL, et al. (2006). Mood switch in bipolar depression: comparison of adjunctive venlafaxine, bupropion and sertraline. Brit J Psychiatry 189: 124–131.

Qin B, Zhang Y, et al. (2014). Selective serotonin reuptake inhibitors versus tricyclic antidepressants in young patients: a meta-analysis of efficacy and acceptability. Clin Ther 36(7): 1087–1095 e1084.

Quinn GR, Singer DE, et al. (2014). Effect of selective serotonin reuptake inhibitors on bleeding risk in patients with atrial fibrillation taking warfarin. Am J Cardiol 114(4): 583–586.

Quitkin FM, Stewart JW, et al. (1993). Columbia atypical depression. A subgroup of depressives with better response to MAOI than to tricyclic antidepressants or placebo. Brit J Psychiatry. (Suppl 21): 30–34.

Ragguett RM, Rong C, et al. (2019). Rapastinel—an investigational NMDA-R modulator for major depressive disorder: evidence to date. Expert Opin Investig Drugs 28(2): 113–119.

Rahimi R, Nikfar S, et al. (2006). Pregnancy outcomes following exposure to serotonin reuptake inhibitors: a meta-analysis of clinical trials. Reprod Toxicol 22(4): 571–575.

Raskin J, Goldstein DJ, et al. (2003). Duloxetine in the long-term treatment of major depressive disorder. J Clin Psychiatry 64: 1237–1244.

Reddy S, Kane C, et al. (2010). Clinical utility of desvenlafaxine 50 mg/d for treating MDD: a review of two randomized placebo-controlled trials for the practicing physician. Curr Med Res Opin 26(1): 139–150.

Reefhuis J, Devine O, et al. (2015). Specific SSRIs and birth defects: Baysian analysis to interpret new data in the context of previous reports. BMJ 351: h3190.

Reid RL, Soares CN (2018). Premenstrual dysphoric disorder: contemporary diagnosis and management. J Obstet Gynaecol Can 40(2): 215–223.

Reis M, Kallen B (2010). Delivery outcome after maternal use of antidepressant drugs in pregnancy: an update using Swedish data. Psychol Med 40(10): 1723–1733.

Renoux, C, Vahey S, et al. (2017). Association of Selective Serotonin Reuptake Inhibitors With the Risk for Spontaneous Intracranial Hemorrhage. JAMA Neurol 74(2): 173–180.

Richelson E (2003). Interactions of antidepressants with neurotransmitter transporters and receptors and their clinical relevance. J Clin Psychiatry 64(Suppl 13): 5–12.

Rickels K, Athanasiou M, et al. (2009). Evidence for efficacy and tolerability of vilazodone in the treatment of major depressive disorder: a randomized, double-blind, placebo-controlled trial. J Clin Psychiatry 70(3): 326–333.

Rihmer Z, Dome P, et al. (2013). Antidepressant response and subthreshold bipolarity in "unipolar" major depressive disorder: implications for practice and drug research. J Clin Psychopharmacol 33(4): 449–452.

Rizvi SJ, Kennedy SH (2013). Management strategies for SSRI-induced sexual dysfunction. J Psychiatry Neurosci 38(5): E27–E28.

Roose SP, Rutherford BR (2016). Selective serotonin reuptake inhibitors and operative bleeding risk: a review of the literature. J Clin Psychopharmacol 36(6): 704–709.

Rosenbaum JF, Arana GW, et al. (2005). Handbook of Psychiatric Drug Therapy, 5th Edition. Philadelphia, PA: Lippincott Williams & Wilkins.

Ross EL, Zivin K, et al. (2018). Cost-effectiveness of electroconvulsive therapy vs pharmacotherapy/psychotherapy for treatment-resistant depression in the United States. JAMA Psychiatry 75(7): 713–722.

Ruepert L, Quartero AO, et al. (2011). Bulking agents, antispasmodics and antidepressants for the treatment of irritable bowel syndrome. Cochrane Database Syst Rev 8: CD003460.

Rush AJ, Trivedi MH, et al. (2006). Acute and longer-term outcomes in depressed outpatients requiring one or several treatment steps: a STAR*D report. Am J Psychiatry 163(11): 1905–1917.

Rush AJ, Trivedi MH, et al. (2011). Combining medications to enhance depression outcomes (CO-MED): acute and long-term outcomes of a single-blind randomized study. Am J Psychiatry 168(7): 689–701.

Saarto T, Wiffen PJ (2007). Antidepressants for neuropathic pain. Cochrane Database Syst Rev Issue 4 CD005454.

Sarris J, Murphy J, et al. (2016). Adjunctive nutraceuticals for depression: a systematic review and meta-analyses. Am J Psychiatry 173(6): 575–587.

Schefft, C, Kilarski LL, et al. (2017). Efficacy of adding nutritional supplements in unipolar depression: a systematic review and meta-analysis. Eur Neuropsychopharmacol 27(11): 1090–1109.

Schueler YB, Koesters M, et al. (2011). A systematic review of duloxetine and venlafaxine in major depression, including unpublished data. Acta Psychiatr Scand 123(4): 247–265.

Serretti A, Chiesa A (2009). Treatment-emergent sexual dysfunction related to antidepressants: a meta-analysis. J Clin Psychopharmacol 29(3): 259–266.

Serretti A, Mandelli L (2010). Antidepressants and body weight: a comprehensive review and meta-analysis. J Clin Psychiatry 71(10): 1259–1272.

Sharma A, Gerbarg P, et al. (2017). S-Adenosylmethionine (SAMe) for neuropsychiatric disorders: a clinician-oriented review of research. J Clin Psychiatry 78(6): e656–e667.

Sheehan DV, Croft HA, et al. (2009). Extended-release trazodone in major depressive disorder: a randomized, double-blind, placebo-controlled study. Psychiatry (Edgmont) 6(5): 20–33.

Sheeler RD, Ackerman MJ, et al. (2012). Considerations on safety concerns about citalopram prescribing. Mayo Clin Proc 87(11): 1042–1045.

Shen ZQ, Gao SY, et al. (2017). Sertraline use in the first trimester and risk of congenital anomalies: a systemic review and meta-analysis of cohort studies. Br J Clin Pharmacol 83(4): 909–922.

Sheu YH, Lanteigne A, et al. (2015). SSRI use and risk of fractures among permenopausal women without mental disorders. Inj Prev 21(6): 397–403.

Shi L, Wang J, et al. (2016). Efficacy and tolerability of vilazodone for major depressive disorder: evidence from phase III/IV randomized controlled trials. Drug Des Devel Ther 10: 3899–3907.

Shi Z, Atlantis E, et al. (2017). SSRI antidepressant use potentiates weight gain in the context of unhealthy lifestyles: results from a 4-year Australian follow-up study. BMJ Open 7(8): e016224.

Sindrup SH, Holbech JV, et al. (2017). The impact of serum drug concentration on the efficacy of imipramine, pregabalin, and their combination in painful polyneuropathy. Clin J Pain 33(12): 1047–1052.

Smit M, Dolman KM, et al. (2016). Mirtazapine in pregnancy and lactation—A systematic review. Eur Neuropsychopharmacol 26(1): 126–135.

Smit M, Wennink H, et al. (2015). Mirtazapine in pregnancy and lactation: data from a case series. J Clin Psychopharmacol 35(2): 163–167.

Spielmans GI (2008). Duloxetine does not relieve painful physical symptoms in depression: a meta-analysis. Psychother Psychosom 77(1): 12–16.

Stanciu CN, Glass OM, et al. (2017). Use of buprenorphine in treatment of refractory depression: a review of current literature. Asian J Psychiatr 26: 94–98.

Stahl SM, Grady MM (2003). Differences in mechanism of action between current and future antidepressants. J Clin Psychiatry 64(Suppl 13): 13–17.

Sterke CS, Ziere G, et al. (2012). Dose-response relationship between selective serotonin reuptake inhibitors and injurious falls: a study in nursing home residents with dementia. Br J Clin Pharmacol 73(5): 812–820.

Stubner S, Grohmann R, et al. (2018). Suicidal ideation and suicidal behavior as rare adverse events of antidepressant medication: current report from the AMSP Multicenter Drug Safety Surveillance Project. Int J Neuropsychopharmacol 21(9): 814–821.

Sung SC, Haley CL, et al. (2012). The impact of chronic depression on acute and long-term outcomes in a randomized trial comparing selective serotonin reuptake inhibitor monotherapy versus each of 2 different antidepressant medication combinations. J Clin Psychiatry 73(7): 967–976.

Suri R, Lin AS, et al. (2014). Acute and long-term behavioral outcome of infants and children exposed in utero to either maternal depression or antidepressants: a review of the literature. J Clin Psychiatry 75(10): e1142–1152.

Sylvester C, Menke M, et al. (2019). Selective serotonin reuptake inhibitors and fertility: considerations for couples trying to conceive. Harv Rev Psychiatry 27(2): 108–118.

Tack J, Broekaert D, et al. (2006). A controlled crossover study of the selective serotonin reuptake inhibitor citalopram in irritable bowel syndrome. Gut 55(8): 1095–1103.

Tak CR, Job KM, et al. (2017). The impact of exposure to antidepressant medications during pregnancy on neonatal outcomes: a review of retrospective database cohort studies. Eur J Clin Pharmacol 73(9): 1055–1069.

Tang SW, Helmeste D, et al. (2012). Is neurogenesis relevant in depression and in the mechanism of antidepressant drug action? A critical review. World J Biol Psychiatry 13(6): 402–412.

Tang M, Osser DN (2012). The Psychopharmacology Algorithm Project at the Harvard South Shore Program: 2012 update on psychotic depression. J Mood Dis 2(4): 168–179.

Taylor MJ, Freemantle N, et al. (2006). Early onset of selective serotonin reuptake inhibitor antidepressant action: systematic review and meta-analysis. Arch Gen Psychiatry 63(11): 1217–1223.

Taylor MJ, Rudkin L, et al. (2013). Strategies for managing sexual dysfunction induced by antidepressant medication. Cochrane Database Syst Rev 5: CD003382.

Thase ME (2012). The role of monoamine oxidase inhibitors in depression treatment guidelines. J Clin Psychiatry 73(Suppl 1): 10–16.

Tripp AC (2010). Bupropion, a brief history of seizure risk. Gen Hosp Psychiatry 32(2): 216–217.

Trivedi MH, Rush AJ, et al. (2001). Do bupropion SR and sertraline differ in their effects on anxiety in depressed patients? J Clin Psychiatry 62(10): 776–781.

Trivedi M, Thase ME, et al. (2008). Adjunctive aripiprazole in major depressive disorder: analysis of efficacy and safety in patients with anxious and atypical features. J Clin Psychiatry 69: 1928–1936.

Turner EH, Matthews AM, et al. (2008). Selective publication of antidepressant trials and its influence on apparent efficacy. N Engl J Med 358(3): 252–260.

Turner EH, Rosenthal R (2008). Efficacy of antidepressants. BMJ 336(7643): 516–517.

Uguz F, Sahingoz M, et al. (2015). Weight gain and associated factors in patients using newer antidepressant drugs. Gen Hosp Psychiatry 37(1): 46–48.

Uher R, Huezo-Diaz P, et al. (2009). Genetic predictors of response to antidepressants in the GENDEP project. Pharmacogenomics J 9(4): 225–233.

Undurraga J, Baldessarini RJ (2017). Direct comparison of tricyclic and serotonin-reuptake inhibitor antidepressants in randomized head-to-head trials in acute major depression: systematic review and meta-analysis. J Psychopharmacol 31(9): 1184–1189.

Vasilakis-Scaramozza C, Aschengrau A, et al. (2013). Antidepressant use during early pregnancy and the risk of congenital anomalies. Pharmacotherapy 33(7): 693–700.

Verdel BM, Souverein PC, et al. (2010). Use of antidepressant drugs and risk of osteoporotic and non-osteoporotic fractures. Bone 47(3): 604–609.

Vermeiden M, Kamperman AM, et al. (2015). Early improvement as a predictor of eventual antidepressant treatment response in severely depressed inpatients. Psychopharmacology (Berl) 232(8): 1347–1356.

Wagner G, Schultes MT, et al. (2018). Efficacy and safety of levomilnacipran, vilazodone and vortioxetine compared with other second-generation antidepressants for major depressive disorder in adults: a systematic review and network meta-analysis. J Affect Disord 228: 1–12.

Wagner S, Engel A, et al. (2017). Early improvement as a resilience signal predicting later remission to antidepressant treatment in patients with Major Depressive Disorder: systematic review and meta-analysis. J Psychiatr Res 94: 96–106.

Walsh BT, Seidman SN, et al. (2002). Placebo response in studies of major depression: variable, substantial, and growing. JAMA 287(14): 1840–1847.

Walther A, Breidenstein J, et al. (2018). Association of testosterone treatment with alleviation of depressive symptoms in men: a systematic review and meta-analysis. JAMA Psychiatry 76(1): 31–40.

Weissman AM, Levy BT, et al. (2004). Pooled analysis of antidepressant levels in lactating mothers, breast milk, and nursing infants. Am J Psychiatry 161(6): 1066–1078.

Welsch P, Uceyler N, et al. (2018). Serotonin and noradrenaline reuptake inhibitors (SNRIs) for fibromyalgia. Cochrane Database Syst Rev 2: CD010292.

White MA, Grilo CM (2013). Bupropion for overweight women with binge-eating disorder: a randomized, double-blind, placebo-controlled trial. J Clin Psychiatry 74(4): 400–406.

Wilkinson ST, Ballard ED, et al. (2018). The effect of a single dose of intravenous ketamine on suicidal ideation: a systematic review and individual participant data meta-analysis. Am J Psychiatry 175(2): 150–158.

Williams LM, Debattista C, et al. (2016). Childhood trauma predicts antidepressant response in adults with major depression: data from the randomized international study to predict optimized treatment for depression. Transl Psychiatry 6: e799.

Williams NR, Heifets BD, et al. (2018). Attenuation of antidepressant effects of ketamine by opioid receptor antagonism. Am J Psychiatry 175(12): 1205–1215.

Wisniewski SR, Fava M, et al. (2007). Acceptability of second-step treatments to depressed outpatients: a STAR*D report. Am J Psychiatry 164: 753–760.

Wisniewski SR, Rush AJ, et al. (2009). Can phase III trial results of antidepressant medications be generalized to clinical practice? A STAR*D report. Am J Psychiatry 166(5): 599–607.

Wohlreich MM, Mallinckrodt CH, et al. (2007). Duloxetine for the treatment of major depressive disorder: safety and tolerability associated with dose escalation. Depression Anxiety 24: 41–52.

World Health Organization (2019). World Health Organization model list of essential medicines, 21st list. https://apps.who.int/iris/bitstream/handle/10665/325771/WHO-MVP-EMP-IAU-2019.06-eng.pdf?ua=1

Xie C, Tang Y, et al. (2015). Efficacy and safety of antidepressants for the treatment of irritable bowel syndrome: a meta-analysis. PLoS One 10(8): e0127815.

Xin LM, Chen L, et al. (2019). Prevalence and clinical features of atypical depression among patients with major depressive disorder in China. J Affect Disord 1(246): 285–289.

Xu XM, Zou DZ, et al. (2016). Efficacy and feasibility of antidepressant treatment in patients with post-stroke depression. Medicine (Baltimore) 95(45): e5349.

Yesavage JA, Fairchild JK, et al. (2018). Effect of repetitive transcranial magnetic stimulation on treatment-resistant major depression in US veterans: a randomized clinical trial. JAMA Psychiatry 75(9): 884–893.

Yildiz A, Gonul, AS, Tamam L (2002). Mechanism of actions of antidepressants: beyond the receptors. Bull Clin Psychopharmacol 12: 194–200.

Yonkers KA, Wisner KL, et al. (2009). The management of depression during pregnancy: a report from the American Psychiatric Association and the American College of Obstetricians and Gynecologists. Gen Hosp Psychiatry 31(5): 403–413.

Zaluska M, Dyduch A (2011). Bupropion in the treatment of depression in Parkinson's disease. Int Psychogeriatr 23(2): 325–327.

Zarate CA Jr., Singh JB, et al. (2006). A randomized trial of an N-methyl-D-aspartate antagonist in treatment-resistant major depression. Arch Gen Psychiatry 63(8): 856–864.

Zarrouf FA, Artz S, et al. (2009). Testosterone and depression: systematic review and meta-analysis. J Psychiatr Pract 15(4): 289–305.

Zhou X, Keitner GI, et al. (2015). Atypical antipsychotic augmentation for treatment-resistant depression: a systematic review and network meta-analysis. Int J Neuropsychopharmacol 18(11): pyv060.

Zhu J, Klein-Fedyshin M, et al. (2017). Serotonin transporter gene polymorphisms and selective serotonin reuptake inhibitor tolerability: review of pharmacogenetic evidence. Pharmacotherapy 37(9): 1089–1104.

Ziere G, Dieleman JP, et al. (2008). Selective serotonin reuptake inhibiting antidepressants are associated with an increased risk of nonvertebral fractures. J Clin Psychopharmacol 28(4): 411–417.

Zimmer B, Daly F, Benjamin L (1984). More on combination antidepressant therapy. Arch Gen Psychiatry 41(5): 527–528.

Zimmerman M, Posternak MA, et al. (2005). Why isn't bupropion the most frequently prescribed antidepressant? J Clin Psychiatry 66(5): 603–610.

Zimmermann-Viehoff F, Kuehl LK, et al. (2014). Antidepressants, autonomic function and mortality in patients with coronary heart disease: data from the Heart and Soul study. Psychol Med 44(14): 2975–2984.

Zivin K, Pfeiffer PN, et al. (2013). Evaluation of the FDA warning against prescribing citalopram at doses exceeding 40 mg. Am J Psychiatry 170(6): 642–650.

2

Anti-Anxiety Medicines and Hypnotics

The pharmacological treatment of anxiety symptoms is both simple and complicated. On the one hand, medications such as benzodiazepines can have a relatively immediate effect on distressing anxiety symptoms. On the other hand, the use of such medications may lead to cognitive impairments, physical dependence, and rebound exacerbations, as well as the risks of psychological dependence or inappropriate use by some patients.

It is not clear that episodic anxiety that is associated with situational stressors should be treated with medications. Anxiety per se may be a normal response to distressing real-life events and a signal that may enhance a person's motivation to address these events. As such, it may be better understood and addressed through psychotherapy rather than pharmacologically. Students and clinicians should be aware of cultural (and managed care) pressures that push for "popping a pill" rather than somewhat more costly counseling to improve coping strategies, much less formal psychotherapy, to address the underlying causes of the patient's anxiety.

In contrast to anxiety as a sole symptom, anxiety disorders are characterized by persisting patterns of anxiety and associated syndromal symptoms that impair functioning. Examples include panic disorder, social anxiety disorder, and generalized anxiety disorder (GAD). Obsessive-compulsive disorder (OCD) and post-traumatic stress disorder (PTSD) also involve symptoms of anxiety, although they are no longer classified as anxiety disorders in the fifth edition of the *Diagnostics and Statistical Manual of Mental Disorders*. The first-line medication treatments for most of these anxiety-related disorders are selective serotonin reuptake inhibitors (SSRIs; or other antidepressants with serotonergic effects—these are listed in Table 1.1). A time period of several weeks may be necessary before clear response. During this time, anxiolytics with more immediate effects (e.g., benzodiazepines) may be used for early symptom control, although their role in OCD and PTSD is more controversial.

Benzodiazepines

Benzodiazepines were first developed in the 1960s and are now the most commonly used anxiolytics in the world. **Alprazolam, lorazepam, diazepam, clonazepam, chlordiazepoxide, temazepam, and oxazepam** are examples of benzodiazepines. Their mechanism of action is through their binding on γ-aminobutyric acid (GABA) receptors (Nutt and Malizia 2001). GABA is the primary inhibitory neurotransmitter in the brain. Benzodiazepines bind to one type of GABA receptor ($GABA_A$) thereby increasing the receptor's affinity for GABA. Increased GABA effect then increases the frequency of chloride channel openings allowing this ion's influx into the cell, which, in turn, decreases normal cell firing. The benzodiazepine binding site is composed of multiple subunits; binding to the alpha-1 subunit may explain sedative effects of benzodiazepines whereas alpha-2 subunit binding may be needed for anxiolytic effects (Nestler, Hyman et al. 2015). In clinical practice, benzodiazepines have been used for the short-term treatment of anxiety and insomnia, as anticonvulsants, and in the treatment of alcohol withdrawal symptoms.

Benzodiazepines are associated with multiple adverse effects. They are sedating, can impair concentration, memory (Buffett-Jerrott and Stewart 2002), and coordination (e.g., as needed for motor vehicle operations), can lead to falls in the elderly (especially at initiation of treatment and after dose increases; Wagner, Zhang et al. 2004), and can cause respiratory depression. They are contraindicated in acute narrow or angle-closure glaucoma and may worsen glaucoma by possibly increasing intraocular pressure (Fritze, Schneider et al. 2002).

The choice of which benzodiazepine to use is often based on its pharmacokinetic properties. Diazepam, chlordiazepoxide, and clonazepam have relatively long half-lives. Diazepam and chlordiazepoxide are hepatically metabolized to desmethyldiazepam, itself a long-acting psychoactive compound. The use of these medications in hepatically compromised or older patients is problematic. In medically ill patients and in the elderly, benzodiazepines that do not require hepatic metabolism and have shorter half-lives such as lorazepam and oxazepam are preferred, especially when the risk of respiratory depression is a concern (e.g., patients with chronic obstructive pulmonary disease or sleep apnea). Alprazolam has a shorter half-life than lorazepam and oxazepam. It is, however, also associated with significant rebound anxiety because of the rapid drop from peak serum level after each dose. Despite its current widespread use (especially in primary care), alprazolam should generally be avoided in patients who may require frequent or daily administration of an anxiolytic drug.

Perhaps the greatest drawback of benzodiazepines, however, is that they can lead to misuse in patients with a history of alcohol or other drug use disorders. *Physiological dependence* is characterized by increased tolerance to these drugs and the development of significant withdrawal symptoms upon discontinuation; this occurs with long-term and/or high-dose use of benzodiazepines and is not necessarily a sign of misuse (although patients should be made aware of the need for very gradual taper of these medications if used long term). A *benzodiazepine use disorder*, on the other hand, is characterized by maladaptive behavioral changes leading to medication misuse. Benzodiazepines (along with barbiturates which were used more often in the past and are discussed later in this chapter) are controlled substances that should be prescribed judiciously and cautiously and only when adequate follow-up is available to ensure appropriate use. Adequate follow-up, however, is not often feasible in some primary care settings. Benzodiazepines should generally be avoided in any patient with a history of a substance or alcohol use disorder: as noted, most benzodiazepine misuse occurs in these individuals. There are circumstances in which a patient with a history of substance abuse may require benzodiazepines (e.g., a patient with a severe debilitating panic disorder who has been refractory to all other nonbenzodiazepine medications, and patients who have a long history of abstinence from the substances they abused and are functioning on a high level)—these circumstances, however, should be considered infrequent (Osser, Renner Bayog 1999).

The following considerations should also be taken into account:

(1) As previously noted, the use of benzodiazepines can increase the risk of falls, especially in the elderly. A review of the association between benzodiazepine use and hip fractures across five Western European countries and the United States showed that an estimated 1.8% to 8.2% of hip fractures may be attributable to benzodiazepine use, with variations based on differences in benzodiazepine use in these countries (Khong, de Vries et al. 2012). Short-acting benzodiazepines can increase the risk of falls in the elderly (van Strien, Koek et al. 2013), as can long-acting benzodiazepines. In another large study of older Veterans Administration outpatients, the number of inpatient and outpatient treatment encounters for physical "injuries" was significantly increased in outpatient benzodiazepine users when compared with the matched cohort (French, Spehar et al. 2005). A more recent review again supported the association between exposure to benzodiazepines and

an elevated risk of falls in the elderly (Diaz-Gutierrez, Martinez-Cengotitabengoa et al. 2017).

(2) Memory and cognitive impairments that can occur with short-term use are also seen with long-term use. A review of literature studying long-term benzodiazepines users (mean of 9.9 years) found evidence of significant cognitive impairment across multiple domains (such as information processing, memory, and attention) when compared to controls, with some indication that impairment may worsen with increased duration of use (Barker, Greenwood et al. 2004). A study of young adults also confirmed an association between long-term use of benzodiazepines and impairment in long-term memory in women (Boeuf-Cazou, Bongue et al. 2011). Long-term impairments may not subside entirely after benzodiazepine discontinuation (Barker, Greenwood et al. 2004).

Although the use of benzodiazepines may be associated with cognitive impairments (including delirium) in the elderly, it is not clear that their use hastens the development of dementia or other types of gradual cognitive decline (Mura, Proust-Lima et al. 2013; Picton, Marino & Nealy 2018). A recent large prospective study failed to show a causal relationship between long-term cumulative benzodiazepines use and the risk of developing or worsening dementia (Gray, Dublin et al. 2016). Nevertheless, due to the risk of falls and delirium, benzodiazepines should be avoided whenever possible in the elderly.

(3) Exposure to benzodiazepines appears to increase the risk of traffic accidents. The risk appears higher with the use of long-acting benzodiazepines, at initiation of use, and with higher doses (Smink, Egberts et al. 2010). As expected, in drivers who are found to be impaired and have a positive toxicology screen for benzodiazepines, the degree of impairment directly correlates with the benzodiazepine

blood level (Bramness, Skurtveit et al. 2002). The profiles of those who drive under the influence may be changing from those who use illicit drugs to an increasing number who use prescription drugs (including benzodiazepines) while driving (Rudisill, Zhao et al. 2014).

Barbiturates

Discovered more than 100 years ago and developed in the 1940s and 1950s, barbiturates are now rarely used for the treatment of anxiety due to a higher risk of dependence and dangerousness in overdose when compared to benzodiazepines. Whereas benzodiazepine binding increases the receptor's affinity for GABA and indirectly affects chloride channels, barbiturates (and alcohol), binding on a different site on $GABA_A$ receptors, can increase chloride influx into neurons even when GABA is not present (Loscher and Rogawski 2012). **Chloral hydrate**, a weaker barbiturate but with the same risks, is still occasionally used in certain settings for the treatment of refractory insomnia or for sedation prior to anxiety provoking medical studies (e.g., magnetic resonance imaging). Other barbiturates such as **phenobarbital**, **pentobarbital**, and **butalbital** are still occasionally used for treatment of conditions (e.g., seizure disorder, migraine) other than anxiety disorders.

Medicines Without Abuse Potential Used for the Treatment of Anxiety

Buspirone is a 5-HT1A receptor partial agonist (primarily, but not exclusively, on presynaptic autoreceptors) that may affect serotonin release from serotonergic neurons. Buspirone has no effect on GABA receptors and, as such, cannot immediately replace benzodiazepines. It has no immediate anxiolytic effects. On the other hand, it has no potential for abuse, and does not impair cognition or motor coordination. Side effects, however, may include headache, insomnia, mental "fogginess," sedation, jitteriness, and nausea. It is efficacious for the treatment of GAD. When buspirone is considered as an alternative to serotonergic antidepressants for GAD, it has the added benefits of not being associated with sexual side effects or treatment-emergent suicidality; treatment-emergent mania should be very rare.

Propranolol is a beta-adrenergic antagonist. Although it is primarily used medically for its effect on heart rate and blood pressure, its "off-label" use in psychiatry is based on its ability to reduce overall sympathetic activation. It is particularly helpful in circumstances where a sympathetic reaction to an anxiety-provoking stimulus can occur, such as in instances of performance anxiety. Musicians or public speakers, for example, may take a dose one hour prior to their appearance on stage, where it may decrease somatic manifestations of anxiety such as tremulousness and tachycardia. It does not, however, help alleviate symptoms associated with generalized social phobia or GAD. Propranolol should be avoided if the patient has congestive heart failure or significant asthma. Despite earlier concerns that beta-blockers may cause depression (Waal 1967) this is not supported by later studies (Ko, Hebert et al. 2002; Ranchord, Spertus et al. 2016).

Propranolol has also been studied for the prevention of PTSD. A review of the few available studies did not indicate any efficacy for the prevention of PTSD when propranolol was administered after exposure to a traumatic event (Amos, Stein & Ipser 2014). A new area of study, however, has been focused on whether propranolol, administered before traumatic memory *reactivation*, can inhibit memory reconsolidation and reduce the fear response (Kindt, Soeter & Sevenster 2014). Recent studies have shown some promise in this regard (Soeter and Kindt 2015; Brunet, Saumier et al. 2018). A single treatment followed by sleep may be enough to reduce trauma related fears (Kindt and Soeter 2018).

Clonidine, initially developed as an antihypertensive, is an alpha-2-adrenergic autoreceptor agonist, which serves to decrease sympathetic drive in the locus ceruleus. Clonidine may decrease hyperarousal (e.g., anxiety, insomnia, nightmares) in patients with PTSD (Boehnlein and Kinzie 2007) and in other conditions associated with autonomic hyperactivity (e.g., rebound hyperactivity in opioid withdrawal states).

Prazosin is an alpha-1-adrenergic receptor antagonist. Like clonidine, it is an antihypertensive, which seems to decrease anxiety symptoms and insomnia associated with posttraumatic states. It usually has no sedative properties but it can help decrease PTSD symptoms during the day and decrease nightmares and disturbed awakenings at night (Taylor, Lowe et al. 2006; Raskind, Peskind et al. 2007; Miller 2008; Taylor, Martin et al. 2008). Subsequent studies have added to the evidence supporting the efficacy of prazosin in the treatment of PTSD-related nightmares, hyperarousal, and insomnia, while being generally well-tolerated despite the possibility of lowering blood pressure (Byers, Allison et al. 2010; Calohan, Peterson et al. 2010; Germain, Richardson et al. 2012; Hudson, Whiteside et al. 2012; Kung, Espinel et al. 2012; Raskind, Peterson et al. 2013; Simon and Rousseau 2017). Effect sizes (differences from placebo) were substantial in some of these studies. Surprisingly, however, the most recent, largest, and the only multicenter randomized study of veterans with PTSD failed to confirm efficacy for prazosin. This may have been due to the study's recruitment of clinically stable patients, exclusion of patients who were on trazodone for help falling asleep, and higher than expected placebo response rates (Raskind, Peskind et al. 2018). Still, some have called prazosin the "penicillin for PTSD" because it works so well in many patients. However, it requires slow titration, to allow time to develop tolerance to the antihypertensive effect, starting with 1 mg at bedtime and increasing gradually up to a mean dose of 16 mg at bedtime in some male veterans with PTSD (Raskind, Peterson et al. 2013). This usually takes many weeks so some clinicians will try clonidine instead despite its minimal evidence-base. There is one small pilot placebo-controlled trial of **doxazosin**, an alpha-antagonist very similar to prazosin but with a much longer half-life

(15–19 hours), in PTSD (Rodgman, Verrico et al. 2016). One of the two primary outcome measures indicated efficacy. More study is needed, but some clinicians prefer it instead of prazosin because of a simpler titration and less effect on blood pressure. Initial doses are 2 to 4 mg with increases every 4 days to a maximum of 16 mg.

Hydroxyzine, a sedating antihistamine that can cross the blood brain barrier, acts as an antagonist (or possibly an inverse agonist) at H-1 histamine receptors on hypothalamic neurons (Nestler, Hyman et al. 2015). (In contrast, nonsedating antihistamines used to treat allergies and H-2 histamine receptor blockers used to reduce gastric acid production are nonsedating because they do not cross the blood brain barrier). Hydroxyzine has less affinity for muscarinic and alpha-1-adrenergic receptors than other sedating antihistamines.

Because it does not cause dependence and has no abuse potential, hydroxyzine is useful for treating anxiety symptoms in patients with a history of substance use disorders. Available since the 1950s, hydroxyzine's role in the treatment of anxiety was initially overshadowed by the benzodiazepines. Currently, however, it has had a re-emergence as a versatile drug in the psychiatric armamentarium (Dowben, Grant et al. 2013). It has been shown to have efficacy in the treatment of GAD (Ferreri, Hantouche et al. 1994; Darcis et al. 1995; Lader and Scotto 1998; Llorca, Spadone et al. 2002; Guaiana, Barbui et al. 2010). Also, it is frequently used (particularly as an "as needed" medication on inpatient settings) for the treatment of anxiety and insomnia in patients for whom the use of other anxiolytics or sedating medications (e.g., benzodiazepines or sedating antipsychotics) is problematic. Hydroxyzine's antihistaminic, antiemetic, and possible (but not confirmed) pain-reducing potentiation effects can render it very useful for many patients with comorbid anxiety.

Pregabalin is a GABA analog that binds to the alpha2-delta subunit on calcium channels, thereby inhibiting these channels and reducing the release of other neurotransmitters (Taylor, Angelotti & Fauman 2007). It was initially developed as an anticonvulsant but appears to have some efficacy in the treatment of GAD. Its efficacy appears to be comparable to that of benzodiazepines for GAD, but it may be better tolerated (Generoso, Trevizol et al. 2017). Preliminary data suggest that it may be similarly comparable to sertraline (an SSRI) in response and tolerability, but with a quicker onset of action (Cvjetkovic-Bosnjak, Soldatovic-Stajic et al. 2015). Response appears to be sustainable over the longer term (Montgomery, Emir et al. 2013). Dizziness, drowsiness, headache and fatigue may be prominent adverse effects. Pregabalin has been approved for the treatment of anxiety in Europe, but not in the United States. The manufacturer twice submitted it to the Food and Drug Administration (FDA) for approval for GAD, and twice it was refused. The reasons for the disapproval have never been made public. The "nonapprovable letter" was sent to the manufacturer, but there is no requirement to release it. Speculations have been published that the reason was the differences from placebo, although statistically significant, were not clinically meaningful (less than three points on the Hamilton Anxiety scale; Wensel, Powe & Cates 2012). In the United States, pregabalin is a scheduled controlled substance, as it may have some abuse potential (and more so than gabapentin discussed later), particularly in patients with a history of substance abuse (Schjerning, Rosenzweig et al. 2016; Bonnet and Scherbaum 2017).

Gabapentin is similar to pregabalin in structure, function, and shares some of the FDA indications, but it is not a scheduled controlled substance, although there is some evidence that it might deserve that designation (Schifano, D'Offizi et al. 2011). It is a generic product at this time and, hence, much less expensive than pregabalin. However, there are no placebo-controlled studies of gabapentin in GAD. It has been found useful in several other kinds of anxiety including pre-operative anxiety and anxiety in breast cancer survivors (Ravindran and Stein 2010; Clarke, Kirkham et al. 2013).

Quetiapine, a second-generation antipsychotic, is primarily used as an antipsychotic and a mood stabilizer (as discussed in subsequent chapters). It also appears to have efficacy for the treatment of GAD (Maneeton, Maneeton et al. 2016). Adverse metabolic risks and QT prolongation, however, preclude its use as a first- or second-line treatment for GAD. Because of its toxicity both the FDA and the European regulatory agency did not approve quetiapine for any use in GAD. Quetiapine may have a role to play, however, for infrequent use in the rapid alleviation of severe anxiety or insomnia during brief crises or in acute care settings (e.g., during brief hospitalizations) in patients for whom benzodiazepines are contraindicated.

Hypnotics

Zolpidem, zaleplon, and **eszopiclone** (enantiomer of racemic zopiclone, a hypnotic not available in the United States) are non-benzodiazepine hypnotics that bind to alpha-1 subunits on the benzodiazepine binding site on GABA receptors (Sanger 2004). These "z-drugs" cause sedation but lack anxiolytic effects despite some cross-reactivity with benzodiazepines. Although their abuse potential is purportedly less than benzodiazepines, they are not free from the risk of dependence and withdrawal symptoms upon discontinuation (Liappas, Malitas et al. 2003; Sethi and Khandelwal 2005; Cubala and Landowski 2007; Victorri-Vigneau, Dailly et al. 2007). Even single doses of these hypnotics can result in rebound worsening of sleep on the second night: the sleep on the second night is more disturbed than if the patient took a placebo for both nights (Walsh 2002). There is insufficient evidence that these hypnotics are either more effective or safer than benzodiazepines. However, successful marketing resulted in widespread use when more cost-effective treatments could have been considered (Glass, Lanctot et al. 2005; Siriwardena, Qureshi et al. 2006). A review of FDA data suggests that although nonbenzodiazepine hypnotics may reduce sleep latency, their effects on polysomnographic sleep latency and subjective sleep latency are relatively small (Huedo-Medina, Kirsch et al. 2012).

More recently, multiple additional concerns have been raised about the safety of these hypnotics (especially about the safety of zolpidem for which there are more available data). Although many of these concerns and risks may also apply to benzodiazepines, increasingly both medical and behavioral side effects of nonbenzodiazepines hypnotics have been reported:

(1) Zolpidem increased the risk for hip fractures up to twofold in patients over 65 years old after controlling for multiple possible covariates (Lin, Chen et al. 2014). Its use can significantly increase falls in inpatients settings. Patients who were treated with zolpidem had an over fourfold increase in falls compared to those who were prescribed the drug but did not take it (Kolla, Lovely et al. 2013).

(2) The FDA (2013) issued warnings in 2013 that the use of higher doses of zolpidem "can increase the risk of next-day impairment of driving and other activities that require full alertness" and suggested a lowering of recommended doses especially in women. It also warned that when taking extended-release zolpidem, patients "should not drive or engage in other activities that require complete mental alertness the day after taking the drug because zolpidem levels can remain high enough the next day to impair these activities" (PDR 2019). The use of z-drugs (as well as benzodiazepines) has been associated with an increase in road traffic accidents (Gustavsen, Bramness et al. 2008; Hansen, Boudreau et al. 2015; Orriols, Philip et al. 2011).

(3) Sleep-related behavioral changes have been observed after taking z-drugs (mostly zolpidem) for sleep (Logan and Couper 2001; Morgenthaler and Silber 2002; Doane and Dalpiaz 2008; Dolder and Nelson 2008). These behaviors could include, but are not limited to, sleep-walking, sleep-eating, sleep-conversations, and sleep-driving. Although these are considered to be rare side effects, one small retrospective study found that slightly over 5% of patients

taking zolpidem reported changes in sleep-related behaviors (Tsai, Yang et al. 2009). The occurrence of these behaviors is likely to be underreported given that the behaviors are usually accompanied by amnesia.

Ramelteon is a fairly new hypnotic that is an MT1 and MT2 melatonin receptor agonist that may have modest efficacy in shortening sleep latency but not in increasing total sleep duration (Roth, Seiden et al. 2006; Sateia, Kirby-Long et al. 2008; Liu and Wang 2012). It does not bind to the benzodiazepine-GABA receptor and seems to have no risk of dependency. It is generally well-tolerated (Johnson, Suess et al. 2006; Mets, van Deventer et al. 2010), but there are no studies to suggest it should be favored over more cost-effective alternatives. The European approval agency rejected it, concluding that benefits were too small in relation to possible risks, including prolactin elevation. It is also not clear if ramelteon is any more effective for sleep than the less costly and over the counter melatonin. Another melatonin receptor agonist, **tasimelteon**, is FDA-approved for the treatment of non-24-hour sleep wake disorder in blind patients only (PDR 2019).

Suvorexant and the newly released **lemborexant** are orexin receptor antagonists and the latest drugs to be approved by the FDA for the treatment of insomnia. Orexins are neuropeptides secreted by the neurons of the hypothalamus that act to regulate wakefulness and arousal; an antagonist at orexin receptors would, therefore, likely inhibit wakefulness and facilitate sleep (Ebrahim, Howard et al. 2002; Bennett, Bray et al. 2014). There is still insufficient clinical experience to support their use. Next day residual sedative effects may be a risk at higher doses (Sun, Kennedy et al. 2013). Suvorexant is a schedule IV controlled substance; further studies are needed to assess the abuse potential of orexin receptor antagonists.

A report in the lay press stirred controversy in asserting that during the FDA approval process, the manufacturer of suvorexant argued that their studies found it to be ineffective at a dose of 10 mg in subjective improvement in sleep. They urged the FDA to approve it with a standard dose of 20 mg. However, the FDA thought the side effects at 20 mg and above were much greater and approved 10 mg as the standard dose (Parker 2013).

Complementary, Alternative, and Other Pharmacotherapies

Available studies and reviews suggest that **kava** (*Piper methysticum*), **passion flower** (*Passiflora incarnate*), **chamomile** extract, and **lavender** oil may be effective for the short-term treatment of anxiety (Pittler and Ernst 2003; Miyasaka, Atallah & Soares 2007; Amsterdam, Li et al. 2009; Kasper, Gastpar et al. 2014; Mao, Xie et al. 2016; Asher, Gerkin & Gaynes 2017; Baric, Dordevic et al. 2018). Chamomile extract may improve sleep quality in the elderly (Adib-Hajbaghery and Mousavi 2017). Reviews of studies for **valerian** root (*Valeriana officinalis*) for insomnia have shown mixed results (Bent, Padula et al. 2006; Taibi, Landis et al. 2007).

The long-term safety of herbal medications has not been established. There are case reports of Kava causing hepatotoxicity (Brown 2017).

Endogenous **melatonin** is produced in the pineal gland and its secretion at night is thought to promote sleep onset and maintenance. Exogenous melatonin is sold in the United States as an over-the-counter supplement. Its use can have very mild effects on sleep onset latency (by 3–4 minutes) and sleep duration (by 13–14 minutes; Brzezinski, Vangel et al. 2005). It generally appears to be well tolerated in clinical practice. Low doses are generally recommended as there is a concern (from animal studies) that high doses of exogenous melatonin may lead to desensitization of melatonin receptors (Gerdin, Masana & Dubocovich 2004). In recent years, the dose of melatonin sold in pharmacies has risen tenfold. It used to be marketed in 0.3 mg doses, and now 3 mg is more usual, and 5 and 10 mg tablets are available for sale. A review of the literature failed to disclose any significant new studies supporting superior efficacy and/or safety of these higher doses.

3,4-methylinedioxymethamphetamine (MDMA), the active drug in "ecstasy" and Molly, is an amphetamine derivative that may enhance the release of norepinephrine, dopamine, and serotonin. It has been studied for the treatment of PTSD. MDMA administered during psychotherapy may reduce PTSD symptoms, with benefits possibly lasting up to a year (Mithoefer, Mithoefer et al. 2018). Changes in memory reconsolidation (as noted with propranolol described earlier) have been proposed as a mechanism of action (Feduccia and Mithoefer 2018). It is still too early to know if MDMA will show any promise for the routine treatment of PTSD.

Purified **cannabidiol (CBD)** is available for sale as an FDA-approved anticonvulsant in the United States (Lexicomp 2019). Reviews of available, but poorly controlled, studies have suggested that CBD may have some potential benefit for anxiety symptoms (Blessing, Steenkamp et al. 2015; Mandolini, Lazzaretti et al. 2018; Shannon, Lewis et al. 2019), but large confirmatory controlled studies are lacking. Drowsiness, lethargy, and sedation are potential adverse effects of the FDA-approved formulation. Potential interactions may occur through effects on CYP450 enzymes (e.g., CBD as a CYP2C19 inhibitor may increase citalopram blood levels; Lexicomp 2019). Potential hepatotoxicity is also a concern.

Further Notes on the Clinical Use of Anxiolytics and Hypnotics

Anxiety Disorders

As previously noted, serotonergic antidepressants such as SSRIs (followed by serotonin-norepinephrine reuptake inhibitors [SNRIs]) are the primary treatments for anxiety disorders. Reviews of existing evidence support the use of these antidepressants for the treatment of GAD (Baldwin, Waldman & Allgulander 2011;

Allgulander and Baldwin 2013; Strawn, Geracioti et al. 2018), panic disorder (Bandelow, Baldwin & Zwanzger 2013; Freire, Machado et al. 2014; Bighelli, Castellazzi et al. 2018), social anxiety disorder (Blanco, Bragdon et al. 2013; Williams, Hattingh et al. 2017), OCD (Soomro, Altman et al. 2008; Fineberg, Reghunandanan et al. 2013; Pittenger and Bloch 2014), and, to a lesser extent, for PTSD (Lee, Schnitzlein et al. 2016).

The risks of benzodiazepines should preclude their use as first-line long-term treatments, even though their effect size may be greater than those of SSRIs and SNRIs for GAD and social anxiety disorder (Gomez, Barthel & Hofmann 2018; Davidson, Potts et al. 1993). The use of an adjunctive benzodiazepine for anxiety may be appropriate in the first few weeks of treatment while the patient waits to respond to the antidepressant, after which the benzodiazepine can be tapered off.

Despite their many potential risks, however, benzodiazepines continue to be commonly prescribed for the treatment of anxiety disorders. Because they are highly effective in relieving short-term anxiety, they are often continued either due to patient request or because the prescribing clinician does not believe that adequately effective alternative medications are available. However as noted in this chapter, effective alternatives do exist for the treatment of most anxiety disorders and these should be considered.

When benzodiazepines are continued over the long run, short-term adverse risks are perpetuated and possibly even compounded over time. Many of these short-term risks have already been discussed above. The combination of benzodiazepines with other hypnotics, barbiturates, and opioids carries higher risks than those associated with each of these substances alone. The adverse physical, psychological, and cognitive effects that have been previously discussed can also be significantly compounded—possibly even to lethal levels as in the case of the increased risk of respiratory depression. Black box warnings have recently been issued for all benzodiazepines noting the risks of combining them with opioids. The risk of physical injury can also significantly increase (French, Chirikos et al. 2005).

Although some patients may combine benzodiazepines with other substances, such as opioids, to enhance the expected euphoria

(Jones, Mogali et al. 2012), for many patients the combination of medications begins as an honest effort by their prescribing clinician to treat the various presenting symptoms. Unfortunately, it is not rare to see a patient who has been concurrently prescribed a daily benzodiazepine for anxiety, a z-drug for insomnia, an opioid for pain, and possibly a migraine medication that includes butalbital (*and* who frequently chooses to add alcohol or cannabis to the mix), who then continues this regimen over the long term. Even if these medications are taken "as prescribed," the risks for dangerous events to occur (as has been seen recently in certain celebrity deaths) is very high. An appropriate role of the psychiatric clinician may be to attempt to help the patient and the primary prescribing clinician gradually lower the overall medication load and to explore factors that have may have led to this polytherapy in the first place.

Given the previously described concerns, efforts should be made to limit benzodiazepines to short-term use whenever possible. Those who have been on long-term treatment and are not doing well should be considered for tapering and replacement of these medications. Gradual dose reduction, in combination with psychological treatments, appears effective in helping patients discontinue benzodiazepine use (Parr, Kavanagh et al. 2009). Surprisingly, simple and "minimal" interventions such as a single letter sent from a family physician recommending dose reduction or discontinuation has been shown to considerably reduce long-term use of benzodiazepines in some patients (Gorgels, Oude Voshaar et al. 2005; Mugunthan, McGuire et al. 2011). Additionally, the majority of patients who had stopped use after receiving a discontinuation letter from their general practitioner were not using benzodiazepines at 10-year follow up. Clearly, given the evidence, there is a likelihood of succeeding in decreasing overall risk and side effect burden if clinicians placed a stronger emphasis on reducing long-term benzodiazepine use in their patients.

Insomnia

As is the case for benzodiazepines, before prescribing nonbenzodiazepine z-drugs for insomnia, clinicians should ask themselves if the proposed medication offers any benefits over other available agents. Risks (including risks of dependence) and benefits should be discussed with patients. It is fairly simple to start these medications but very difficult to stop them in many patients. The underlying causes of acute insomnia should always be identified: often there is a psychiatric or medical disorder that requires treatment with something other than a benzodiazepine or z-drug.

When considering treatment of chronic insomnia, prescribing clinicians should thoroughly review the differential diagnosis of possible contributing factors (Schutte-Rodin, Broch et al. 2008) and not overlook the benefits that may be derived from nonpharmacological (e.g., behavioral) therapies (Sivertsen, Omvik et al. 2006). None of the benzodiazepines or the z-drugs are approved specifically for the treatment of chronic insomnia. Alternatives such as a low dose of a sedating antidepressant like trazodone (for non-bipolar patients) or an antihistamine such as hydroxyzine should be considered. In patients with concurrent psychiatric disorders, such as schizophrenia or bipolar disorder, adjustments in the dose or timing of the current standing antipsychotic, mood stabilizer, or other adjunctive medications, may be sufficient to enhance sleep.

Finally, it should be kept in mind that some patients with chronic insomnia may have a treatable sleep disorder (e.g., obstructive sleep apnea) and referral to a sleep specialist or arranging for a sleep study may be more appropriate than continuing to try multiple sedating medications.

Treatment-Resistant Anxiety and Insomnia

If SSRIs and SNRIs are not helpful for anxiety disorders (or unacceptable due to their sexual side effects) then buspirone, hydroxyzine, and pregabalin can be considered instead. Clonidine or prazosin should be considered for PTSD if not yet tried. Chronic benzodiazepine and antipsychotic use should only be considered for patients who are refractory to first- and second-line treatments. Adding psychotherapy, if not already in place, should also be considered.

Alternative medications for chronic insomnia have been previously mentioned.

Use in Women of Childbearing Potential, Pregnancy, and Breastfeeding

Pregnancy

The decision as to whether anxiolytics should be prescribed during pregnancy often depends on the severity of anxiety symptoms. Untreated severe anxiety or prolonged insomnia may directly affect maternal self-care and have potential adverse effects on the fetus. (The risks and benefits of serotonergic antidepressants during pregnancy were already discussed in the previous chapter.)

Despite earlier concerns that benzodiazepines administered during the first trimester may increase the risk of cleft lip and palate, more recent studies do not confirm that the overall risk of malformations is increased with these medications (Bellantuono, Tofani et al. 2013). Another earlier review noted that although diazepam and chlordiazepoxide (but not alprazolam) appear to be safe during pregnancy, risks could still be minimized by avoiding all benzodiazepines during the first trimester (Iqbal, Sobhan & Ryals 2002). Given limited evidence, an increased risk of congenital malformations cannot be ruled out entirely with benzodiazepines, nor can it be assumed that all benzodiazepines are equivalent in their degree of risk. Still, they are not absolutely contraindicated in pregnancy if maternal anxiety or insomnia are severe.

The use of benzodiazepines may also increase the risk of preterm birth, cesarean delivery, and low birth weight (Wikner, Stiller et al. 2007; Yonkers, Gilstad-Hayden et al. 2017). A recent large study found that the risk of spontaneous abortions may be almost doubled in women who had filled one or more prescriptions of short- or long-acting benzodiazepines in the first trimester (Sheehy, Zhao & Berard 2019). Finally, neonatal sedation and associated symptoms such as muscular hypotonia, hypothermia, and neurological depression on the one hand, or benzodiazepine withdrawal symptoms on the other, may occur after birth (Ram and Gandotra 2015).

There is insufficient evidence to support the use of buspirone, pregabalin, and z-drugs during pregnancy. There is some evidence that H1 antihistamines in general, and hydroxyzine in particular, may not be associated with increased malformations in humans (Einarson, Bailey et al. 1997; Etwel, Faught et al. 2017); still, it is difficult to support hydroxyzine use during pregnancy, given that it can cross the placenta, and animal studies have shown an increase in fetal abnormalities (FDA 2014).

Breastfeeding

Infants may be exposed to benzodiazepines from breast milk, although the amounts are usually low. If benzodiazepines are necessary, shorter-acting agents and single doses are favored. The nursing infant should be monitored for any signs of lethargy, sedation, or respiratory distress (Kronenfeld, Berlin et al. 2017).

Table of Non-Antidepressant Medicines for Anxiety and Insomnia

Table 2.1 summarizes the characteristics of selected non-antidepressant medicines for the treatment of anxiety and insomnia (Ansari and Osser 2015; WHO 2019; PDR 2019; Lexicomp 2019). Antidepressants used in the treatment of anxiety disorders are listed in Table 1.1.

TABLE 2.1 Non-Antidepressant Medicines for Anxiety and Insomnia

Medication[a]	Adult Dosing[b]	Comments/FDA *Indication*
Clonazepam (Benzodiazepine) (Klonopin®, Clonazepam Orally Disintegrating Tablets®)	Start: 0.25–0.5 mg po bid for panic disorder, increase as needed, use lowest effective dose. Equivalence: 0.25 mg equals lorazepam 1 mg. Tmax = 1–4 hrs t ½ = 19–50 hrs Reduce dose for hepatic or renal impairment; avoid if significant liver disease	Benzodiazepine with convenient pharmacokinetics for the treatment of panic disorder (30–50 hours half-life); has treatment-emergent suicide risk warning in package insert as do all antiepileptic drugs; CYP3A4 substrate. Black Box Warning: Risks from concomitant use with opioids *Panic disorder/Specific seizure disorders (see package insert)*
Diazepam (Benzodiazepine) (Valium®, Diastat®, Diazepam Injection®)	For oral diazepam, Valium®: Start: 2 mg po bid-tid for anxiety, increase as needed, use lowest effective dose. Equivalence: 5 mg equals lorazepam 1 mg. Tmax = 1–1.5 hrs t ½ = 48–100 hrs (if including t ½ of active metabolite). Reduce dose for hepatic or renal impairment; avoid if significant liver disease	Rapid onset of action due to lipid solubility followed by rapid distribution to lipid compartment, long elimination half-life because of metabolite. IM absorption is less reliable. Substrate of multiple CYP450 enzymes. On WHO Essential Medicines List for anxiety disorders. Black Box Warning: Risks from concomitant use with opioids *Anxiety disorders and short-term relief of anxiety symptoms/Acute alcohol withdrawal symptoms/Adjunctive treatment for convulsive disorders/Adjunctive therapy in skeletal muscle spasms*
Chlordiazepoxide (Benzodiazepine) (Librium®)	Start: 10 mg po tid-qid for anxiety, increase as needed, use lowest effective dose. Equivalence: 25 mg equals lorazepam 1 mg. Tmax = 1–4 hrs t ½ = 48–100 hrs (if including t ½ of active metabolites) Avoid if hepatic impairment due to risks of drug and metabolite accumulation; reduce dose if renal impairment	Frequently used in inpatient detoxification for severe alcohol withdrawal symptoms when there is no hepatic dysfunction; multiple psychoactive metabolites. CYP3A4 substrate. Black Box Warning: Risks from concomitant use with opioids *Anxiety disorders and short-term relief of anxiety symptoms/Acute alcohol withdrawal symptoms/Preoperative anxiety and apprehension*

(continued)

TABLE 2.1 Continued

Medication[a]	Adult Dosing[b]	Comments/FDA Indication
Oxazepam (Benzodiazepine) (Serax®)	Start: 10 mg po tid for anxiety, increase as needed, use lowest effective dose. Equivalence: 15 mg equals lorazepam 1 mg. Tmax = 3 hrs (5 hours in elderly, not practical as a "prn") t ½ = 5–15 hrs	Used in inpatient detoxification when hepatic impairment is present; slowest onset of action among benzodiazepines. Black Box Warning: Risks from concomitant use with opioids *Anxiety disorders and short-term relief of anxiety symptoms/ Anxiety associated with depression/Management of anxiety in the elderly/Acute alcohol withdrawal*
Lorazepam (Benzodiazepine) (Ativan®, Ativan Injection®)	For oral lorazepam, Ativan: Start: 0.5 mg po bid-tid for anxiety, increase as needed, use lowest effective dose. Tmax = 2 hrs t ½ = 12 hrs For oral dosing: Reduce dose and use with caution if severe hepatic impairment	Most widely used in inpatient setting for "as needed" treatment of anxiety, agitation, and withdrawal states; only benzodiazepine available IM (except for diazepam which is available but not reliably absorbed IM). Black Box Warning: Risks from concomitant use with opioids *Anxiety disorders and short-term relief of anxiety symptoms or anxiety associated with depressive symptoms/Status epilepticus (for injection)/Preanesthetic medication for adults (for injection)*
Alprazolam (Benzodiazepine) (Xanax®, Xanax XR®, Niravam®)	For immediate release alprazolam, Xanax®: Usual starting dose is 0.25 mg po tid, change to other benzodiazepine if ongoing treatment is needed. Equivalence: 0.5 mg equals lorazepam 1 mg. Tmax = 1–2 hrs t ½ = 6–11 hrs Use caution in patients with hepatic or renal impairment	Most addictive benzodiazepine—greatest euphoric effect in alcoholic patients; infrequent "as needed" use may be appropriate; CYP3A4 substrate. Black Box Warning: Risks from concomitant use with opioids *Anxiety disorders and short-term relief of anxiety symptoms/Panic disorder*

TABLE 2.1 Continued

Medication[a]	Adult Dosing[b]	Comments/FDA *Indication*
Buspirone (Atypical anxiolytic—5-HT1A partial agonist) (Buspar®)	Start: 5 mg po bid-tid; increase every 2–3 days by 5 mg to 30–40 mg/day in 2–3 divided doses, maximum dose is 60 mg/day. Use with caution and reduce dose in patients with mild to moderate hepatic or renal impairments, respectively; avoid if hepatic or renal impairments are severe.	Alcoholics with anxiety may require near maximum doses; use for symptoms corresponding to generalized anxiety disorder (not as helpful for short-term relief of anxiety symptoms despite FDA indication); CYP3A4 substrate. *Generalized Anxiety Disorder and short-term relief of anxiety symptoms*
Propranolol (Beta-blocker) (Inderal®, Inderal LA®, Innopran XL®)	For immediate release propranolol, Inderal®: Start: test dose of 10 mg po 30–60 minutes before anxiety provoking event for performance anxiety, then increase if needed gradually up to 40 mg dose. Use with caution if with hepatic or renal impairments.	Used in psychiatry to treat performance anxiety, akathisia, lithium-induced tremor and clozapine-induced tachycardia. When taken daily requires gradual taper if stopping use, given cardiac risks upon abrupt discontinuation. CYP2D6, CYP1A2, CYP2C19 substrate. Black Box Warning: Cardiac ischemia after abrupt discontinuation *Migraine prophylaxis/ Hypertension/Essential tremor/ Other cardiac conditions (see package insert)*
Clonidine (Antihypertensive— Alpha 2 agonist) (Catapres®, Catapres-TTS®)	For oral clonidine, Catapres®: Start: 0.1 mg po bid or qhs, increase as needed and tolerated. Reduce doses in patients with renal impairment	May be helpful for hyperarousal associated with PTSD. Also used for opioid withdrawal. Monitor for sedation and hypotension, especially at higher doses. Black Box Warning: Risks associated with epidural clonidine *Attention-deficit/hyperactivity disorder/ Hypertension/ Pain management (as epidural)*

(continued)

108 | PSYCHOPHARMACOLOGY

TABLE 2.1 Continued

Medication[a]	Adult Dosing[b]	Comments/FDA Indication
Prazosin (Antihypertensive— Alpha 1 antagonist) (Minipress®)	Per clinical studies for PTSD: Start dose for males and titrate as tolerated: 1 mg po qhs, after 2 days increase to 2 mg po qhs, after 5 more days increase to 4 mg po qhs, if no response after 7 days then increase to 6 mg po qhs for a week, then 10 mg po qhs for a week then to 15 mg po qhs for a week then to 20 mg po qhs if needed and tolerated. Mean optimally effective dose was 16 mg for men, 7 mg for women in the Raskind et al. 2013 study. Max dose for hypertension is 20 mg/day. Dosage for women was lower, with max of 12 mg po qhs. Lower doses may be needed in patients with hepatic impairment	Helpful for insomnia, nightmares, and disturbed awakenings associated with PTSD. Also some patients may benefit from titration gradually up to 5 mg daily for daytime PTSD symptoms in men, and 2 mg daily for women, as tolerated. Monitor for hypotension. *Hypertension*
Hydroxyzine (Antihistamine—H1 antagonist) (Atarax®, Vistaril®)	Start: 10–12.5 mg po morning and midday and 20–25 mg po qhs for anxiety symptoms or generalized anxiety disorder. Anecdotal usage at higher doses: Higher doses of up to 100 mg po qhs may be beneficial for insomnia. Total daily dose should not exceed 100 mg because of QT prolongation above that dose. Dose reductions may be necessary in patients with hepatic or renal impairment	May also have analgesic effects; muscle relaxation properties, bronchodilator activity, antiemetic, antihistamine, may help with insomnia. *Anxiety symptoms/Multiple other indications (see package insert)*

TABLE 2.1 Continued

Medication[a]	Adult Dosing[b]	Comments/FDA *Indication*
Pregabalin (GABA analogue) (Lyrica ®, Lyrica CR®)	For pregabalin, (Lyrica®): Start at 75 mg po bid. If tolerated, increase after 7 days to 150 mg po bid. Max dose: 450 mg/day in divided doses (but studies have indicated doses up to 300 mg po bid may be beneficial). Reduce dose in patients with renal impairment, avoid in severe renal impairment	Provides alternative to buspirone and serotonergic antidepressants for GAD. Has treatment-emergent suicidality warning in package insert as do all antiepileptic drugs. Abuse potential; a scheduled drug. *Partial seizures/ Diabetic peripheral neuropathic pain, postherpetic neuralgia, fibromyalgia, neuropathic pain associated with spinal cord injury*
Zolpidem (Hypnotic) (Ambien®, Ambien-CR®, Edluar®, Intermezzo®, ZolpiMist® (mouth spray))	For immediate release zolpidem, Ambien®: Start: 5 mg po qhs, may increase to 10 mg po qhs if needed but be aware of risk of next day impairment; take 7–8 hours before needing to be awake (see package insert for other formulations). Max 10 mg po qhs. (lower doses whenever possible in women). Tmax = 1.6 hrs t ½ = 2–3 hrs (but duration of action may last up to 8 hours) Use lower doses for patients with mild to moderate hepatic impairment, avoid in severe hepatic impairment	Rapid onset; reported cases of amnesia and sleep-related behaviors; sertraline may increase serum level. FDA alert in 2013 recommending lower nightly doses to decrease risk of next day impairment with increased risk of impairment seen in women and with Ambien-CR. FDA also warns that patients taking Ambien-CR at night should not drive the next morning. Avoid combining with other sedatives. Primarily metabolized by CYP3A4 but also by multiple other CYP450 enzymes. Black Box Warning: Complex sleep behaviors while not fully awake *Short-term treatment of insomnia characterized by difficulties with sleep initiation*—also *sleep maintenance* for CR formulation—see package insert.

(continued)

TABLE 2.1 Continued

Medication[a]	Adult Dosing[b]	Comments/FDA *Indication*
Zaleplon (Hypnotic) (Sonata®)	Start: 5 mg po qhs, may increase to 10 mg qhs, maximum 20 mg po qhs. Tmax = 1 hour t ½ = 1 hour Lower doses for patients with mild to moderate hepatic impairments, avoid in severe hepatic impairment	Amnesia may occur as it does with benzodiazepines; ultra-short half-life; expensive; CYP3A4 substrate. Black Box Warning: Complex sleep behaviors while not fully awake *Short-term treatment of insomnia*
Eszopiclone (Hypnotic) (Lunesta®)	Start: 1 mg po qhs, maximum 3 mg po qhs— but 2–3 mg doses increase next day impairment Tmax = 1 hour t ½ = 6 hours Reduce doses for patients with severe hepatic impairment	Amnesia may occur; similar dependence potential and A.M. driving impairment to zolpidem—but may last up to 11 hours; expensive with no advantages; CYP3A4 substrate. Black Box Warning: Complex sleep behaviors while not fully awake *Treatment of insomnia*
Ramelteon (melatonin receptor agonist) (Rozerem®)	Start: 8 mg po within 30 minutes of bedtime, do not take with fatty meal. Max is 8 mg po qhs. Tmax = 0.75 hrs t ½ = 1–2 hrs (metabolite up to 5 hours) Use with caution in patients with mild to moderate hepatic impairment, avoid in patients with severe hepatic impairment	No DEA restriction; very short half-life; expensive; Unclear if any different in effect from over the counter melatonin. CYP1A2, CYP2C9, and CYP3A4 substrate. *Treatment of insomnia characterized by difficulty with sleep onset*

SEE PACKAGE INSERT FOR DOSING AND OTHER INFORMATION BEFORE PRESCRIBING MEDICATIONS. Dosing should be adjusted downwards ("start low, go slow" strategy) for the elderly and/or the medically compromised. Abbreviations: bid (bis in die), twice a day; COPD, chronic obstructive pulmonary disease; CYP, cytochrome P450 enzyme; DEA, Drug Enforcement Administration; FDA, Food and Drug Administration; IM, intramuscular; mg, milligram; po (per os), orally; PTSD, posttraumatic stress disorder; qhs (quaque hora somni), at bedtime; qid (quater in die), four times a day; tid (ter in die), three times a day; Tmax, time from administration to maximum serum concentration; t ½, medication half-life; WHO-World Health Organization.

[a]Generic and U.S. brand name(s).

[b]Doses are provided for educational purposes only.

References

Adib-Hajbaghery M, Mousavi SN (2017). The effects of chamomile extract on sleep quality among elderly people: a clinical trial. Complement Ther Med 35: 109–114.

Allgulander C, Baldwin DS (2013). Pharmacotherapy of generalized anxiety disorder. Mod Trends Pharmacopsychiatry 29: 119–127.

Amos T, Stein DJ, Ipser JC (2014). Pharmacological interventions for preventing post-traumatic stress disorder (PTSD). Cochrane Database Syst Rev 7: CD006239.

Amsterdam JD, Li Y, et al. (2009). A randomized, double-blind, placebo-controlled trial of oral Matricaria recutita (chamomile) extract therapy for generalized anxiety disorder. J Clin Psychopharmacol 29(4): 378–382.

Ansari A, Osser DN (2015). Psychopharmacology, A Concise Overview for Students and Clinicians, 2nd Edition. North Charleston, SC: CreateSpace.

Asher GN, Gerkin J, Gaynes BN (2017). Complementary Therapies for Mental Health Disorders. Med Clin North Am 101(5): 847–864.

Baldwin DS, Waldman S, Allgulander C (2011). Evidence-based pharmacological treatment of generalized anxiety disorder. Int J Neuropsychopharmacol 14(5): 697–710.

Bandelow B, Baldwin DS, Zwanzger P (2013). Pharmacological treatment of panic disorder. Mod Trends Pharmacopsychiatry 29: 128–143.

Baric H, Dordevic V, et al. (2018). Complementary and alternative medicine treatments for generalized anxiety disorder: systematic review and meta-analysis of randomized controlled trials. Adv Ther 35(3): 261–288.

Barker MJ, Greenwood KM, et al. (2004). Cognitive effects of long-term benzodiazepine use: a meta-analysis. CNS Drugs 18(1): 37–48.

Barker MJ, Greenwood KM, et al. (2004). Persistence of cognitive effects after withdrawal from long-term benzodiazepine use: a meta-analysis. Arch Clin Neuropsychol 19(3): 437–454.

Bellantuono C, Tofani S, et al. (2013). Benzodiazepine exposure in pregnancy and risk of major malformations: a critical overview. Gen Hosp Psychiatry 35(1): 3–8.

Bennett T, Bray D, et al. (2014). Suvorexant, a dual orexin receptor antagonist for the management of insomnia. P T 39(4): 264–266.

Bent S, Padula A, et al. (2006). Valerian for sleep: a systematic review and meta-analysis. Am J Med 119(12): 1005–1012.

Bighelli I, Castellazzi M, et al. (2018). Antidepressants versus placebo for panic disorder in adults. Cochrane Database Syst Rev 4: CD010676.

Blanco C, Bragdon LB, et al. (2013). The evidence-based pharmacotherapy of social anxiety disorder. Int J Neuropsychopharmacol 16(1): 235–249.

Blessing EM, Steenkamp MM, et al. (2015). Cannabidiol as a Potential Treatment for Anxiety Disorders. Neurotherapeutics 12(4): 825–836.

Boehnlein JK, Kinzie JD (2007). Pharmacologic reduction of CNS noradrenergic activity in PTSD: the case for clonidine and prazosin. Journal of Psychiatric Practice 13: 72–78.

Boeuf-Cazou O, Bongue B, et al. (2011). Impact of long-term benzodiazepine use on cognitive functioning in young adults: the VISAT cohort. Eur J Clin Pharmacol 67(10): 1045–1052.

Bonnet U, Scherbaum N (2017). How addictive are gabapentin and pregabalin? A systematic review. Eur Neuropsychopharmacol 27(12): 1185–1215.

Bramness JG, Skurtveit S, et al. (2002). Clinical impairment of benzodiazepines—relation between benzodiazepine concentrations and impairment in apprehended drivers. Drug Alcohol Depend 68(2): 131–141.

Brown AC (2017). Liver toxicity related to herbs and dietary supplements: online table of case reports. Part 2 of 5 series. Food Chem Toxicol 107(Pt A): 472–501.

Brunet A, Saumier D, et al. (2018). Reduction of PTSD symptoms with pre-reactivation propranolol therapy: a randomized controlled trial. Am J Psychiatry 175(5): 427–433.

Brzezinski A, Vangel MG, et al. (2005). Effects of exogenous melatonin on sleep: a meta-analysis. Sleep Med Rev 9(1): 41–50.

Buffett-Jerrott SE, Stewart SH (2002). Cognitive and sedative effects of benzodiazepine use. Current Pharmaceutical Design 8: 45–58.

Byers MG, Allison KM, et al. (2010). Prazosin versus quetiapine for nighttime posttraumatic stress disorder symptoms in veterans: an assessment of long-term comparative effectiveness and safety. J Clin Psychopharmacol 30(3): 225–229.

Calohan J, Peterson K, et al. (2010). Prazosin treatment of trauma nightmares and sleep disturbance in soldiers deployed in Iraq. J Trauma Stress 23(5): 645–648.

Clarke H, Kirkham KR, et al. (2013). Gabapentin reduces preoperative anxiety and pain catastrophizing in highly anxious patients prior to major surgery: a blinded randomized placebo-controlled trial. Can J Anaesth 60(5): 432–443.

Cubala WJ, Landowski J (2007). Seizure following sudden zolpidem withdrawal. Progr Neuropsychopharmacol Biol Psychiatry 31: 539–540.

Cvjetkovic-Bosnjak M, Soldatovic-Stajic B, et al. (2015). Pregabalin versus sertraline in generalized anxiety disorder: an open label study. Eur Rev Med Pharmacol Sci 19(11): 2120–2124.

Darcis T, Scotto JC (1995). A multicentre double-blind placebo-controlled study investigating the anxiolytic efficacy of hydroxyzine in patients with generalized anxiety. Hum Psychopharmacol: Clin Experim, 10(3): 181–187.

Davidson JR, Potts N, et al. (1993). Treatment of social phobia with clonazepam and placebo. J Clin Psychopharmacol 13(6): 423–428.

Diaz-Gutierrez MJ, Martinez-Cengotitabengoa M, et al. (2017). Relationship between the use of benzodiazepines and falls in older adults: a systematic review. Maturitas 101: 17–22.

Doane JA, Dalpiaz AS (2008). Zolpidem-induced sleep-driving. Am J Med 121(11): e5.

Dolder CR, Nelson MH (2008). Hypnosedative-induced complex behaviours: incidence, mechanisms and management. CNS Drugs 22(12): 1021–1036.

Dowben JS, Grant JS, et al. (2013). Biological perspectives: hydroxyzine for anxiety: another look at an old drug. Perspect Psychiatr Care 49(2): 75–77.

Ebrahim IO, Howard RS, et al. (2002). The hypocretin/orexin system. J R Soc Med 95(5): 227–230.

Einarson A, Bailey B, et al. (1997). Prospective controlled study of hydroxyzine and cetirizine in pregnancy. Ann Allergy Asthma Immunol 78(2): 183–186.

Etwel F, Faught LH, et al. (2017). The risk of adverse pregnancy outcome after first trimester exposure to H1 antihistamines: a systematic review and meta-analysis. Drug Saf 40(2): 121–132.

Feduccia AA, Mithoefer MC (2018). MDMA-assisted psychotherapy for PTSD: are memory reconsolidation and fear extinction underlying mechanisms? Prog Neuropsychopharmacol Biol Psychiatry 84(Pt A): 221–228.

Fineberg NA, Reghunandanan S, et al. (2013). Pharmacotherapy of obsessive-compulsive disorder: evidence-based treatment and beyond. Aust N Z J Psychiatry 47(2): 121–141.

Ferreri M, Hantouche EG, et al. (1994). Value of hydroxyzine in generalized anxiety disorder: controlled double-blind study versus placebo. L' Encephale 20: 785–791.

Food and Drug Administration. (2013). FDA drug safety communication: FDA approves new label changes and dosing for zolpidem products and a recommendation to avoid driving the day after using Ambien CR. http://www.fda.gov/Drugs/DrugSafety/ucm352085.htm

Food and Drug Administration. (2014). Vistaril® (hydroxyzine pamoate) capsules and oral suspension. https://www.accessdata.fda.gov/drugsatfda_docs/label/2014/011459s048,011795s025lbl.pdf

Freire, RC, Machado S, et al. (2014). Current pharmacological interventions in panic disorder. CNS Neurol Disord Drug Targets 13(6): 1057–1065.

French DD, Chirikos TN, et al. (2005). Effect of concomitant use of benzodiazepines and other drugs on the risk of injury in a veterans population. Drug Saf 28(12): 1141–1150.

French DD, Spehar AM, et al. (2005). Outpatient benzodiazepine prescribing, adverse events, and costs. In K Henriksen, JB Battles, ES Marks, DI

Lewin (Eds.), *Advances in Patient Safety: From Research to Implementation* (Vol 1: Research Findings). Rockville, MD. Agency for Healthcare Research and Quality (US). Pages: 185–198.

Fritze J, Schneider B, et al. (2002). Benzodiazepines and benzodiazepine-like anxiolytics and hypnotics: the implausible contraindication of closed angle glaucoma. Nervenarzt 73(1): 50–53.

Generoso MB, Trevizol AP, et al. (2017). Pregabalin for generalized anxiety disorder: an updated systematic review and meta-analysis. Int Clin Psychopharmacol 32(1): 49–55.

Gerdin MJ, Masana MI, Dubocovich ML (2004). Melatonin-mediated regulation of human MT(1) melatonin receptors expressed in mammalian cells. Biochem Pharmacol 67(11): 2023–2030.

Germain A, Richardson R, et al. (2012). Placebo-controlled comparison of prazosin and cognitive-behavioral treatments for sleep disturbances in US military veterans. J Psychosom Res 72(2): 89–96.

Glass J, Lanctot KL, et al. (2005). Sedative hypnotics in older people with insomnia: meta-analysis of risks and benefits. Brit Med J 331: 1169.

Gomez AF, Barthel AL, Hofmann SG (2018). Comparing the efficacy of benzodiazepines and serotonergic anti-depressants for adults with generalized anxiety disorder: a meta-analytic review. Expert Opin Pharmacother 19(8): 883–894.

Gorgels WJ, Oude Voshaar RC, et al. (2005). Discontinuation of long-term benzodiazepine use by sending a letter to users in family practice: a prospective controlled intervention study. Drug Alcohol Depend 78(1): 49–56.

Gray SL, Dublin S, et al. (2016). Benzodiazepine use and risk of incident dementia or cognitive decline: prospective population based study. BMJ 352: i90.

Guaiana G, Barbui C, et al. (2010). Hydroxyzine for generalised anxiety disorder. Cochrane Database Syst Rev 12: CD006815.

Gustavsen I, Bramness JG, et al. (2008). Road traffic accident risk related to prescriptions of the hypnotics zopiclone, zolpidem, flunitrazepam and nitrazepam. Sleep Med 9(8): 818–822.

Hansen RN, Boudreau DM, et al. (2015). Sedative hypnotic medication use and the risk of motor vehicle crash. Am J Public Health 105(8): e64–69.

Hudson SM, Whiteside TE, et al. (2012). Prazosin for the treatment of nightmares related to posttraumatic stress disorder: a review of the literature. Prim Care Companion CNS Disord 14(2): PCC.11r01222.

Huedo-Medina TB, et al. (2012). Effectiveness of non-benzodiazepine hypnotics in treatment of adult insomnia: meta-analysis of data submitted to the Food and Drug Administration. BMJ 345: e8343.

Iqbal MM, Sobhan T, Ryals T (2002). Effects of commonly used benzodiazepines on the fetus, the neonate, and the nursing infant. Psychiatr Serv 53(1): 39–49.

Johnson MW, Suess PE, et al. (2006). Ramelteon: a novel hypnotic lacking abuse liability and sedative adverse effects. Arch Gen Psychiatry 63: 1149–1157.

Jones JD, Mogali S, et al. (2012). Polydrug abuse: a review of opioid and benzodiazepine combination use. Drug Alcohol Depend 125(1–2): 8–18.

Kasper S, Gastpar M, et al. (2014). Lavender oil preparation Silexan is effective in generalized anxiety disorder—a randomized, double-blind comparison to placebo and paroxetine. Int J Neuropsychopharmacol 17(6): 859–869.

Khong TP, de Vries F, et al. (2012). Potential impact of benzodiazepine use on the rate of hip fractures in five large European countries and the United States. Calcif Tissue Int 91(1): 24–31.

Kindt M, Soeter M (2018). Pharmacologically induced amnesia for learned fear is time and sleep dependent. Nat Commun 9(1): 1316.

Kindt M, Soeter M, Sevenster D (2014). Disrupting reconsolidation of fear memory in humans by a noradrenergic beta-blocker. J Vis Exp 94. doi:10.3791/52151

Ko DT, Hebert PR, et al. (2002). Beta-blocker therapy and symptoms of depression, fatigue, and sexual dysfunction. JAMA 288: 351–357.

Kolla BP, Lovely JK, et al. (2013). Zolpidem is independently associated with increased risk of inpatient falls. J Hosp Med 8(1): 1–6.

Kronenfeld N, Berlin M, et al. (2017). Use of psychotropic medications in breastfeeding women. Birth Defects Res 109(12): 957–997.

Kung S, Espinel Z, et al. (2012). Treatment of nightmares with prazosin: a systematic review. Mayo Clin Proc 87(9): 890–900.

Lader M, Scotto JC (1998). A multicenter double-blind comparison of hydroxyzine, buspirone and placebo in patients with generalized anxiety disorder. Psychopharmacology 139: 402–406.

Lee DJ, Schnitzlein CW, et al. (2016). Psychotherapy versus pharmacotherapy for posttraumatic stress disorder: systemic review and meta-analyses to determine first-line treatments. Depress Anxiety 33(9): 792–806.

Lexicomp. (2019). https://www.wolterskluwercdi.com/lexicomp-online/

Liappas IA, Malitas PN, et al. (2003). Zolpidem dependence case series: possible neurobiological mechanisms and clinical management. J Psychopharmacology 17: 131–135.

Lin FY, Chen PC, et al. (2014). Retrospective population cohort study on hip fracture risk associated with zolpidem medication. Sleep 37(4): 673–679.

Liu J, Wang LN (2012). Ramelteon in the treatment of chronic insomnia: systematic review and meta-analysis. Int J Clin Pract 66(9): 867–873.

Llorca PM, Spadone C, et al. (2002). Efficacy and safety of hydroxyzine in the treatment of generalized anxiety disorder: a 3-month double blind study. J Clin Psychiatry 63: 1020–1027.

Logan BK, Couper FJ (2001). Zolpidem and driving impairment. J Forensic Sci 46(1): 105–110.

Loscher W, Rogawski MA (2012). How theories evolved concerning the mechanism of action of barbiturates. Epilepsia 53(Suppl 8): 12–25.

Mandolini GM, Lazzaretti M, et al. (2018). Pharmacological properties of cannabidiol in the treatment of psychiatric disorders: a critical overview. Epidemiol Psychiatr Sci 27(4): 327–335.

Maneeton N, Maneeton B, et al. (2016). Quetiapine monotherapy in acute treatment of generalized anxiety disorder: a systematic review and meta-analysis of randomized controlled trials. Drug Des Devel Ther 10: 259–276.

Mao JJ, Xie SX, et al. (2016). Long-term chamomile (*Matricaria chamomilla L.*) treatment for generalized anxiety disorder: a randomized clinical trial. Phytomedicine 23(14): 1735–1742.

Mets MA, van Deventer KR, et al. (2010). Critical appraisal of ramelteon in the treatment of insomnia. Nat Sci Sleep 2: 257–266.

Miller LJ (2008). Prazosin for the treatment of posttraumatic stress disorder sleep disturbances. Pharmacotherapy 28: 656–666.

Mithoefer MC, Mithoefer AT, et al. (2018). 3,4-methylene-dioxymethamphetamine (MDMA)-assisted psychotherapy for post-traumatic stress disorder in military veterans, firefighters, and police officers: a randomised, double-blind, dose-response, phase 2 clinical trial. Lancet Psychiatry 5(6): 486–497.

Miyasaka LS, Atallah AN, Soares BG (2007). Passiflora for anxiety disorder. Cochrane Database Syst Rev 1: CD004518.

Montgomery S, Emir B, et al. (2013). Long-term treatment of anxiety disorders with pregabalin: a 1 year open-label study of safety and tolerability. Curr Med Res Opin 29(10): 1223–1230.

Morgenthaler TI, Silber MH (2002). Amnestic sleep-related eating disorder associated with zolpidem. Sleep Med 3(4): 323–327.

Mugunthan K, McGuire T, et al. (2011). Minimal interventions to decrease long-term use of benzodiazepines in primary care: a systematic review and meta-analysis. Br J Gen Pract 61(590): e573–578.

Mura T, Proust-Lima C, et al. (2013). Chronic use of benzodiazepines and latent cognitive decline in the elderly: results from the Three-city study. Eur Neuropsychopharmacol 23(3): 212–223.

Nutt DJ, Malizia AL (2001). New insights into the role of the GABA(A)-benzodiazepine receptor in psychiatric disorder. Brit J Psychiatry 179: 390–396.

Nestler EJ, Hyman SE, et al. (2015). *Molecular Neuropharmacology, A Foundation for Clinical Neuroscience, 3rd Edition*. New York, NY: McGraw-Hill.

Orriols L, Philip P, et al. (2011). Benzodiazepine-like hypnotics and the associated risk of road traffic accidents. Clin Pharmacol Ther 89(4): 595–601.

Osser DN, Renner JA, Bayog R (1999). Algorithms for the pharmacotherapy of anxiety disorders in patients with chemical abuse and dependence. Psychiatric Annals 29(5): 285–301.

Parker I (2013, December 9). The big sleep. *The New Yorker*, pp. 50–63.

Parr JM, Kavanagh DJ, et al. (2009). Effectiveness of current treatment approaches for benzodiazepine discontinuation: a meta-analysis. Addiction 104(1): 13–24.

PDR (2019). Prescriber's digital reference. http://www.pdr.net

Picton JD, Marino AB, Nealy KL (2018). Benzodiazepine use and cognitive decline in the elderly. Am J Health Syst Pharm 75(1): e6–e12.

Pittenger C, Bloch MH (2014). Pharmacological treatment of obsessive-compulsive disorder. Psychiatr Clin North Am 37(3): 375–391.

Pittler MH, Ernst E (2003). Kava extract for treating anxiety. Cochrane Database Syst Rev 1: CD003383.

Ram D, Gandotra S (2015). Antidepressants, anxiolytics, and hypnotics in pregnancy and lactation. Indian J Psychiatry 57(Suppl 2): S354–371.

Ranchord AM, Spertus JA, et al. (2016). Initiation of beta-blocker therapy and depression after acute myocardial infarction. Am Heart J 174: 37–42.

Raskind MA, Peskind ER, et al. (2007). A parallel group placebo controlled study of prazosin for trauma nightmares and sleep disturbance in combat veterans with post-traumatic stress disorder. Biol Psychiatry 61: 928–934.

Raskind MA, Peskind ER, et al. (2018). Trial of prazosin for post-traumatic stress disorder in military veterans. N Engl J Med 378(6): 507–517.

Raskind MA, Peterson K, et al. (2013). A trial of prazosin for combat trauma PTSD With nightmares in active-duty soldiers returned from Iraq and Afghanistan. Am J Psychiatry 170(9): 1003–1010.

Ravindran LN, Stein MB (2010). The pharmacologic treatment of anxiety disorders: a review of progress. J Clin Psychiatry 71(7): 839–854.

Rodgman C, Verrico CD, et al. (2016). Doxazosin XL reduces symptoms of posttraumatic stress disorder in veterans with PTSD: a pilot clinical trial. J Clin Psychiatry 77(5): e561–565.

Roth T, Seiden D, et al. (2006). Effects of ramelteon on patient-reported sleep latency in older adults with chronic insomnia. Sleep Medicine 7: 312–318.

Rudisill TM, Zhao S, et al. (2014). Trends in drug use among drivers killed in U.S. traffic crashes, 1999–2010. Accid Anal Prev. 70: 178–187.

Sanger DJ (2004). The pharmacology and mechanisms of action of new generation, non-benzodiazepine hypnotic agents. CNS Drugs 18(Suppl 1): 9–15.

Sateia MJ, Kirby-Long P, et al. (2008). Efficacy and clinical safety of ramelteon: an evidence-based review. Sleep Medicine Reviews 12: 319–332.

Schifano F, D'Offizi S, et al. (2011). Is there a recreational misuse potential for pregabalin? Analysis of anecdotal online reports in comparison with related gabapentin and clonazepam data. Psychother Psychosom 80(2): 118–122.

Schjerning O, Rosenzweig M, et al. (2016). Abuse potential of pregabalin: a systematic review. CNS Drugs 30(1): 9–25.

Schutte-Rodin S, Broch L, et al. (2008). Clinical guideline for the evaluation and management of chronic insomnia in adults. J Clin Sleep Med 4(5): 487–504.

Sethi PK, Khandelwal DC (2005). Zolpidem at supratherapeutic doses can cause drug abuse, dependence and withdrawal seizure. J Assoc Physicians India 53: 139–140.

Shannon S, Lewis N, et al. (2019). Cannabidiol in anxiety and sleep: a large case series. Perm J 23: 18–041.

Sheehy O, Zhao JP, Berard A (2019). Association between incident exposure to benzodiazepines in early pregnancy and risk of spontaneous abortion. JAMA Psychiatry 76(9): 948–957.

Simon PY, Rousseau PF (2017). Treatment of post-traumatic stress disorders with the alpha-1 adrenergic antagonist prazosin. Can J Psychiatry 62(3): 186–198.

Siriwardena AN, Qureshi Z, et al. (2006). GPs' attitudes to benzodiazepines and "z-drug" prescribing: a barrier to implementation of evidence and guidance on hypnotics. Brit J Gen Practice 56: 964–967.

Sivertsen B, Omvik S, et al. (2006). Cognitive behavioral therapy vs. zopiclone for treatment of chronic primary insomnia in older adults: a randomized controlled trial. JAMA 295: 2851–2858.

Smink BE, Egberts AC, et al. (2010). The relationship between benzodiazepine use and traffic accidents: a systematic literature review. CNS Drugs 24(8): 639–653.

Soeter M, Kindt M (2015). An abrupt transformation of phobic behavior after a post-retrieval amnesic agent. Biol Psychiatry 78(12): 880–886.

Soomro GM, Altman D, et al. (2008). Selective serotonin re-uptake inhibitors (SSRIs) versus placebo for obsessive compulsive disorder (OCD). Cochrane Database Syst Rev 1: CD001765.

Strawn JR, Geracioti L, Rajdev N, et al. (2018). Pharmacotherapy for generalized anxiety disorder in adult and pediatric patients: an evidence-based treatment review. Expert Opin Pharmacother 19(10): 1057–1070.

Sun H, Kennedy WP, et al. (2013). Effects of suvorexant, an orexin receptor agonist, on sleep parameters as measured by polysomnography in healthy men. Sleep 36(2): 259–267.

Taibi DM, Landis CA, Petry H, et al. (2007). A systematic review of valerian as a sleep aid: safe but not effective. Sleep Med Rev 11(3): 209–230.

Taylor CP, Angelotti T, Fauman E (2007). Pharmacology and mechanism of action of pregabalin: the calcium channel alpha2-delta (alpha2-delta) subunit as a target for antiepileptic drug discovery. Epilepsy Res 73(2): 137–150.

Taylor FB, Lowe K, et al. (2006). Daytime prazosin reduces psychological distress to trauma specific cues in civilian trauma posttraumatic stress disorder. Biological Psychiatry 59: 577–581.

Taylor FB, Martin P, et al. (2008). Prazosin effects on objective sleep measures and clinical symptoms in civilian trauma posttraumatic stress disorder: a placebo-controlled study. Biol Psychiatry 63: 629–632.

Tsai JH, Yang P, et al. (2009). Zolpidem-induced amnesia and somnambulism: rare occurrences? Eur Neuropsychopharmacol 19(1): 74–76.

van Strien AM, Koek HL, van Marum RJ, et al. (2013). Psychotropic medications, including short acting benzodiazepines, strongly increase the frequency of falls in elderly. Maturitas 74(4): 357–362.

Victorri-Vigneau C, Dailly E, et al. (2007). Evidence of zolpidem abuse and dependence: results of the French Centre for Evaluation and Information on Pharmacodependence (CEIP) network survey. Brit J Clin Pharmacol 64: 198–209.

Waal HJ (1967). Propranolol-induced depression. Brit Med J 2: 50.

Wagner AK, Zhang F, et al. (2004). Benzodiazepine use and hip fractures in the elderly: who is at greatest risk? Arch Intern Med 164: 1567–1572.

Walsh JK (2002). Zolpidem "as needed" for the treatment of primary insomnia: a double-blind, placebo-controlled study. Sleep Med Rev 6(Suppl 1): S7–S10; discussion S10–S11, S31–S13.

Wensel TM, Powe KW and Cates ME (2012). Pregabalin for the treatment of generalized anxiety disorder. Ann Pharmacother 46(3): 424–429.

Wikner BN, Stiller CO, Bergman U, et al. (2007). Use of benzodiazepines and benzodiazepine receptor agonists during pregnancy: neonatal outcome and congenital malformations. Pharmacoepidemiol Drug Saf 16(11): 1203–1210.

Williams T, Hattingh CJ, Kariuki CM, et al. (2017). Pharmacotherapy for social anxiety disorder (SAnD). Cochrane Database Syst Rev 10: CD001206.

World Health Organization. (2019). World Health Organization model list of essential medicines, 21st list. https://apps.who.int/iris/bitstream/handle/10665/325771/WHO-MVP-EMP-IAU-2019.06-eng.pdf?ua=1

Yonkers KA, Gilstad-Hayden K, Forray A, et al. (2017). Association of panic disorder, generalized anxiety disorder, and benzodiazepine treatment during pregnancy with risk of adverse birth outcomes. JAMA Psychiatry 74(11): 1145–1152.

3

Antipsychotics

Antipsychotics are used to treat schizophrenia and schizoaffective disorder. They are effective medicines that can significantly improve the lives of patients with chronic psychotic disorders and are often indispensable for most of these patients. However, they have the potential to cause serious and severe adverse effects. Since many affected patients are at risk of having psychotic symptoms for the rest of their lives, judicious use over the long run while monitoring for and managing adverse effects are required aspects of treatment with these medications.

Antipsychotics may also play a role in the treatment of several other psychiatric disorders (including most notably bipolar disorder) or may help resolve short-term psychosis in patients without chronic psychotic illnesses. As such, they have multiple uses, and their use has increased significantly over the past decade—while potential adverse effects continue to pose ongoing risks to patients who need them.

First-Generation Antipsychotics

The first antipsychotic, chlorpromazine, was developed in the 1950s (Meyer and Simpson 1997). Subsequently other antipsychotics were developed that shared similarities in their mechanisms of action and in their side effect profiles. **Chlorpromazine,** thioridazine, perphenazine, thiothixene, pimozide, fluphen-azine, and haloperidol are examples of these medications that are now characterized as first-generation antipsychotics (FGAs). Alternative names for this class of medications include: "neuro-leptics" (for their propensity to cause adverse neurological effects), "major tranquilizers" (as opposed to the later designated "minor tranquilizers" such as benzodiazepines and barbiturates), "typical" antipsychotics, and "conventional" antipsychotics.

All FGAs are believed to exert their antipsychotic effects through postsynaptic D2 dopamine receptor antagonism, thereby reducing the effect of endogenous dopamine released by presynaptic dopa-minergic neurons (Nestler, Hyman et al. 2015). In doing so, they bind more tightly to the D2 receptor than dopamine itself (Seeman 2002). In terms of clinical use, it has been shown that the optimal D2 receptor occupancy level for maximizing antipsychotic effect while minimizing adverse effects is 60% to 70% (Farde, Nordstrom et al. 1992). The D2 receptor occupancy level for eliciting extrapy-ramidal (neuroleptic) symptoms is about 80% (Seeman 2002).

Dopaminergic neurons originate from three distinct nuclei and project to other areas of the brain through four distinct pathways. One group of dopaminergic neurons projects from the ventral tegmental area of the midbrain to the nucleus accumbens, cingulate cortex and prefrontal cortex (the mesolimbic and mesocortical pathways); these affect emotions and cognition and as such are the targets for the therapeutic effects of antipsychotic drugs. Dopaminergic neurons also arise from the substantia nigra and project to the striatum (the nigrostriatal pathway); these are implicated in the neurological side effects of antipsychotics. And finally, hypothalamic dopaminergic neurons project to the pituitary gland and serve to regulate the release of prolactin (the tuberoinfundibular pathway); disruption of this system with D2 blockade can result in hyperprolactinemia associated with the use of antipsychotics.

FGAs have traditionally been divided into low potency (e.g., chlorpromazine, thioridazine), mid-potency (e.g., perphenazine, thiothixene), and high potency (e.g., haloperidol, fluphenazine) antipsychotics, based on the number of milligrams of each drug needed to show comparable efficacy. For example, chlorpromazine 300 mg (low potency) may have the same therapeutic effect as perphenazine 24 mg (mid-potency) and haloperidol 6 mg (high potency). FGAs are often listed as a spectrum from low to high potency.

The low-potency antipsychotics usually exhibit tricyclic antidepressant (TCA)-like side effects such as anticholinergic, antihistaminic, and orthostatic effects (see section on antidepressants) but have a lower risk of causing acute muscle dystonias. At the other end of the spectrum, high-potency FGAs have lower risks of TCA-like adverse effects but a much higher risk of causing acute dystonias. Mid-potency antipsychotics share all these side effects but less so than those of either pole. Clinicians today use the FGAs less often; still they should become familiar with using at least one antipsychotic from each potency class to be able to match the side effect profile to the patient's pre-existing vulnerabilities. Their efficacy, overall, is at least comparable to the newer antipsychotics.

When dosing FGAs, it is important to consider that although in most efficacy studies the presumed therapeutic dose of haloperidol is 10 mg/day or more, the ideal dose may be much lower: haloperidol 2 mg/day in neuroleptic-naïve patients and 4 mg in nonneuroleptic-naïve patients may be sufficient to produce a "neuroleptic threshold"—the dose at which cogwheel rigidity, a sign of more-than-sufficient D2 receptor blockade, first appears (McEvoy, Stiller et al. 1986).

The propensity of FGAs to cause neurological symptoms such as acute muscle dystonias, parkinsonism, akathisia, and tardive dyskinesia (TD) significantly limits their use in current practice. *Acute dystonias*, which are more likely to occur if the patient is young, male, has a history of substance abuse, and/or a prior history of dystonias, are primarily seen in patients taking FGAs, although they can also occur in patients on any antipsychotic with significant D2 receptor antagonism (see following discussion of risperidone). Use of anticholinergic medications, such as benztropine or diphenhydramine (or promethazine, used more often outside the United States) can decrease the occurrence of early dystonias or treat them acutely. *Parkinsonism*, characterized by bradykinesia, tremor, rigidity, and masked facies, can develop after one to four weeks of treatment with FGAs. Anticholinergic medications or a dopamine releasing agent such as amantadine may be helpful, although changing the antipsychotic may be required. *Akathisia*, which is an unpleasant subjective sense of inner restlessness relieved by movement, is also commonly seen in patients treated with FGAs. Identifying akathisia as a cause of agitation (or even worsening psychosis or suicidality) is important because treatment would include decreasing, rather than increasing, the antipsychotic dose. Akathisia is treated with beta-blockers, anticholinergic agents, and benzodiazepines (although ongoing use of benzodiazepines is not favored given that their use may be associated with cognitive impairments and increased mortality in this population; Fontanella, Campo et al. 2016; Fond, Berna et al. 2018). TD, a potentially irreversible syndrome of abnormal involuntary movements, can develop with extended use of antipsychotics, especially if high doses are used for long periods of time. Patients with prolonged antipsychotic treatment, a history of affective disorders, and a history of parkinsonian side effects with initial antipsychotic treatment, as well as women and the elderly, are at a higher risk for developing TD. Once TD has developed, withdrawal of the antipsychotic (especially if this is precipitous) may unmask worsened abnormal movements. Resumption of antipsychotic treatment may suppress these symptoms for a period of time, but progression of the underlying movement disorder toward permanence may continue.

Historically, treatments for TD have been only partially effective (Soares-Weiser and Fernandez 2007). In clinical settings, treatments that have been considered include antipsychotic dose reduction or switching to a second-generation antipsychotic (SGA) with low affinity to the D2 receptor (especially clozapine but possibly quetiapine—see following discussion; van Harten and Tenback 2011). Many medications have been studied as possible add-on treatments for TD, but most the studies have been contradictory or too small to reach a firm conclusion regarding efficacy. Examples of possibly promising agents include vitamin E (mostly for use early in the course of the symptoms), vitamin B6, ginkgo biloba, thiamine, diltiazem, amantadine, clonazepam, and tetrabenazine. (Soares-Weiser, Maayan et al. 2011; Bhidayasiri, Fahn et al. 2013; Bhidayasiri, Jitkritsadakul et al. 2018). However more recently, two new medications, valbenazine and deutetrabenazine, both vesicular monoamine 2 transporter inhibitors similar to tetrabenazine, have been found to be significantly effective in reducing involuntary movements associated with TD (Fernandez, Factor et al. 2017; Hauser, Factor et al. 2017; Touma and Scarff 2018). Although clinicians still have minimal experience with these treatments, they are both Food and Drug Administration (FDA)-approved and are becoming first-line therapies for TD. However, they are extremely costly and may not be affordable depending on insurance coverage. It may be necessary to first try one or more of the older, less-evidenced, but generic and therefore inexpensive options. Decreasing tardive symptoms by switching to the cost-effective and highly clinically effective antipsychotic clozapine (discussed in the following text) at the onset of TD is supported by a recent observational study (Lee, Baek et al. 2019).

Neuroleptic malignant syndrome (NMS) is a poorly understood, rare, but potentially fatal complication of treatment with FGAs and other antipsychotics. NMS is characterized by a constellation of symptoms that may include delirium, lead-pipe rigidity, autonomic instability, and high fevers. It can develop very early in the course of antipsychotic treatment. A high serum creatine phosphokinase and elevated white blood cell count are supportive of the diagnosis of NMS. If NMS appears likely, then the offending antipsychotic should be immediately discontinued. Medical hospitalization is necessary and treatment may include the use of a dopamine ago-nist (e.g., bromocriptine), a muscle relaxant (e.g., dantrolene), aggressive hydration, and the use of benzodiazepines if needed for behavioral agitation (Hu and Frucht 2007). Once the patient has been medically stabilized, the offending agent should be avoided. Rechallenge with another (optimally low-potency) antipsychotic may be possible two weeks after all symptoms of NMS have abated.

Second-Generation Antipsychotics

Most SGAs—sometimes called "atypical antipsychotics" because of having fewer extrapyramidal symptoms (EPS) than the FGAs, although that is not always true—are believed to exert their anti-psychotic effects through the similar mechanism of action of FGAs (i.e., dopamine antagonism) but have profiles of receptor activity that frequently produce different side effects than FGAs. Although their antipsychotic effect is believed to be due to D2 receptor antag-onism, most SGAs, in contrast to FGAs, bind less tightly to these receptors than dopamine (Seeman 2002); they also more rapidly dissociate from the D2 receptors (Stahl 2001). SGAs also bind to 5-HT2 serotonin receptors, which may have some effect in indirectly reducing their neuroleptic risks, while not altering their antipsy-chotic effects (Stahl 2001; Nestler, Hyman et al. 2015).

The first SGA to be developed was **clozapine**, which was fol-lowed by the sequential introduction of **risperidone, olanzapine, quetiapine, ziprasidone**, and **aripiprazole** in the United States (and amisulpride and zotepine among others, in other countries). Subsequently, four newer SGAs—namely, **paliperidone, iloperi-done, asenapine**, and **lurasidone**—were introduced in the United States, and most recently, two others, **brexpiprazole** and **caripra-zine**, have been made available for use.

Whereas the high potency FGAs were known to (a) possi-bly worsen (or possibly not improve) the negative symptoms of schizophrenia and (b) cause EPS including TD, SGAs were hoped to be more effective in treating negative symptoms and less likely to cause movement disorders. It is true that, by and large, SGAs do not worsen negative symptoms of schizophrenia (Darba, Minoves et al. 2011). They also have a much lower risk of causing TD (Correll, Leucht et al. 2004; Tarsy, Lungu et al. 2011; O'Brien 2016). One more recent meta-analysis found that the yearly incidence of TD in patients taking SGAs was 2.6%, compared to 6.5% in patients taking FGAs (Carbon, Kane et al. 2018). Although most other EPS are relatively uncommon with SGAs (except in high doses), akathisia is still common with some. NMS can rarely occur with SGAs and may present similarly as in FGAs (although it may present differently with clozapine [discussed later], where it may exhibit with less muscle rigidity; Trollor, Chen et al. 2009).

Questions, however, regarding the differential effectiveness of SGAs as compared with FGAs and the SGAs' greater risks of inducing other (nonneurological) adverse effects have served to dampen the optimistic expectations initially associated with these newer medications. Nevertheless, in most of the world where they are available, SGAs are considered to be the first line for treatment of psychotic disorders primarily because of the reduced risk of TD.

Risperidone, one of the earliest SGAs to be developed, was released in 1994. It is similar to FGAs in that it is a potent D2 receptor antagonist, but like many other SGAs, it is also a postsynaptic serotonin 5-HT2A antagonist. This is thought to mitigate the D2 receptor-mediated neurological side effects. Because of its D2 blocking potency, it is likely to have a higher risk of causing EPS and hyperprolactinemia than other SGAs (except for paliperidone [see following text]; Komossa, Rummel-Kluge et al. 2011). Nevertheless, at doses lower than 6 mg/day (i.e., at usual therapeutic doses), risperidone carries a low risk of causing EPS; at higher doses, stronger D2 blockade effects predominate and the risk of EPS increases significantly. EPS are usually not present at risperidone 3 mg/day—a dose at which 72% of D2 receptors are occupied

(Nyberg, Eriksson et al. 1999). The optimal dose derived from clinical studies appears to be 3 to 6 mg daily (Osser and Sigadel 2001). Although generally a well-tolerated antipsychotic, other side effects of risperidone include possible hypotension, and in children and adolescents, it produces considerable weight gain (Sikich, Frazier et al. 2008). It is a hepatic CYP2D6 enzyme substrate and therefore its metabolism can be slowed by (a) inhibitors such as fluoxetine and paroxetine (Spina, Scordo et al. 2003) or (b) the CYP2D6 variant gene for slow metabolism, which results in a less active form of the CYP2D6 enzyme (found more often in Chinese and other East Asian individuals) (Bertilsson 1995; Bradford 2002). Another gene variant that causes "poor" metabolism is found in 5% to 10% of Whites and results in severe side effects, especially EPS (Pi and Gray 2000). Risperidone has a medium propensity to cause adverse metabolic effects in adults (see following discussion). On the positive side, it may have a somewhat more rapid onset of action compared to other SGAs (Osser and Sigadel 2001).

Olanzapine was introduced in 1996. It has less affinity for D2 receptors than risperidone and a greater affinity for 5-HT2A and 5-HT2C serotonin receptors. Olanzapine also has significant antihistaminic and anticholinergic effects. Although it is an effective antipsychotic for the treatment of schizophrenia (Komossa, Rummel-Kluge et al. 2010) especially at doses equal to or greater than 15 mg/day (Osser and Sigadel 2001), it is (along with clozapine as discussed later) a frequent cause of weight gain, insulin resistance, and hyperlipidemia (i.e., "metabolic syndrome"). Concern about the increased morbidity and mortality associated with the metabolic syndrome has led to a reduction of the use of olanzapine in recent years. Many practice guidelines have proposed that it be avoided as a first-line agent because of these adverse effects (Osser, Roudsari et al. 2013; Mohammad and Osser 2014). Side effects increase when olanzapine is used at higher than recommended doses (e.g., 40 mg/day vs. the package insert maximum dose of 20–30 mg/day, depending on route of administration) with no additional antipsychotic benefit at much higher doses (Kinon, Volavka et al. 2008; Citrome, Stauffer et al. 2009; Osser, Roudsari et al. 2013). Liver transaminases can also become transiently elevated (more often with olanzapine than with risperidone).

Quetiapine shows weak binding affinity at both dopamine and 5-HT2 serotonin receptors, but with overall similar receptor occupancy profile to the more potent SGAs (Seeman 2002). It has alpha-adrenergic antagonism and antihistaminic effects, causing orthostasis and sedation, respectively. Quetiapine is less likely than olanzapine and clozapine, but more likely than most FGAs, risperidone, and other SGAs to cause metabolic side effects. Quetiapine at low doses, which may still be associated with weight gain (Williams, Alinejad et al. 2010), is widely (and too readily) used in psychiatric practice for the treatment of insomnia and acute anxiety in a wide range of patients with personality and/or substance abuse disorders for whom benzodiazepine use may be problematic. This "off-label" use should only be considered after a thoughtful review of risks, benefits, and alternative treatments, especially evidence-supported treatments, for the patient's diagnosed condition. Clinicians should be aware also of reports of abuse and "street value" for this medication (Hanley and Kenna 2008); abuse of quetiapine is not uncommon (Klein, Bangh et al. 2017). Use of quetiapine for anxiety symptoms may be more appropriate in acute care settings such as during hospitalizations, or for infrequent use during short-term exacerbation of symptoms. Quetiapine's effectiveness in psychotic disorders may be less than that of olanzapine and risperidone (McCue, Waheed et al. 2006; Suzuki, Uchida et al. 2007), and it has among the lowest success rates in preventing future episodes (Kreyenbuhl, Slade et al. 2011). Hence, it is not favored as a first-line treatment for schizophrenia, given that prevention of the next episode is one of the important clinical priorities for newly diagnosed patients. Using quetiapine at doses higher than usual approved doses (i.e., greater than 800 mg/day) does not appear to provide any added benefit and is not recommended (Lindenmayer, Citrome et al. 2011; Honer, MacEwan et al. 2012). Quetiapine produces significant QT prolongation and a package insert warning added in 2011 cites 12 medications with which it should not be combined. Quetiapine may have a stronger role in treating patients with bipolar disorders (see discussion later in this chapter and in the chapter on mood stabilizers).

Ziprasidone is an SGA with moderate D2 antagonism and significant 5-HT2A antagonism (i.e., a high 5-HT2A–D2 ratio). Although it is not clear if it is as effective as olanzapine and risperidone in the acute treatment of schizophrenia (McCue, Waheed et al. 2006), it does not cause metabolic changes and may even improve lipid profile, especially if the patient was previously on a weight gain-inducing agent (Lieberman, Stroup et al. 2005). A major issue with using ziprasidone is the necessity of taking it with food, or it will not be well-absorbed. A 500-calorie meal is needed with each of the twice-daily doses (Miceli, Glue et al. 2007). The optimal dose for ziprasidone is 80 mg twice daily: lower doses may not be different from placebo in schizophrenia (Citrome, Yang et al. 2009).

Ziprasidone has the potential to prolong QT more than other SGAs. Although a pretreatment ECG is not required in every patient, those who are deemed, based on history or age, to be at higher cardiac risk would benefit from an ECG (and medical consultation if cardiac disease or arrhythmias are present) before starting ziprasidone. Like most other antipsychotics, it should be avoided if baseline QTc is greater than or equal to 500 msec. Electrolyte disturbances such as hypomagnesemia and hypokalemia should be corrected. Other QT prolonging medications should not be used in combination with ziprasidone. Despite concerns regarding this effect, post-marketing studies (e.g., Clinical Antipsychotics Trials of Intervention Effectiveness [CATIE] trial) did not show any clinically significant QT prolongation with ziprasidone use (Lieberman, Stroup et al. 2005).

Clinicians should be aware that most antipsychotics (with the possible exceptions of aripiprazole and lurasidone discussed later) could have significant effects on cardiac conduction, potentially delaying conduction enough to lead to fatal arrhythmias. There is an association between the use of antipsychotics (as well as TCAs) and sudden cardiac death (Ray, Chung et al. 2009; Ray, Meredith et al. 2004; Straus, Bleumink et al. 2004). An increased risk of unexpected deaths has also been observed in young patients taking antipsychotics (Ray, Stein et al. 2019). As discussed in the chapter on antidepressants, prolonged QTc is associated with torsades de pointes, a potentially fatal arrhythmia. The QT interval includes both the QRS interval as well as the ST segment. Whereas TCAs and some FGAs with tricyclic structure (e.g., chlorpromazine) may lengthen the QRS interval by interfering with sodium channels and depolarization, most other antipsychotics, including SGAs, may lengthen the ST interval by affecting potassium channels and the repolarization phase (Glassman and Bigger 2001). Both effects would be reflected in the QT interval. Although it is not clear if QT prolongation is always a reliable indicator of the risk of torsades, measuring this interval is the simplest way to estimate this risk (Shah 2005; Nielsen, Graff et al. 2011). Therefore, increases in the QTc above normal requires ECG monitoring; a QTc of 500 msec or higher necessitates antipsychotic discontinuation (Nielsen, Graff et al. 2011). In either case, any underlying hypokalemia or hypo-magnesemia should be corrected. Personal or family history of cardiac arrhythmias, cardiomyopathy, congenital prolonged QT, or syncope may also alert the clinician to those at higher risk of cardiac effects from the use of antipsychotics (Nielsen, Graff et al. 2011). In addition to **ziprasidone**, the FGAs **thioridazine, mesoridazine, pimozide**, and **droperidol** are among the antipsychotics with the highest propensity to prolong the QT interval (Fayek, Kingsbury et al. 2001).

Aripiprazole, in contrast to earlier SGAs, is a high affinity partial agonist at the D2 receptor (Mamo, Graff et al. 2007). It is proposed that aripiprazole decreases overall dopamine effect in dopamine rich environments (e.g., in mesolimbic pathways—thereby ameliorating psychosis) and increases dopamine effect in dopamine depleted environments (e.g., in mesocortical pathways to the prefrontal cortex—thereby potentially improving negative symptoms such as social withdrawal; Stahl 2008). At therapeutic doses, it highly saturates the targeted dopamine receptors and shows very slow dissociation from the receptors upon discontinuation (Goff 2008; Grunder, Fellows et al. 2008). It also exhibits D3 dopamine receptor partial agonism and moderate 5-HT2A and 5-HT2C antagonism (Frankel and Schwartz 2017). However, the theoretical ramifications of this pharmacodynamic profile (i.e., dopaminergic effect) do not seem to have been fully realized: efficacy appears to be only average (Osser, Roudsari et al. 2013). Aripiprazole's side effect profile is relatively mild, however. It is free from significant anticholinergic and antihistaminic effects. It has only small effects on QT and cardiac function (El-Sayeh, Morganti et al. 2006; Chung and Chua 2011) and only mild weight gain in chronic patients (Fava, Wisniewski et al. 2009). However, in adolescents and others receiving first time treatment with an antipsychotic, weight gain can be significant (e.g., 10 lbs. over 11 weeks; Correll, Manu et al. 2009).

Aripiprazole carries a low risk of EPS, likely due to its partial agonism rather than full antagonism, at D2 receptors (Takahata, Ito et al. 2012). Although it is less likely to cause EPS in general, it has been observed in practice to cause akathisia more readily than other SGAs. This may occur early in treatment and is usually only mild to moderate in severity (Kane, Barnes et al. 2010). Akathisia may be more common if the patient was recently on a strong D2 antagonist such as an FGA or risperidone and consequently has an upregulated or hypersensitive population of D2 receptors (Raja 2007).

Aripiprazole at 15 mg/day may be more efficacious than 30 mg/day in schizophrenia, although full response may take longer than with a comparable dose of haloperidol (Kane, Carson et al. 2002). Higher doses (e.g., 30 mg/day) may be more useful in treatment-resistant schizophrenia (TRS; Kane, Meltzer et al. 2007). Relapse rates may be somewhat higher with aripiprazole than with some other SGAs (Pigott, Carson et al. 2003).

Clozapine, the first and, in some respects, the most impressive of the SGAs, binds broadly to different dopamine receptors. It binds weakly to the D2 receptor but shows relatively greater net antagonism at D4 dopamine receptors (Seeman 1992; Brunello, Masotto et al. 1995). It has moderate affinity for 5-HT2A and 5-HT2C receptors. It is often effective when other antipsychotics are not (Lewis, Barnes et al. 2006) and has been found to have superior antisuicidal effects in patients with schizophrenia or schizoaffective disorder in comparison with olanzapine (Meltzer, Alphs et al. 2003). However, because of an approximately 0.4% to 2% risk of agranulocytosis, most of which occurs between the first six weeks to six months of treatment (Honigfeld, Arellano et al. 1998; Meltzer 2012), it is indicated primarily for schizophrenia and schizoaffective patients who have failed to respond adequately to at least two other antipsychotics. It also has FDA approval for non-TRS patients with active suicidal ideation. Strict monitoring and blood draws—initially weekly for the first six months, then every two weeks for the next six months, and then every four weeks—are required to monitor the absolute neutrophil count. The clinician should consult the package insert and strictly follow the monitoring guidelines that are periodically revised. Clozapine should not be combined with other medications (e.g., carbamazepine) that may also cause leukopenia.

Clozapine can also cause multiple other adverse effects, which include (but are not limited to) an increased risk of seizures, rare myocarditis, eosinophilia, anticholinergic and antihistaminic effects, orthostasis, weight gain, and adverse metabolic effects (Lamberti, Olson et al. 2006). Given the complicated nature of clozapine treatment, the clinician should refer to a more in-depth discussion of this drug before use (Meyer and Stahl 2020). Clozapine has multiple other potential side effects including severe constipation (because it is strongly anticholinergic) leading to paralytic ileus, toxic megacolon, and death, as well as sedation, hypersaliva-tion, tachycardia, and a low-grade fever. It is interesting to note that a retrospective chart review found that gastrointestinal and pulmonary illnesses were the most likely reasons for medical hos-pitalizations for patients taking clozapine; this may be a testament to psychiatrists' successful monitoring for this medicine's other serious adverse effects (e.g., agranulocytosis and myocarditis; Leung, Hasassri et al. 2017). The pulmonary illnesses may include aspiration pneumonia from hypersalivation, made more likely by respiratory depression from ill-advised concomitant treatment with benzodiazepines.

Among the SGAs, clozapine and olanzapine are the most likely (and aripiprazole, ziprasidone, asenapine, and lurasidone discussed later may be the least likely) to cause adverse metabolic effects. These would include weight gain, hyperglycemia and diabetes (with or without weight gain), and hyperlipidemia (American Diabetes Association 2004). A 2 to 3 kg weight gain within the first three weeks of treatment often predicts the risk of significant weight gain over the long term (Lipkovich, Citrome et al. 2006). Another more recent study of olanzapine also found that a 1 kg weight gain at two weeks reliably predicted more significant weight gain later (Lin, Lin et al. 2018). Decreased insulin secretion and increased tri-glycerides (i.e., the lipids most affected by SGAs; Osser, Najarian & Dufresne 1999) can also be seen within one to two weeks of treat-ment (Chiu, Chen et al. 2006) or even after a single dose of olan-zapine (Hahn, Wolever et al. 2013). These changes are an additional burden on schizophrenic patients who, even prior to antipsychotic treatment, may be at a higher baseline risk for glucose and insulin dysregulation (Pillinger, Beck et al. 2017). Antipsychotic-induced metabolic changes are additional cardiac risk factors for patients with schizophrenia.

Prior to starting olanzapine or clozapine, measurements of base-line weight, serum glucose, and lipid profile should be obtained. If the patient has pre-existing diabetes, other antipsychotics should be considered. Once treatment is initiated, serum glucose and weight should be monitored, and if glucose levels become elevated, a glucose tolerance test—which can predict up to 96% of patients who would develop diabetes—should be done (van Winkel, De Hert et al. 2006). If metabolic problems do arise during treatment, switching to another antipsychotic should be considered. Treatment with the glucose-lowering medication metformin, especially if combined with lifestyle changes, may reduce antipsychotic-induced weight gain and metabolic effects (Baptista, Rangel et al. 2007; Wu, Zhao et al. 2008; Maayan, Vakhrusheva et al. 2010; Praharaj, Jana et al. 2011; Caemmerer, Correll et al. 2012; Correll, Sikich et al. 2013). Pharmacogenomic findings, such as an association between 5-HT2C polymorphisms and antipsychotic induced weight gain (Sicard, Zai et al. 2010) as well as multiple other polymorphisms, may allow for better screening and personalization of treatment in the future.

Clozapine may cause orthostatic hypotension. Patients who are elderly, have cardiac histories, or who are taking antihypertensives are at higher risk for this side effect. Clozapine should be started at a very low dose and increased gradually (starting at 12.5 mg for the first dose and increasing the dose by 25 mg daily as tolerated). Usually, patients adjust and become tolerant to the hypotensive effects of this medication. However, this tolerance may not last longer than 48 hours. If, during active treatment, a patient discontinues clozapine therapy for more than 48 hours, treatment should be restarted with a 12.5 mg dose. After that, the dose may be more quickly raised to the previous dose as tolerated. It is important for the physician who may be admitting a psychiatric patient to the medical or surgical ward of the hospital to stop and think before continuing clozapine at its prior dose: recent compliance needs to be verified first.

Due to its many potential adverse effects and the time required to monitor and manage these effects, clozapine is underutilized in the United States. Even though it is often effective when patients are treatment-refractory to other antipsychotics, many clinicians choose to delay its appropriate use. When two or more adequate trials of antipsychotics have been ineffective in treating a patient's schizophrenia, it is often the case that psychiatrists opt for other, often unsuccessful, antipsychotic trials or combination antipsychotic therapies (for which there is very little supportive evidence), rather than considering clozapine (for which there is a significant evidence base). Consequently, multiple failed trials and polypharmacy then may burden patients with increased adverse effects and, more important, fail to adequately treat their psychotic illness. Clinicians should keep in mind that for many patients clozapine is likely to (a) be more effective than other antipsychotics for treatment-resistant psychosis, (b) reduce suicidality, (c) have a low risk for TD, (d) improve quality of life, and (e) decrease the risk of relapse (Meltzer 2012). Along with long-acting injectible antipsychotics discussed later, clozapine appears to have the lowest risks of relapse and hospitalization compared to other antipsychotics in patients with schizophrenia (Tiihonen, Mittendorfer-Rutz et al. 2017).

Newer Second-Generation Antipsychotics

Several years after the first group of SGAs was made available, four newer antipsychotics—**paliperidone, iloperidone, asenapine,** and **lurasidone**—were introduced in the United States. Their mechanism of action is generally considered to be similar to those of the previously discussed D2 antagonists. Paliperidone, as noted later, behaves clinically in a similar manner to risperidone, its parent compound. The remaining three exhibit some variations in their effects on serotonin receptor subtypes, but it is still not clear if any of these variations confer any added clinical benefit in either efficacy (in schizophrenia or schizoaffective disorder) or tolerability when compared to older less costly SGAs. Differences do exist, however, among them in terms of side effect profiles. Iloperidone, asenapine, and lurasidone all appear to have relatively favorable metabolic risk profiles compared to olanzapine and clozapine. However, lurasidone and asenapine appear to have a significant risk of treatment-emergent akathisia. Lurasidone is now also FDA-approved for adolescents with schizophrenia.

Paliperidone is the major active metabolite of risperidone and has similar efficacy and side effects. Because it is not metabolized by CYP2D6 and is mostly renally excreted, it is likely to have fewer drug–drug interactions (Wang, Han et al. 2012). However, it may have a higher risk of QT prolongation (Suzuki, Fukui et al. 2012), more tachycardia, and possibly more EPS (although with similar propensity to increase prolactin) than risperidone (Nussbaum and Stroup 2012). Paliperidone is often favored when a long-acting injectable (LAI) antipsychotic is being considered, with competition from aripiprazole and its new LAI formulations (see following discussion).

Iloperidone (not a metabolite or analogue of paliperidone or risperidone) is a D2 and 5-HT2A receptor antagonist. It also has a high affinity for D3 and noradrenergic alpha-1 receptors, and moderate affinity for D4, 5-HT6 and 5-HT7 receptors. Alpha-1 blockade results in a significant propensity to cause orthostasis, thereby requiring slow dose titration. It is thought to carry a very low risk of causing EPS or akathisia and has little effect on prolactin levels, but the evidence is mixed (Weiden, Manning et al. 2016; Subeesh, Maheswari et al. 2019). Moderate weight gain (more than risperidone but without significant change in glucose or lipids), mild sedation, peripheral edema, and priapism may also occur (Subeesh, Maheswari et al. 2019). QT prolongation may be higher than with some other antipsychotics (Citrome 2010; Weiden 2012).

Asenapine, another D2 and 5-HT2 antagonist, is also a partial agonist at the 5-HT1A receptor. It also shows high affinity and antagonism for a broad range of other 5-HT and dopamine receptors, the clinical relevance of which is unclear. Asenapine is

associated with low metabolic risks, low risk of prolactin elevation, and mild EPS risk; however, dose-dependent akathisia may
occur. It is the first sublingually administered antipsychotic and
is administered in twice daily doses, but if swallowed too quickly,
absorption will be poor. Usage is associated with oral numbing,
which may also affect compliance (Potkin 2011; Stoner and Pace
2012; Tarazi and Stahl 2012). Subsequently, a transdermal patch
has been approved by the FDA, making asenapine the first antipsychotic to be approved in the United States for use as a patch. Severe
and potentially lethal allergic reactions may occur with asenapine,
even after the first dose (FDA 2011a).

Lurasidone is a potent D2 and 5-HT2A antagonist. It also
acts as a potent 5-HT7 antagonist and a 5-HT1A agonist. It is
not yet clear how these receptor effects might influence clinical
efficacy (although based on animal studies, effects on cognition,
depression, and anxiety have been proposed; Ishibashi, Horisawa
et al. 2010; Risbood, Lee et al. 2012). It is associated with minimal weight gain and appears to have a low risk of metabolic side
effects, and it may have no significant effect on QT prolongation
(Kantrowitz and Citrome 2012; Risbood, Lee et al. 2012). Prolactin
elevation may occur, and a dose-dependent increase in parkinsonism, akathisia, and somnolence may be observed (McIntyre, Cha
et al. 2012; Risbood, Lee et al. 2012). It should be taken once a day
with a 350-calorie meal. Given its efficacy and tolerability in bipolar depression, lurasidone is often considered for this indication
(Fornaro, De Berardis et al. 2017; Ansari and Osser 2010), with the
added benefit of causing less weight gain than alternatives such as
quetiapine and olanzapine (Ostacher, Ng-Mak et al. 2018).

Newest Second-Generation Antipsychotics

Most recently two new SGAs, **brexpiprazole** and **cariprazine**,
have become available that, like aripiprazole, are D2 and D3

receptor partial agonists. Together these three antipsychotics may be emerging as a subtype of SGAs or "atypical" SGAs, which some have viewed as "dopamine stabilizers." In addition these antipsychotics are antagonists with varying degrees of effect at serotonin, histamine, and cholinergic receptors (Frankel and Schwartz 2017).

In addition to all three having FDA approval for use in schizophrenia, brexpiprazole has been approved as adjunctive therapy for major depression, and cariprazine has been approved for the treatment of mania or mixed episodes and for bipolar depression. These are indications that they share with several other antipsychotics. It is too early to know if these new (and costly) antipsychotics provide any added benefits to previously available SGAs.

Both brexpiprazole and cariprazine are thought to have a low risk of causing metabolic syndrome (Citrome 2013; Kane, Skuban et al. 2016).

Emerging Antipsychotic

Pimavanserin, a selective 5-HT2A receptor inverse agonist/antagonist with lesser effect on 5-HT2C, is a new FDA-approved medication for the treatment of psychosis associated with Parkinson's disease (PD; Kitten, Hallowell et al. 2018; Sahli and Tarazi 2018). At this time, it is extremely costly and therefore may be out of reach for many patients. Although SGAs with weaker D2 antagonism potency (e.g., quetiapine, olanzapine, and clozapine) have been traditionally used in patients with PD, only clozapine (at relatively low doses) appears to have any benefit over placebo, and none have FDA approval for this indication (Jethwa and Onalaja 2015).

Pimavanserin may also have some effect on dementia related psychosis (Ballard, Banister et al. 2018), although none of the other SGAs have received FDA approval for this indication despite extensive testing. It carries the same warnings about increased risk of death and stroke in patients with dementia, and QT prolongation is still a concern (PDR 2019). Pimavanserin's potential role, if any, in the treatment of primary psychotic illnesses has not yet emerged; it has not yet been studied as a stand-alone treatment for schizophrenia (also see the following section on TRS).

Complementary, Alternative, and Other Pharmacotherapies

Although **omega 3 fatty-acids, vitamin** D, and **vitamin A** have been studied in patients with schizophrenia, there is insufficient evidence to recommend their use for the treatment of psychosis, even if nutritional deficiencies may be common in this population (Balanza Martinez 2017). **Vitamin B and L-methylfolate** supplementation, however, may reduce some psychiatric symptoms in patients with schizophrenia (Firth, Stubbs et al. 2017; Roffman, Petruzzi et al. 2018).

Despite recent interest in microbiota–brain–gut axis and potential recommendations for dietary manipulations and **probiotic** interventions (Nemani, Hosseini Ghomi et al. 2015; Karakula-Juchnowicz, Dzikowski et al. 2016), there is insufficient evidence to make any specific recommendations in support of these strategies.

More recently, there has been greater interest in the effects of **cannabinoids** on psychosis. A large multicenter study concluded that a greater incidence of psychotic disorders may be linked to higher rates of high potency cannabis use (i.e., increased use of cannabis with higher concentrations of delta9-tetrahydrocannabinol; Di Forti, Quattrone et al. 2019). Furthermore, patients who already have a psychotic disorder are at a greater risk of a psychotic relapse with ongoing cannabis use, especially if higher potency cannabis is used (Schoeler, Petros et al. 2016). It has been proposed, however, that **cannabidiol**, which is found in low concentrations in marketed cannabis, may counteract the psychotogenic effects of delta9-tetrahydrocannabinol and, therefore, may have independent antipsychotic effects (Leweke, Mueller et al. 2016). Although findings from several small studies have supported the notion that cannabidiol may normalize brain function in those at high risk for psychosis (Bhattacharyya, Wilson et al. 2018; Hahn 2018; Slomski 2019), there are insufficient controlled clinical data to support recommending it as an antipsychotic in patients with schizophrenia.

Further Notes on the Clinical Use of Antipsychotics in Psychotic Disorders

Choice of Antipsychotic

All antipsychotics are indicated for the treatment of schizophrenia and are considered to be reasonably safe and effective treatments for this debilitating disorder. SGAs (with the exception of clozapine, which is reserved for refractory psychosis) may be considered as first-line treatments. SGAs that have been around longer (i.e., those for which there is more clinical experience) are considered more often that the newest agents.

However, there has been much debate about whether there are efficacy differences among these medications or whether the side effect differences, which are considerable, should be the primary basis for selecting a medication for a particular patient. Regarding efficacy, a meta-analysis of 78 head-to-head comparisons in the literature through 2007 concluded that the efficacy differences are small, but there was some superiority to olanzapine and risperidone, when compared with aripiprazole, quetiapine, and ziprasidone (Leucht, Komossa et al. 2009). A problem with this meta-analysis, however, was that almost all of the studies were industry-sponsored. Such studies invariably find outcomes in favor of the sponsor's product, and olanzapine and risperidone have sponsored the largest number of studies. Similarly, but with the same reservations, a more recent meta-analysis in early onset schizophrenia supported the slight superior efficacy of olanzapine and risperidone compared to quetiapine, ziprasidone, and aripiprazole in early-onset psychosis (Harvey, James et al. 2016). The authors of these reviews emphasize that the side effects differ considerably, especially over the long term, and this must be balanced against the small differences in efficacy when selecting antipsychotics for patients. For first-episode patients, it may be best to choose from among the antipsychotics with the least weight, metabolic side effects, and EPS even if those options have slightly less efficacy, such as aripiprazole and lurasidone. The argument would be that whichever one is selected, the patient is likely to have to live with it and its side effects for a long time, and thus it would be worthwhile to find out if the patient can respond to a milder agent. However, if the patient fails to respond to the first trial, efficacy would become more important for the second trial, and risperidone or olanzapine could be favored. In one important randomized trial, risperidone was compared with aripiprazole in 198 patients receiving their first antipsychotic trial (Robinson, Gallego et al. 2015). Effectiveness on positive symptoms was similar (63% with aripiprazole; 57% with risperidone), but there was significantly better response on negative symptoms with aripiprazole (due probably to secondary negative symptoms generated by risperidone's EPS). Aripiprazole seemed like the better choice for patients getting first treatment with an antipsychotic.

Another consideration in early selection is that the medication should have good evidence of ability to prevent the next episode. As noted earlier, quetiapine has not done well in meta-analyses of maintenance efficacy and hence would not be a good early choice even though some of its side effects (e.g., EPS) are milder (Kreyenbuhl, Slade et al. 2011; Tiihonen, Mittendorfer-Rutz et al. 2017).

Another meta-analysis focused on 150 studies that directly compared FGAs with SGAs (Leucht, Corves et al. 2009). The authors found that clozapine (which is reserved for refractory psychosis) was clearly superior to the others especially for positive symptoms of hallucinations and delusions. Olanzapine and risperidone were superior to the rest, but with a small effect size. After that, there were no differences in efficacy. The side effect profiles differed markedly, with no pattern to the differences.

Many clinicians put more reliance on the few comparison outcome studies that were independently funded, such as the CATIE study (Lieberman, Stroup et al. 2005), funded by the U.S. National Institute of Mental Health. This study prospectively compared the FGA perphenazine, with SGAs (clozapine, olanzapine, risperidone, quetiapine, ziprasidone) and found generally no differences in effectiveness except that clozapine was superior. There were no differences in the ability to improve impaired cognition, despite prior claims for SGA superiority from studies sponsored by the SGA pharmaceutical firms (Keefe, Bilder et al. 2007). None worked well for this, and there was thus no evidence of a "neuroprotective effect" of SGAs.

Some experts have interpreted CATIE as showing olanzapine to be superior to the other nonclozapine antipsychotics, but this seems likely to be due to peculiar results with the cohort of patients who were on olanzapine prior to entering the CATIE study. These patients (22% of the sample) were randomly assigned to either continue on olanzapine or be switched to one of the other options in CATIE (perphenazine, risperidone, quetiapine, or ziprasidone). The patients who were assigned to remain on olanzapine did better than those who were abruptly switched to any of the other options (Essock, Covell et al. 2006). By contrast, the patients who entered the study on risperidone (the second largest group with 19%) showed no advantage to staying on risperidone compared to switching to another agent. Notably, there was no advantage to switching to olanzapine. Hence, the superiority of olanzapine seen in CATIE may be due to the study having a large sample of patients who had been previously stabilized on olanzapine and who clearly responded only to olanzapine or who may have been more prone to a withdrawal-induced exacerbations when taken off of olanzapine.

As noted earlier, since olanzapine has a very unfavorable side effect profile with its tendency to promote weight gain, insulin resistance, and the metabolic syndrome, this would appear to make it undesirable as a first-line choice even if it does have slightly superior efficacy.

Other findings from CATIE could be summarized as follows: (a) the FGA perphenazine was generally at least as effective as the SGAs quetiapine, risperidone, and ziprasidone and was the most cost-effective; however, more patients on perphenazine had EPS; (2) those who discontinued the FGA perphenazine subsequently did better on olanzapine or quetiapine rather than on risperidone, the SGA with the strongest D2 affinity; (3) olanzapine and risperidone were generally more effective than quetiapine and ziprasidone (although see previous caveats for olanzapine); (4) in terms of side effects, patients on olanzapine had the most metabolic side effects, risperidone was associated with hyperprolactinemia, and ziprasidone did not show any clinically relevant QT prolongation; and (5) clozapine worked best in treatment-resistant patients. These findings suggest that antipsychotics are not equally effective and tolerability profiles are variable. As always, treatment of patients with schizophrenia should be customized to meet each patient's individual needs and profiles (Keefe, Bilder et al. 2007; Swartz, Stroup et al. 2008; Lieberman and Stroup 2011).

Time to Response

Antipsychotics, whether first or second generation, do not have immediate full antipsychotic effect. Sedation, which can be a nonspecific side effect of most but not all antipsychotics, may immediately decrease assaultiveness and agitation should these be present. Hallucinations and disorganization may then begin to improve over the next few weeks, and delusions may take much longer to become less prominent (or they may persist despite ongoing treatment). As previously noted, patients with first-episode psychosis (i.e., those who are treatment naïve) may improve with lower than usual recommended doses of an antipsychotic (Buchanan, Kreyenbuhl et al. 2010). Historically, when antipsychotics first became available, significant improvement was observed over many months. A therapeutic sequence of initially diminished assaultiveness and increased cooperation (within the first week), followed by gradual socialization while psychosis persisted (within four to six weeks), followed sometimes by the elimination of thought disorder over many months, was observed when FGAs were first used (Lehman 1964).

Today, managed care organizations often choose to presume that significant improvement (e.g., improvement that would allow discharge from the hospital) could be expected in as soon as a week. This is likely to be too optimistic. It may be reasonable to expect that a quarter of treated first-episode schizophrenia patients could show a modest 20% or greater improvement in rating scales within the first week; however, a third of the patients may require four to eight weeks for similar response (Emsley, Rabinowitz et al. 2006). However, the lack of any response within the first two weeks of treatment, a period within which some clear response is often noted (Jager, Riedel et al. 2010), predicts poor response within three months. No response in two weeks may therefore suggest the need for change in dose or type of antipsychotic (Leucht, Busch et al. 2007). Clinicians should keep in mind, however, that antipsychotics vary in their speed of response (e.g., quicker response may be seen with risperidone; Osser and Sigadel 2001). Use of adjunctive benzodiazapines to decrease agitation in the short term may also be a reasonably safe way to speed progress to dischargeability (Osser, Roudsari et al. 2013). Treatment-resistant patients may require a longer time to respond.

Treatment Continuation

Once a patient with schizophrenia has responded adequately to an antipsychotic during the acute phase, the same medication is continued for maintenance. The dose needed for initial response is often continued, but adverse effects (or the potential risks associated with a higher dose over time) may necessitate a reduction in dose. Once satisfactory maintenance is achieved, however, continuous antipsychotic treatment (in contrast to intermittent treatment or no treatment) helps to reduce the risk of relapse (Leucht, Tardy et al. 2012; De Hert, Sermon et al. 2015; Hui, Honer et al. 2018). Maintenance antipsychotic treatment is usually lifelong.

Antipsychotics for Acute Behavioral Control

Both SGAs and FGAs are used in psychiatric practice to treat *behavioral agitation.* In acutely psychotic and/or manic patients, FGAs, such as oral or intramuscular haloperidol (invariably combined with lorazepam and/or benztropine or diphenhydramine to decrease the risk of acute dystonias), remain the mainstay of treatment (Ansari, Osser et al. 2009; Osser, Roudsari et al. 2013). Intramuscular fluphenazine can also be considered in place of haloperidol if the patient has a haloperidol allergy. SGAs, such as olanzapine and ziprasidone, are also available in short-acting intramuscular form but seem to have no advantage in effectiveness or side effects when compared with the previously noted combination therapy (Satterthwaite, Wolf et al. 2008) and, in a controlled study, were inferior in one or the other of these respects (Mantovani, Labate et al. 2013). When considering antipsychotics for behavioral agitation, clinicians should be advised not to use (a) intramuscular droperidol due to a high risk of QT prolongation, (b) intramuscular chlorpromazine due to risk of severe hypotension and no greater effectiveness versus haloperidol (Ahmed, Jones et al. 2010), (c) intramuscular ziprasidone if the patient is taking other medications that can also prolong QT including oral ziprasidone, or (d) intramuscular olanzapine in combination with lorazepam or other benzodiazepines due to the risk of hypotension, other cardiovascular effects, or respiratory depression (Zacher and

Roche-Desilets 2005; Marder, Sorsaburu et al. 2010). Similarly, emergency department use of intravenous olanzapine, with or without a benzodiazepine (e.g., midazolam), is not recommended. The use of antipsychotics for the treatment of behavioral agitation in elderly patients with *dementia* is problematic both in terms of effectiveness and tolerability. First, in terms of effect, they do not appear to provide more than minimal benefit in targeting symptoms of agitation (Cheung and Stapelberg 2011); SGAs may not be different from placebo in this regard (Yury and Fisher 2007). The National Institute of Mental Health–sponsored CATIE-AD study, which studied the effectiveness of olanzapine, quetiapine, and risperidone in the treatment of symptoms of psychosis, aggression, and agitation in patients with Alzheimer's disease, also found that even when these symptoms did improve with treatment, the antipsychotic did not improve overall functioning (Sultzer, Davis et al. 2008). Furthermore, any improvement in specific symptoms was offset by adverse effects and led to overall discontinuation rates (when both efficacy and tolerability were considered) that were no different from placebo (Schneider, Tariot et al. 2006). Second, antipsychotics have been found to be associated with an increased risk of stroke in patients with dementia and an overall increased risk of adverse medical events and death in this population (Gill, Rochon et al. 2005; Herrmann and Lanctot 2005; Rochon, Normand et al. 2008; Schneider, Dagerman et al. 2005). Both FGAs and SGAs appear to increase the risk of death in patients with dementia (Schneeweiss, Setoguchi et al. 2007; Wang, Schneeweiss et al. 2005). Nevertheless, it should be noted that despite all these safety concerns, if immediate relief from acutely dangerous behavior is required (as in periods of hospitalization), antipsychotics may still need to be considered in behaviorally dysregulated patients with dementia (Davies, Burhan et al. 2018; Osser, Braun & Fischer 2013). Non-psychopharmacological and non-antipsychotic interventions however should also be concurrently considered. The American Geriatrics Society Beers Criteria®

recommends that antipsychotics should be avoided in elderly patients (except for those with schizophrenia or bipolar disorder) unless non-psychopharmacological interventions have "failed or are not possible" and the patient is "threatening substantial harm to self or others" (American Geriatrics Society 2019).

High-potency FGAs are also often used in the treatment of the behavioral and psychotic manifestations of *delirium* in hospitalized patients (Lonergan, Britton et al. 2007). SGAs such as olanzapine, risperidone, and quetiapine have suggestive efficacy. (Tahir, Eeles et al. 2010; Grover, Mattoo et al. 2011). However, a systematic review of 19 studies concluded that the use of antipsychotics for delirium is not supported by the evidence: they are not effective for reducing delirium duration, severity, length of hospital stay, or mortality, and adverse outcomes were greater than with placebo (Oh, Fong et al. 2017). Delirium is a medical condition that should be treated by addressing the underlying medical cause.

Long-Acting Injectable Antipsychotics

In the United States, six antipsychotics are available for long-acting (i.e., depot) intramuscular administration: **haloperidol decanoate, fluphenazine decanoate, LAI risperidone, olanzapine LAI, paliperidone LAI**, and **aripiprazole LAI**. These long-acting formulations are options for patients who are frequently poorly adherent to oral medication (Olfson, Marcus et al. 2007). A trial of the antipsychotic in oral form is generally prescribed first to assess patients' response to, and tolerance of, the selected agent, although if the patient will not adhere adequately with the oral trial, a change to the LAI of that antipsychotic can allow completion of the trial and a more accurate determination of the effectiveness of that agent. Depending on which agent is used, injections are given every two or four weeks. For example, every four-week injections of haloperidol decanoate or biweekly injections of LAI fluphenazine or risperidone are then continued while the oral agent is gradually tapered.

Two to six weeks (or longer) of the selected oral antipsychotic may be necessary while waiting for the depot to achieve steady state before oral medications should be completely withdrawn (Osser and Sigadel 2001). More recently, paliperidone has gained favor as a long-term injectable because it can be front-loaded and therefore may need less time to achieve steady state; it can also be switched after four monthly injections to the every three-month injectable formulation (Kim, Solari et al. 2012; Morris and Tarpada 2017; Bioque and Bernardo 2018). A new once-monthly subcutaneously administered risperidone injectable is claimed to provide clinically effective serum levels after the first injection (Citrome 2018; Lexicomp 2019), thereby not requiring concurrent oral administration. The effectiveness of this new LAI formulation of risperidone is yet to be confirmed in the clinical setting.

Unfortunately, patients who adhere poorly to oral medications in real-world community settings where follow-up services may be suboptimal are generally nonadherent to depot antipsychotics as well (Olfson, Marcus et al. 2007). Although some studies suggest that depot antipsychotics can reduce relapse, the findings appear to be limited by many of these studies' methodological problems (Leucht, Heres et al. 2011; Osser, Roudsari et al. 2013). Still, more recent reviews have found improvements in real-world outcome measures (e.g., relapse rates, hospitalizations, treatment failure) with injectables relative to oral antipsychotics (Alphs, Benson et al. 2015; Tiihonen, Mittendorfer-Rutz et al. 2017). Although early nonadherence to injections in some patients can undermine treatment, in the patients who continue initial injections and achieve steady state, depots do have a subsequent advantage: if the patient discontinues treatment, the antipsychotic effect can continue for up to several months after the last received dose giving some time for other interventions to be employed and for the patient to be encouraged to resume injections. Finally, long-acting formulations may work best in research subjects and in other populations of relatively cooperative and less firmly nonadherent patients who have good support in the community.

Treatment-Resistant Schizophrenia

TRS (i.e., schizophrenia refractory to two or more antipsychotics) continues to be a clinical challenge. As previously noted, clozapine is the treatment of choice for TRS. If clozapine is insufficiently effective, its augmentation with another antipsychotic is often considered, even though it is difficult to draw any definitive conclusions from available data to support this (Barber, Olotu et al. 2017). The effectiveness of augmentation with antiepileptic drugs is also unclear though a recent review found surprising support for the addition of sodium valproate to clozapine (Zheng, Xiang et al. 2017). Augmentations with risperidone (Kontaxakis, Ferentinos et al. 2006; Weiner, Conley et al. 2010) or lamotrigine (Zoccali, Muscatello et al. 2007; Tiihonen, Wahlbeck & Kiviniemi 2009) are slightly supported (Freudenreich, Henderson et al. 2007; Vayisoglu, Anil Yagcioglu et al. 2013), and are therefore considered when psychosis continues despite clozapine therapy. More recently a large cohort study found that the combination of clozapine and aripiprazole was superior to clozapine alone in reducing the risk of rehospitalization (Tiihonen, Taipale et al. 2019).

Finally, a recent small study of 10 patients who had continued to have hallucinations and delusions despite clozapine therapy showed that the addition of pimavanserin significantly improved these refractory symptoms (Nasrallah, Fedora & Morton 2019). More studies are needed to further evaluate this effect.

Electroconvulsive therapy (ECT) is often considered when antipsychotic pharmacotherapy is unsuccessful for TRS (Grover, Sahoo et al. 2019; Sinclair, Zhao et al. 2019), although historically the addition of ECT to an antipsychotic has been associated with greater adverse cognitive effects. Continuation ECT may be helpful for clozapine-resistant schizophrenia (Braga, John et al. 2019) or as acute augmentation of clozapine treatment (Wang, Zheng et al. 2018). However, the one sham-controlled trial of ECT added to clozapine because of treatment-resistance found no efficacy (Melzer-Ribeiro, Rigonatti et al. 2017).

Clinical Use of Antipsychotics in Other Psychiatric Disorders

SGAs have been studied for use in nonpsychotic disorders and some have FDA indications for use in these disorders. However, given issues related to the long-term risks associated with antipsychotics, in particular the risk of TD which is greater in patients with mood disorders (Solmi, Pigato et al. 2018), it is important to consider less problematic alternatives prior to considering the use of antipsychotics in most nonpsychotic disorders. The 2.6% yearly incidence of TD with SGAs (Carbon, Kane et al. 2018), is likely to be higher in individuals with mood disorders (and particularly higher if these patients are also elderly), suggesting that these patients should be monitored even more closely for TD than patients who are taking these medications for schizophrenia.

Depending on the diagnosis, therefore, they should generally be considered for short-term use only in nonpsychotic patients and should be tapered off when no longer needed. Still, they do have an important role in the treatment of bipolar disorder that is discussed later and in the chapter on mood stabilizers.

Anxiety

SGAs, particularly quetiapine as previously noted, may help with symptomatic relief of anxiety symptoms and have been studied for generalized anxiety disorder (Bandelow, Chouinard et al. 2010; Depping, Komossa et al. 2010; Katzman, Brawman-Mintzer et al. 2011; Khan, Joyce et al. 2011). Risperidone and aripiprazole may also add some benefit as augmentation treatments (i.e., added to a selective serotonin reuptake inhibitor) for the treatment of refractory obsessive-compulsive disorder (Veale, Miles et al. 2014). None of the SGAs however have been approved by the FDA for obsessive-compulsive disorder or anxiety-related disorders due to their more severe side effects compared to other effective agents.

Unipolar Depression

Several SGAs have been studied for augmentation of antidepressants in treatment-resistant unipolar depression (Spielmans, Berman et al. 2013). Aripiprazole at lower than usual doses (average 10 mg per day) may be efficacious when added to an antidepressant and tolerable in the short run (Berman, Marcus et al. 2007; Khan 2008; Marcus, McQuade et al. 2008; Nelson, Thase et al. 2012). Brexpiprazole, olanzapine, quetiapine (extended release), and risperidone may also reduce depressive symptoms when added to an antidepressant (Spielmans, Berman et al. 2013; Yoon, Jeon et al. 2017). In general, about nine patients must be treated with SGA augmentation before one patient's improvement is noted that would not have occurred on placebo. However, the risk of serious side effects (e.g., weight gain) is much higher than placebo. Older augmentation strategies such as the addition of a second antidepressant such as bupropion, buspirone, or thyroid hormone to a partially effective antidepressant should be considered prior to considering SGA augmentation—intense marketing associated with the SGAs notwithstanding. Switching to a different antidepressant (bupropion) is nearly as effective and produces fewer side effects than augmenting with aripiprazole according to a recent large (1,500 subject) study in veterans (Mohamed, Johnson et al. 2017).

Bipolar Disorder

Antipsychotics are frequently used in the treatment of patients with bipolar disorder. Traditionally, FGAs have been used for their sedative effects on acutely agitated manic patients, but they are no longer in favor because, compared to SGAs, they produce higher rates of patients switching to depression after resolution of the mania (Mohammad and Osser 2014). SGAs are effective, and most are FDA-approved for the acute treatment of mania (Perlis, Welge et al. 2006; Cipriani, Barbui et al. 2011). They are also frequently used in conjunction with other mood stabilizers such as lithium, carbamazepine, or valproate. It usually takes three to four weeks for improvement and more time for remission in mania.

Of note, however, in the depressive phase of bipolar disorder, not all SGAs are equally efficacious. Quetiapine is well-established as effective in bipolar depression and may be considered as one of the first-line treatments for this condition (Ansari and Osser 2010). Olanzapine (only in combination with fluoxetine) has also been found to have efficacy in treating bipolar depression. However, poorer longer-term tolerability of the olanzapine component limits its use. Lurasidone is also efficacious and is approved for acute bipolar depression (Loebel, Cucchiaro et al. 2014; Fornaro, De Berardis et al. 2017), although it has not yet been studied for mania. In 2019 cariprazine received FDA approval for the treatment of acute bipolar depression with three out of four studies showing a positive response (Durgam, Earley et al. 2016; Earley, Burgess et al. 2019). It joins quetiapine as one of only two SGAs that are approved for both acute bipolar depression and acute mania.

No FGAs or SGAs are FDA-approved for maintenance treatment of bipolar disorder as monotherapies, but several SGAs are approved for adjunctive use with lithium or valproate for acute and maintenance treatment. Such combinations should be limited to situations where monotherapy has failed to avoid generating unnecessary side effects.

In summary, antipsychotics are frequently considered and used in a wide variety of mood and anxiety disorders either as augmentations when antidepressants produce unsatisfactory results or as primary treatments for bipolar disorders. Still, data indicating that

SGAs and FGAs are associated with double to triple the rate of sudden cardiac death (presumably from electrophysiological effects related to QT prolongation) suggest that these agents should not be first-line ongoing treatments in many of these clinical situations (Ray, Chung et al. 2009). However, antipsychotics are powerful and important options in the treatment of schizophrenia and severe bipolar disorders, and these cardiac concerns should not deter clinicians for prescribing them appropriately for patients with these disorders.

Eating Disorders

In general, antipsychotics do not have a role to play in the treatment of eating disorders. However, olanzapine has been found to have modest beneficial effects on weight for patients with anorexia nervosa (Attia, Kaplan et al. 2011; Attia, Steinglass et al. 2019). The effect is usually on weight only, about one pound a month more than placebo, and other psychological symptoms are often unchanged. Given the cardiac and glucose dysregulation effects of this medication, olanzapine may be best reserved for patients who are not responding to other interventions.

Personality Disorders

Although nonpharmacological therapies should remain the mainstay of treatment for patients with personality disorders, antipsychotics are sometimes considered when severe stress-related symptoms, such as acute increases in transient perceptual distortions, impulsivity, anger, and affective dysregulation, put the overwhelmed patient at risk of self-injury or other harm. Published reviews suggest that antipsychotics may be helpful for these symptoms (Mercer, Douglass & Links 2009; Ingenhoven, Lafay et al. 2010; Lieb, Vollm et al. 2010). Antipsychotics, if considered for reducing potentially dangerous personality-driven behaviors, should be used cautiously and at low doses to minimize risks.

Clinical Use of Antipsychotics in Nonpsychiatric Disorders

Antipsychotics can decrease nausea and vomiting by D2 antagonism at the chemorecepter trigger zone in the brain. Chlorpromazine and perphenazine are FDA-approved for this indication, and prochlorperazine (structurally similar to chlorpromazine but not used as antipsychotic) has historically been used for the same symptoms (e.g., for nausea associated with migraines). Among the SGAs, olanzapine has been the most widely studied in this regard and found to have some utility in preventing chemotherapy-induced nausea (Yang, Liu et al. 2017; Yoodee, Permsuwan & Nimworapan 2017). Antipsychotics, however, should not be used as first-line treatments for nausea.

Chlorpromazine is also FDA-approved for the treatment of hiccups. Other psychotropics including haloperidol have also been studied for intractable hiccups, but no clear recommendations can be made about their use (Polito & Fellow 2017).

Finally, several antipsychotics, namely pimozide, haloperidol, and aripiprazole, have FDA approval for the control of tics associated with Tourette syndrome. The adverse side effect profiles of antipsychotics, however, may argue for the use of alternative non-antipsychotic therapies for this disorder (Quezada and Coffman 2018).

Use in Women of Childbearing Potential, Pregnancy, and Breastfeeding

Pregnancy

The risks of harm to the mother and fetus are significant if maternal schizophrenia is untreated (Robinson 2012). Most pregnant patients are therefore continued on their daily antipsychotic regimen. Although it is reassuring that observational studies have found that the risk of major malformations with antipsychotics appears to be generally low, the result are not conclusive, and care should be customized to the needs of the individual mother (McKenna, Koren et al. 2005; Einarson and Boskovic 2009; Habermann, Fritzsche et al. 2013). More recent studies and reviews support the relative safety of antipsychotics during pregnancy, but one notes that even though the overall risk of malformations does not appear to be "meaningfully" increased with antipsychotic use, risperidone use may be associated with a small increase in the risk of overall (including cardiac) malformations, indicating the need for further studies for this antipsychotic (Huybrechts, Hernandez-Diaz et al. 2016; Ornoy, Weinstein-Fudim & Ergaz 2017). Another recent study supported the finding that for quetiapine, the risk of major fetal malformations is not increased over the baseline rate (Cohen, Goez-Mogollon et al. 2018).

There are data to suggest that quetiapine and olanzapine during the first 20 weeks of pregnancy may increase the risk of maternal gestational diabetes (Park, Hernandez-Diaz et al. 2018). A more recent review of 10 relevant studies, however, did not confirm these findings (Uguz 2019).

Poor neonatal adaptation may be seen with maternal antipsychotic use (Kulkarni, Storch et al. 2015; Ornoy, Weinstein-Fudim et al. 2017). The FDA warns that there is a potential risk of EPS in newborns if antipsychotics are taken during the third trimester, but it does not advise that all pregnant patients should discontinue their antipsychotic (FDA 2011b). EPS in newborns may manifest as changes in muscle tone, sleep, feeding and breathing, which may last for hours or days or longer.

Although short-term developmental (i.e., motor and speech acquisition) delays have been observed from intrauterine exposure to antipsychotics, it is difficult to draw any definitive conclusions regarding the risk of developing adverse long-term neurodevelopmental effects from such exposure (Gentile and Fusco 2017; Ornoy, Weinstein-Fudim et al. 2017).

Breastfeeding

Breastfeeding is generally supported to help establish and maintain the mother–child relationship. In patients with schizophrenia, the antipsychotic found effective and used during pregnancy is often continued after delivery, but this needs to be balanced against what is safe for the feeding infant.

For olanzapine, risperidone, and quetiapine, the amounts of drug transferred to the infant through breast milk appear to be low, and their use does not appear to be associated with major adverse effects for the infant (Uguz 2016). Based on available data, olanzapine followed by quetiapine may be favored during breastfeeding (Uguz 2016; Kronenfeld, Berlin et al. 2017). Among the FGAs, haloperidol (up to 10 mg/day) and perphenazine (up to 24 mg/day) may be favored during breastfeeding (Kronenfeld, Berlin et al. 2017). As with the administration of other sedating medications, the infant should be monitored for sedation and other adverse effects by the pediatrician (Payne 2017). There are insufficient data to support the use of other antipsychotics during breastfeeding.

Table of Antipsychotics

Table 3.1 summarizes the characteristics of commonly discussed antipsychotics (Ansari and Osser 2015; World Health Organization 2019; Lexicomp 2019; PDR 2019).

TABLE 3.1 Antipsychotics

Medication[a]	Adult Dosing[b]	Comments/FDA Indication
Chlorpromazine (FGA) (Thorazine®)	For oral: Start: 25–50 mg po qhs then increase as tolerated to 300 mg po qhs or in divided doses. Potency: 100 mg po equals haloperidol 2 mg po. Use with caution in patients with renal or hepatic impairments.	Tricyclic structure, therefore with TCA side effects, plus EPS; now rarely used as primary antipsychotic; avoid IM given risk of severe orthostasis. CYP2D6 substrate. On WHO Essential Medicines List for psychotic disorders. Black Box Warning: Stroke, death in elderly with dementia-related psychosis *Psychotic disorders/Bipolar Mania/ Nausea and vomiting/Hiccups/Other indications (see package insert)*
Thioridazine (FGA) (Mellaril®)	Start: 25 mg po q day/bid/ tid, increase the same as chlorpromazine. Potency: 80–100 mg po equals haloperidol 2 mg po. Contraindicated in patients with significant hepatic impairment	Was once the most frequently prescribed antipsychotic; now should avoid use due to the highest risk of QTc prolongation of all FGAs and SGAs; doses over 800 mg/day may cause pigmentary retinopathy; CYP2D6 substrate, avoid combining with CYP2D6 inhibitors, SSRIs, or propranolol. Black Box Warning: QT prolongation. Stroke, death in elderly with dementia-related psychosis. *Schizophrenia in patients not responsive to or intolerant to other antipsychotics*
Perphenazine (FGA) (Trilafon®)	Start: 4 mg po bid then increase by 4–8 mg every 2 days; 20–24 mg/day in divided doses may be sufficient, 40 mg/day in treatment resistant patients, maximum dose 64 mg/day. Potency: 8–10 mg po equals haloperidol 2mg po. Contraindicated in patients with significant hepatic impairment; use with caution in patients with renal impairment	Effective in recent studies in comparison with SGAs; good choice as a first-line FGA if an FGA is considered. CYP2D6 substrate. Black Box Warning: Stroke, death in elderly with dementia-related psychosis *Schizophrenia/Nausea, vomiting*

TABLE 3.1 Continued

Medication[a]	Adult Dosing[b]	Comments/FDA *Indication*
Pimozide (FGA) (Orap®)	Start: 0.5 mg po q day, increase very gradually if needed and maintain low doses (less than stated maximum of 10 mg/day). CYP2D6 genotyping is needed for doses 4 mg/day or higher. Potency: 1 mg po equals haloperidol 2 mg po. Use with caution in patients with renal or hepatic impairments.	Avoid use; historically used for delusional parasitosis but no reason to believe it is better for this than other antipsychotics; high risk of QT prolongation; CYP3A4, CYP1A2, CYP2D6 substrate. Black Box Warning: Stroke, death in elderly with dementia-related psychosis *Suppression of refractory tics secondary to Tourette's Syndrome who failed to respond to standard therapy*
Fluphenazine (FGA) (Prolixin®)	For oral: Start: 0.5–2 mg po bid and increase as tolerated and necessary, usual daily dose is 5–10 mg/day. PO max is 40 mg/day IM max is 20 mg/day Oral dose is equipotent with haloperidol Contraindicated in patients with hepatic impairment; use with caution in patients with renal impairment.	Available in short-acting IM for behavioral control and long-acting injectable depot preparation for maintenance treatment of poorly adherent patients given every 2 weeks (see package insert); CYP2D6 substrate. On WHO Essential Medicines List for psychotic disorders. Black Box Warning: Stroke, death in elderly with dementia-related psychosis *Psychosis*
Haloperidol (FGA) (Haldol®)	For oral: Start: 0.5–2 mg po q day or bid and increase as tolerated and necessary, lower doses for elderly delirious patients and higher doses in patients with schizophrenia, 4–10 mg/day may be sufficient in schizophrenia Use with caution in patients with hepatic impairment. Reduce dose or avoid if with significant hepatic impairment.	Most widely used FGA; also used for secondary symptoms of delirium and behavioral control; available in short-acting IM form for behavioral control and long-acting injectable depot form for maintenance treatment given every 4 weeks (see package insert); CYP2D6, CYP3A4 substrate. On WHO Essential Medicines List for psychotic disorders. Black Box Warning: Stroke, death in elderly with dementia-related psychosis *Schizophrenia/control of tics in Tourette disorder/other indications (see package insert)*

(continued)

TABLE 3.1 Continued

Medication[a]	Adult Dosing[b]	Comments/*FDA Indication*
Risperidone (SGA) (Risperdal®, Risperdal M-Tab®, Risperdal Consta®, Perseris®)	For oral: Start: 0.5–1 mg po bid and increase gradually every 1–2 days to target of 4 mg/day, if no response in 1–2 weeks then increase to 6 mg/day. May lose "atypicality" at higher doses. Unlikely to be used ever at package insert max of 16 mg/day.

Reduce doses in patients with renal or hepatic impairments. | Fairly well-tolerated SGA, usually no significant EPS under 4 mg/day, and medium to low risk of metabolic changes in adults; orthostasis may be a problem initially; hyperprolactinemia is common; may have more rapid action than other SGAs; available in long-acting injectable depot form for maintenance treatment given every 2–4 weeks (see package insert); CYP2D6, CYP3A4 substrate. On WHO Essential Medicines List for psychotic disorders.

Black Box Warning:

Stroke, death in elderly with dementia-related psychosis *Schizophrenia/Psychotic disorders/ Acute mania or mixed episodes/ Adjunctive therapy with lithium or valproate for Bipolar I maintenance (for long-acting IM)/Irritability associated with autistic disorder/ (also see package insert)* |

TABLE 3.1 Continued

Medication[a]	Adult Dosing[b]	Comments/FDA Indication
Olanzapine (SGA) (Zyprexa®, Zydis®, Zyprexa IntraMuscular®, Zyprexa Relprevv®, Symbyax®— olanzapine, fluoxetine combination)	For oral: Start: 5–10 mg daily with initial target dose of 10 mg before further increases. Some clinicians use 15 mg/day for rapid effect in male smokers for schizophrenia; 10 mg in women smokers; 5 mg in non-smoking women. May increase by 5 mg/day at 1 week intervals (although rate of increase may depend on patient acuity) until 10–20 mg/day, the upper end may benefit more severely ill patients; (package insert max is 20 mg/day for oral, and 30 mg/day for short-acting injectable; otherwise see package insert for short-acting intramuscular use). Use cautiously in patients with hepatic impairment. Reduced olanzapine doses needed in patients with hepatic impairment if combined with fluoxetine.	Along with clozapine the highest risk of weight gain and metabolic syndrome among SGAs. Hypotension or respiratory depression may occur at higher doses or in combination with benzodiazepines. May cause transaminitis and liver injury. CYP1A2, CYP2D6 substrate. For long acting injection steady state is achieved after 3 months; "post-injection delirium/sedation syndrome" may occur within 5 hours of injection from inadvertent IV administration. See package insert for long-acting injectable. Black Box Warning: CNS depression, sedation increased if co-administered with other CNS depressants, and also due to post-injection delirium/sedation syndrome from long-acting injectable. Stroke, death in elderly with dementia-related psychosis. Suicidality (if in combination with fluoxetine). *Schizophrenia/Acute treatment of mania or mixed episodes/Bipolar Maintenance/ As adjunct to lithium or valproate for treatment of manic or mixed episodes/ For acute agitation associated with schizophrenia or mania/In combination with fluoxetine for treatment-resistant depression or bipolar depression*

(continued)

TABLE 3.1 Continued

Medication[a]	Adult Dosing[b]	Comments/FDA Indication
Quetiapine (SGA) (Seroquel®, Seroquel XR®)	For non-XR: Start: 25–50 mg po bid and double daily until 100 mg bid then increase by 200 mg/day as tolerated depending on sedation and orthostasis to 600–800 mg/day in schizophrenia or mania. Usual dose for acute bipolar depression is 300 mg per day. XR is once-daily version: As adjunct to antidepressant: 50 mg nightly for 2 days and then 150 mg nightly, may increase to 300 mg nightly. For severely manic patients some clinicians have used 200 mg po qhs on day one, 400 mg po qhs on day 2, 600 mg po qhs on day 3, but hypotension may be a limiting factor. Max dose is 800 mg/day. Reduce doses in patients with hepatic impairment.	Efficacious in bipolar depression; used frequently off-label as anti-anxiety agent in substance use disorders, and in those who are personality disordered; CYP3A4 substrate. Black Box Warning: Suicidality. Stroke, death in elderly with dementia-related psychosis. *Schizophrenia/Acute mania, alone or as adjunct to lithium or valproate/ Bipolar I/II depression/Maintenance treatment of bipolar I disorder as adjunct to lithium or divalproex/ For treatment-resistant depression as adjunct to an antidepressant (for XR formulation)*
Ziprasidone (SGA) (Geodon®, Geodon for Injection®)	For oral: Start: 20 mg po bid and increase dose incrementally every 2 days to 80 mg po bid (need to take with 500 kcal of food for adequate absorption—see text). May start with 40 mg po bid for acute mania. Max is 80 mg bid which is also the best dose for schizophrenia. Use with caution in patients with hepatic impairment. Use IM formulation with caution in patients with renal impairment.	SGA with low risk of weight gain and metabolic side effects; SGA with highest risk of QT prolongation; available in short-acting IM form for behavioral control (see package insert); CYP3A4, CYP1A2 substrate. Black Box Warning: Stroke, death in elderly with dementia-related psychosis. *Schizophrenia/Acute mania or mixed episodes/As an adjunct to lithium or valproate for maintenance for bipolar I/Acute agitation in schizophrenia*

TABLE 3.1 Continued

Medication[a]	Adult Dosing[b]	Comments/FDA Indication
Aripiprazole (SGA) (Abilify®, Abilify Discmelt®, Abilify Maintena®, Abilify Mycite®, Aristada®,)	For oral: in schizophrenia and mania, start and stay at 10–15 mg po q am as tolerated, maximum is 30 mg/day, but 15 mg/day may be more effective in acute schizophrenia; in mania 15 mg and 30 mg appear equally effective. For oral: as adjunct for major depression: start 2–5 mg per day, may adjust at 5 mg intervals each week as needed to 15 mg daily.	SGA with low risk of cardiac and metabolic effects; however, akathisia is common; very long half-life; See package inserts for long-acting injectable forms. CYP2D6 and CYP3A4 substrate. Black Box Warning: Suicidality, stroke, death in elderly with dementia-related psychosis. *Schizophrenia/Acute treatment of mixed/manic episodes/ Maintenance treatment as monotherapy or adjunct to lithium or valproate for Bipolar I/ Adjunctive therapy to antidepressants for acute treatment of MDD/Irritability associated with autistic disorder in ages 6–17. Tourette disorder*
Clozapine (SGA) (Clozaril®, FazaClo®, Versacloz®)	Start: 12.5 mg po once or twice daily then increase by 25 mg/day in divided doses as tolerated to 200–400 mg/day and check for response (check serum level if no response—therapeutic serum level of clozapine is over 350 ng/mL, some studies suggest over 450 ng/mL). Package insert max is 900 mg/day, but lower doses are used based on serum level and response/tolerability. Need to restart at 12.5 mg for the first dose if discontinued 48 hours or more. Dose reductions may be needed in patients with hepatic or renal impairment. Stop treatment if patient develops significant transaminitis during treatment.	Risk of agranulocytosis; need CBC/WBC/ANC count and ECG before treatment. Need ongoing ANC monitoring—see package insert for periodically updated monitoring algorithms; multiple other risks. Along with lithium may be one of only two drugs with antisuicidal effects; use caution when using with benzodiazepines—rare reports of respiratory depression and death; do not combine with carbamazepine; CYP1A2, CYP2D6, CYP3A4 substrate. On WHO Essential Medicines List for psychotic disorders. Black Box Warnings: Agranulocytosis (neutropenia), Risk Evaluation Mitigation Strategy (REMS), hypotension, bradycardia, syncope, QT prolongation, cardiomyopathy/myocarditis, seizures, stroke, death in elderly with dementia-related psychosis. *Treatment resistant severe schizophrenia/Reduction of recurrent suicidal behavior in chronically at risk patients with schizophrenia or schizoaffective disorder* (do not have to be treatment resistant for this latter indication)

(continued)

TABLE 3.1 Continued

Medication[a]	Adult Dosing[b]	Comments/*FDA Indication*
NEWER SECOND-GENERATION ANTIPSYCHOTICS:		
Paliperidone (SGA) (Invega®) (Invega Sustenna®) (Invega Trinza®)	For oral: Start: 6 mg po daily, increase by 3 mg/day every 4 days if needed. Many patients will require up to 12 mg po daily; max is 12 mg/day. Reduce doses in mild to moderate renal impairment; do not use in severe renal impairment.	Major metabolite of risperidone. Available only in extended release capsules; gradual release may have less effect on acute agitation and anxiety; significant risk of EPS with upper end of dosing, higher QT prolongation than risperidone. Favored for long-acting IM over risperidone LAI because it can be front-loaded (see package insert), starting with 2 IM injections one week apart then every 4 weeks. Also available in q 3 month injections. Minimal metabolism by CYP3A4 and CYP2D6 enzymes and primarily excreted by kidneys, therefore has decreased hepatic mediated drug-drug interactions. Black Box Warnings: Stroke, death in elderly with dementia-related psychosis. *Schizophrenia/schizoaffective disorder*
Iloperidone (SGA) (Fanapt®)	Start: 1 mg po bid, increase by 1–2 mg per day increments, target dose is 6–12 mg bid; max is 12 mg bid. Titrate slowly over first 7 days to avoid postural hypotension. Doses may need to be reduced in patients with moderate hepatic impairment; avoid if severe hepatic impairment.	Moderate weight gain, otherwise low metabolic risks, low risks of EPS or akathisia; but with risk of QT prolongation. CYP3A4 and CYP2D6 substrate Black Box Warnings: Stroke, death in elderly with dementia-related psychosis. *Schizophrenia*

TABLE 3.1 Continued

Medication[a]	Adult Dosing[b]	Comments/FDA *Indication*
Asenapine (SGA) (Saphris®) (Secuado®-- transdermal patch)	Start (for oral): 5 mg SL bid for schizophrenia, increase to 10 mg bid if needed after one week; start 5–10 mg bid for mania. Max is 10 mg bid. Sublingual only, not to eat or drink for 10 minutes after each dose. If swallowed only 5% bioavailability because of liver metabolism to inactive compounds. Associated with oral numbing. Contraindicated in patients with severe hepatic impairment.	Low metabolic risks, mild EPS. Risk of dose-dependent akathisia. FDA warning about severe allergic reactions even after first dose. Extensively metabolized by liver. CYP1A2, CYP3A4, and CYP2D6 substrate. Black Box Warnings: Stroke, death in elderly with dementia-related psychosis. *Schizophrenia/Bipolar I disorder, acute mixed or manic episode, monotherapy or as adjunct to lithium or valproate.*
Lurasidone (SGA) (Latuda ®)	Start: 40 mg po daily, usual maximum of 80 mg daily for schizophrenia. Should be taken with (350 calories) food. Although package insert max is 160 mg/day, doses higher than 60–80 mg/day may show no added benefit. For bipolar depression optimal dose may be 60 mg daily after titration. Dose reductions are needed in patients with moderate to severe hepatic impairment and renal impairment.	Low metabolic risk, low QT prolongation risk. Risk of dose-dependent akathisia. CYP3A4 substrate: contraindicated in patients taking strong inhibitors (e.g., ketoconazole, large amount of grapefruit juice), or inducers of this enzyme. Black Box Warnings: Suicidality, stroke, death in elderly with dementia-related psychosis. *Schizophrenia/Bipolar I depression, monotherapy or as adjunct to lithium or valproate*
NEWEST SECOND-GENERATION ANTIPSYCHOTICS:		
Brexpiprazole (SGA) (Rexulti®)	For schizophrenia: Start: 1 mg daily for 4 days, increase by 1 mg per day every 4 days as needed and tolerated, to max of 4 mg per day. For adjunct to antidepressant: Start 0.5–1 mg daily, increase by 0.5–1 mg/day every week as needed, to max of 3 mg per day. Reduced doses are needed in patients with moderate to severe hepatic impairment or renal impairment.	Very new antipsychotic very similar to aripiprazole in clinical effects. Not clear if any benefit over already existing treatments. Akathisia, increased triglycerides and weight gain may occur. CYP3A4 and CYP2D6 substrate. Black Box Warnings: Suicidality, stroke, death in elderly with dementia-related psychosis. *Schizophrenia/Adjunctive treatment of major depression*

(continued)

TABLE 3.1 Continued

Medication[a]	Adult Dosing[b]	Comments/FDA Indication
Cariprazine (SGA) (Vraylar®)	Start: For schizophrenia or mania, 1.5 mg on first day, 3 mg on second day, may increase by 1.5–3 mg, if needed or tolerated, with max of 6 mg/day. For bipolar depression, begin with 1.5 mg and if no response after two weeks may increase to 3 mg though results were better overall at 1.5 mg. Do not use in severe hepatic or renal impairment.	Very new antipsychotic. Not clear if any benefit over already existing treatments for schizophrenia. Long half-life. EPS, akathisia may occur. CYP2D6 and CYP3A4 substrate. (Dose should be halved in those taking a strong CYP3A4 inhibitor). Black Box Warnings: Suicidality, stroke, death in elderly with dementia-related psychosis. *Schizophrenia/Acute mania or mixed episode/ Depression associated with bipolar I disorder*
EMERGING ANTIPSYCHOTIC:		
Pimavanserin (for use in Parkinson Disease only) (Nuplazid®)	May start at 10 mg po daily, although package insert recommends starting at 34 mg po daily and continuing at this dose (which is also max dose). 10 mg/day dose if patient is taking a strong CYP3A4 inhibitor. Use with caution in patients with renal impairment	No data yet to support its use in other psychotic disorders or schizophrenia. May prolong QT. CYP3A4 (primary) and CYP3A5 substrate. Black Box Warnings: Stroke, death in elderly with dementia-related psychosis. *Treatment of hallucinations and delusions associated with Parkinson disease*

SEE PACKAGE INSERT FOR DOSING AND OTHER INFORMATION BEFORE PRESCRIBING MEDICATIONS. Dosing should be adjusted downward, ("start low, go slow" strategy) for the elderly and/or the medically compromised. Abbreviations: ANC, absolute neutrophil count; bid (bis in die), twice a day; CBC, complete blood count; CYP, cytochrome P450 enzyme; ECG, electrocardiogram; EPS, extrapyramidal symptoms; FGA, first-generation antipsychotics; IM, intramuscular; MDD, major depressive disorder; mg, milligram; ng/mL, nanogram per milliliter; po (per os), orally; q (quaque), every; qhs (quaque hora somni), at bedtime; SGA, second-generation antipsychotics; SL, sublingual; SSRI, selective serotonin reuptake inhibitor; TCA, tricyclic antidepressants; WBC, white blood cell; WHO, World Health Organization.

[a]Generic and U.S. brand name(s).

[b]Doses are provided for educational purposes only.

References

American Diabetes Association (2004). American Diabetes Association, American Psychiatric Association, American Association of Clinical Endocrinologists, North American Association for the Study of Obesity: consensus development conference on antipsychotic drugs and obesity and diabetes. J Clin Psychiatry 65: 267–272.

Ahmed U, Jones H, et al. (2010). Chlorpromazine for psychosis induced aggression or agitation. Cochrane Database Syst Rev 4: CD007445.

Alphs L, Benson C, et al. (2015). Real-world outcomes of paliperidone palmitate compared to daily oral antipsychotic therapy in schizophrenia: a randomized, open-label, review board-blinded 15-month study. J Clin Psychiatry 76(5): 554–561.

American Geriatrics Society (2019). American Geriatrics Society 2019 Updated AGS Beers Criteria® for potentially inappropriate medication use in older adults. J Am Geriatr Soc 67(4): 674–694.

Ansari A, Osser DN (2010). The psychopharmacology algorithm project at the Harvard South Shore Program: an update on bipolar depression. Harv Rev Psychiatry 18(1): 36–55.

Ansari A, Osser DN (2015). *Psychopharmacology, A Concise Overview for Students and Clinicians, 2nd Edition*. North Charleston, SC: CreateSpace.

Ansari A, Osser DN, et al. (2009). Pharmacological approach to the psychiatric inpatient, in Ovsiew F, Munich RL Eds., *Principles of Inpatient Psychiatry*. Philadelphia, PA: Lippincott Williams & Wilkins. Pages: 43–69.

Attia E, Kaplan AS, et al. (2011). Olanzapine versus placebo for out-patients with anorexia nervosa. Psychol Med 41(10): 2177–2182.

Attia E, Steinglass JE, et al. (2019). Olanzapine versus placebo in adult outpatients with anorexia nervosa: a randomized clinical trial. Am J Psychiatry 176(6): 449–456.

Balanza Martinez V (2017). Nutritional supplements in psychotic disorders. Actas Esp Psiquiatr 45(Suppl): 16–25.

Ballard C, Banister C, et al. (2018). Evaluation of the safety, tolerability, and efficacy of pimavanserin versus placebo in patients with Alzheimer's disease psychosis: a phase 2, randomised, placebo-controlled, double-blind study. Lancet Neurol 17(3): 213–222.

Bandelow B, Chouinard G, et al. (2010). Extended-release quetiapine fumarate (quetiapine XR): a once-daily monotherapy effective in generalized anxiety disorder. Data from a randomized, double-blind, placebo- and active-controlled study. Int J Neuropsychopharmacol 13(3): 305–320.

Baptista T, Rangel N, et al. (2007). Metformin as an adjunctive treatment to control body weight and metabolic dysfunction during olanzapine administration: a multicentric, double-blind, placebo-controlled trial. Schizophr Res 93: 99–108.

Barber S, Olotu U, et al. (2017). Clozapine combined with different antipsychotic drugs for treatment-resistant schizophrenia. Cochrane Database Syst Rev 3: CD006324.

Berman RM, Marcus RN, et al. (2007). The efficacy and safety of aripiprazole as adjunctive therapy in major depressive disorder: a multicenter, randomized, double-blind, placebo-controlled study. J Clin Psychiatry 68(6): 843–853.

Bertilsson L (1995). Geographical/interracial differences in polymorphic drug oxidation. Current state of knowledge of cytochromes P450 (CYP) 2D6 and 2C19. Clin Pharmacokinetics 29: 192–209.

Bhattacharyya S, Wilson R, et al. (2018). Effect of cannabidiol on medial temporal, midbrain, and striatal dysfunction in people at clinical high risk of psychosis: a randomized clinical trial. JAMA Psychiatry 75(11): 1107–1117.

Bhidayasiri R, Fahn S, et al. (2013). Evidence-based guideline: treatment of tardive syndromes: report of the Guideline Development Subcommittee of the American Academy of Neurology. Neurology 81(5): 463–469.

Bhidayasiri R, Jitkritsadakul O, et al. (2018). Updating the recommendations for treatment of tardive syndromes: a systematic review of new evidence and practical treatment algorithm. J Neurol Sci 389: 67–75.

Bioque M, Bernardo N (2018). The current data on the 3-month paliperidone palmitate formulation for the treatment of schizophrenia. Expert Opin Pharmacother 19(14): 1623–1629.

Bradford LD (2002). CYP2D6 allele frequency in European Caucasians, Asians, Africans and their descendants. Pharmacogenomics 3(2): 229–243.

Braga RJ, John M, et al. (2019). Continuation electroconvulsive therapy for patients with clozapine-resistant schizophrenia: a pilot study. J ECT 35(3): 156–160.

Brunello N, Masotto C, et al. (1995). New insights into the biology of schizophrenia through the mechanism of action of clozapine. Neuropsychopharmacology 13(3): 177–213.

Buchanan RW, Kreyenbuhl J, et al. (2010). The 2009 schizophrenia PORT psychopharmacological treatment recommendations and summary statements. Schizophr Bull 36(1): 71–93.

Caemmerer J, Correll CU, et al. (2012). Acute and maintenance effects of non-pharmacologic interventions for antipsychotic associated weight gain and metabolic abnormalities: a meta-analytic comparison of randomized controlled trials. Schizophr Res 140(1–3): 159–168.

Carbon M, Kane JM, et al. (2018). Tardive dyskinesia risk with first- and second-generation antipsychotics in comparative randomized controlled trials: a meta-analysis. World Psychiatry 17(3): 330–340.

Cheung G, Stapelberg J (2011). Quetiapine for the treatment of behavioural and psychological symptoms of dementia (BPSD): a meta-analysis of randomised placebo-controlled trials. N Z Med J 124(1336): 39–50.

Chiu CC, Chen KP, et al. (2006). The early effect of olanzapine and risperidone on insulin secretion in atypical-naïve schizophrenic patients. J Clin Psychopharmacol 26: 504–507.

Chung AK, Chua SE (2011). Effects on prolongation of Bazett's corrected QT interval of seven second-generation antipsychotics in the treatment of schizophrenia: a meta-analysis. J Psychopharmacol 25(5): 646–666.

Cipriani A, Barbui C, et al. (2011). Comparative efficacy and acceptability of antimanic drugs in acute mania: a multiple-treatments meta-analysis. Lancet 378(9799): 1306–1315.

Citrome L (2010). Iloperidone: chemistry, pharmacodynamics, pharmacokinetics and metabolism, clinical efficacy, safety and tolerability, regulatory affairs, and an opinion. Expert Opin Drug Metab Toxicol 6(12): 1551–1564.

Citrome L (2013). Cariprazine: chemistry, pharmacodynamics, pharmacokinetics, and metabolism, clinical efficacy, safety, and tolerability. Expert Opin Drug Metab Toxicol 9(2): 193–206.

Citrome L (2018). Sustained-release risperidone via subcutaneous injection: a systematic review of RBP-7000 (PERSERIS™) for the treatment of schizophrenia. Clin Schizophr Relat Psychoses 12(3): 130–141.

Citrome L, Stauffer VL, et al. (2009). Olanzapine plasma concentrations after treatment with 10, 20, and 40 mg/d in patients with schizophrenia: an analysis of correlations with efficacy, weight gain, and prolactin concentration. J Clin Psychopharmacol 29(3): 278–283.

Citrome L, Yang R, et al. (2009). Effect of ziprasidone dose on all-cause discontinuation rates in acute schizophrenia and schizoaffective disorder: a post-hoc analysis of 4 fixed-dose randomized clinical trials. Schizophr Res 111(1–3): 39–45.

Cohen LS, Goez-Mogollon L, et al. (2018). Risk of major malformations in infants following first-trimester exposure to quetiapine. Am J Psychiatry 175(12): 1225–1231.

Correll CU, Leucht S, et al. (2004). Lower risk of tardive dyskinesia associated with second-generation antipsychotics: a systematic review of 1-year studies. Am J Psychiatry 161: 414–425.

Correll CU, Manu P, et al. (2009). Cardiometabolic risk of second-generation antipsychotic medications during first-time use in children and adolescents. JAMA 302(16): 1765–1773.

Correll CU, Sikich L, et al. (2013). Metformin for antipsychotic-related weight gain and metabolic abnormalities: when, for whom, and for how long? Am J Psychiatry 170(9): 947–952.

Darba J, Minoves A, et al. (2011). Efficacy of second-generation-antipsychotics in the treatment of negative symptoms of schizophrenia: a meta-analysis of randomized clinical trials. Rev Psiquiatr Salud Ment 4(3): 126–143.

Davies SJ, Burhan AM, et al. (2018). Sequential drug treatment algorithm for agitation and aggression in Alzheimer's and mixed dementia. J Psychopharmacol 32(5): 509–523.

De Hert M, Sermon J, et al. (2015). The use of continuous treatment versus placebo or intermittent treatment strategies in stabilized patients with schizophrenia: a systematic review and meta-analysis of randomized controlled trials with first- and second-generation antipsychotics. CNS Drugs 29(8): 637–658.

Depping AM, Komossa K, et al. (2010). Second-generation antipsychotics for anxiety disorders. Cochrane Database Syst Rev 12: CD008120.

Di Forti M, Quattrone D, et al. (2019). The contribution of cannabis use to variation in the incidence of psychotic disorder across Europe (EU-GEI): a multicentre case-control study. Lancet Psychiatry 6(5): 427–436.

Durgam S, Earley W, et al. (2016). An 8-week randomized, double-blind, placebo-controlled evaluation of the safety and efficacy of cariprazine in patients with bipolar I depression. Am J Psychiatry 173(3): 271–281.

Earley W, Burgess MV, et al. (2019). Cariprazine treatment of bipolar depression: a randomized double-blind placebo-controlled phase 3 study. Am J Psychiatry 176(6): 439–448.

Einarson A, Boskovic R (2009). Use and safety of antipsychotic drugs during pregnancy. J Psychiatr Pract 15(3): 183–192.

El-Sayeh HG, Morganti C, et al. (2006). Aripiprazole for schizophrenia. Systematic review. Br J Psychiatry 189: 102–108.

Emsley R, Rabinowitz J, et al. (2006). Time course for antipsychotic treatment response in first-episode schizophrenia. Am J Psychiatry 163(4): 743–745.

Essock SM, Covell NH, et al. (2006). Effectiveness of switching antipsychotic medications. Am J Psychiatry 163: 2090–2095.

Farde L, Nordstrom AL, et al. (1992). Positron emission tomographic analysis of central D1 and D2 dopamine receptor occupancy in patients treated with classical neuroleptics and clozapine. Relation to extrapyramidal effects. Arch Gen Psychiatry 49: 538–544.

Fava M, Wisniewski SR, et al. (2009). Metabolic assessment of aripiprazole as adjunctive therapy in major depressive disorder: a pooled analysis of 2 studies. J Clin Psychopharmacol 29(4): 362–367.

Fayek M, Kingsbury SJ, et al. (2001). Cardiac effects of antipsychotic medications. Psychiatr Serv 52: 607–609.

Fernandez HH, Factor SA, et al. (2017). Randomized controlled trial of deutetrabenazine for tardive dyskinesia: the ARM-TD study. Neurology 88(21): 2003–2010.

Firth J, Stubbs B, et al. (2017). The effects of vitamin and mineral supplementation on symptoms of schizophrenia: a systematic review and meta-analysis. Psychol Med 47(9): 1515–1527.

Fond G, Berna F, et al. (2018). Benzodiazepine long-term administration is associated with impaired attention/working memory in schizophrenia: results from the national multicentre FACE-SZ data set. Eur Arch Psychiatry Clin Neurosci 268(1): 17–26.

Fontanella CA, Campo JV, et al. (2016). Benzodiazepine use and risk of mortality among patients with schizophrenia: a retrospective longitudinal study. J Clin Psychiatry 77(5): 661–667.

Food and Drug Administration (2011a). FDA Drug Safety Communication: serious allergic reactions reported with the use of Saphris (asenapine maleate). http://www.fda.gov/Drugs/DrugSafety/ucm270243.htm

Food and Drug Administration (2011b). FDA Drug Safety Communication: antipsychotic drug labels updated on use during pregnancy and risk of abnormal muscle movements and withdrawal symptoms in newborns. https://www.fda.gov/Drugs/DrugSafety/ucm243903.htm

Fornaro M, De Berardis D, et al. (2017). Lurasidone in the treatment of bipolar depression: systematic review of systematic reviews. Biomed Res Int 2017: 3084859.

Frankel JS, Schwartz TL (2017). Brexpiprazole and cariprazine: distinguishing two new atypical antipsychotics from the original dopamine stabilizer aripiprazole. Ther Adv Psychopharmacol 7(1): 29–41.

Freudenreich O, Henderson DC, et al. (2007). Risperidone augmentation for schizophrenia partially responsive to clozapine: a double-blind, placebo-controlled trial. Schizophr Res 92(1–3): 90–94.

Gentile S, Fusco ML (2017). Neurodevelopmental outcomes in infants exposed in utero to antipsychotics: a systematic review of published data. CNS Spectr 22(3): 273–281.

Gill SS, Rochon PA, et al. (2005). Atypical antipsychotic drugs and risk of ischemic stroke: population based retrospective cohort study. BMJ 330: 445.

Glassman AH, Bigger JT Jr. (2001). Antipsychotic drugs: prolonged QTc interval, torsade de pointes, and sudden death. Am J Psychiatry 158: 1774–1782.

Goff DC (2008). New insights into clinical response in schizophrenia: from dopamine D2 receptor occupancy to patients' quality of life. Am J Psychiatry 165: 940–943.

Grover S, Mattoo SK, et al. (2011). Usefulness of atypical antipsychotics and choline esterase inhibitors in delirium: a review. Pharmacopsychiatry 44(2): 43–54.

Grover S, Sahoo S, et al. (2019). ECT in schizophrenia: a review of the evidence. Acta Neuropsychiatr 31: 115–127.

Grunder G, Fellows C, et al. (2008). Brain and plasma pharmacokinetics of aripiprazole in patients with schizophrenia: an [18F]fallypride PET study. Am J Psychiatry 165: 988–995.

Habermann F, Fritzsche J, et al. (2013). Atypical antipsychotic drugs and pregnancy outcome: a prospective, cohort study. J Clin Psychopharmacol 33(4): 453–462.

Hahn B (2018). The potential of cannabidiol treatment for cannabis users with recent-onset psychosis. Schizophr Bull 44(1): 46–53.

Hahn MK, Wolever TM, et al. (2013). Acute effects of single-dose olanzapine on metabolic, endocrine, and inflammatory markers in healthy controls. J Clin Psychopharmacol 33(6): 740–746.

Hanley MJ, Kenna GA (2008). Quetiapine: treatment for substance abuse and drug of abuse. Am J Health-Syst Pharm 65: 611–618.

Harvey RC, James AC, Shields GE (2016). A systematic review and network meta-analysis to assess the relative efficacy of antipsychotics for the treatment of positive and negative symptoms in early-onset schizophrenia. CNS Drugs 30(1): 27–39.

Hauser RA, Factor SA, et al. (2017). KINECT 3: a phase 3 randomized, double-blind, placebo-controlled trial of valbenazine for tardive dyskinesia. Am J Psychiatry 174(5): 476–484.

Herrmann N, Lanctot KL (2005). Do atypical antipsychotics cause stroke? CNS Drugs 19: 91–103.

Honer WG, MacEwan GW, et al. (2012). A randomized, double-blind, placebo-controlled study of the safety and tolerability of high-dose quetiapine in patients with persistent symptoms of schizophrenia or schizoaffective disorder. J Clin Psychiatry 73(1): 13–20.

Honigfeld G, Arellano F, et al. (1998). Reducing clozapine-related morbidity and mortality: 5 years of experience with the Clozaril National Registry. J Clin Psychiatry 59(Suppl 3): 3–7.

Hu SC, Frucht SJ (2007). Emergency treatment of movement disorders. Curr Treat Opt Neurology 9: 103–114.

Hui CLM, Honer WG, et al. (2018). Long-term effects of discontinuation from antipychotic maintenance following first-episode schizophrenia and related disorders: a 10 year follow-up of a randomised, double-blind trial. Lancet Psychiatry 5(5): 432–442.

Huybrechts KF, Hernandez-Diaz S, et al. (2016). Antipsychotic use in pregnancy and the risk for congenital malformations. JAMA Psychiatry 73(9): 938–946.

Ingenhoven T, Lafay P, et al. (2010). Effectiveness of pharmacotherapy for severe personality disorders: meta-analyses of randomized controlled trials. J Clin Psychiatry 71(1): 14–25.

Ishibashi T, Horisawa T, et al. (2010). Pharmacological profile of lurasidone, a novel antipsychotic agent with potent 5-hydroxytryptamine 7 (5-HT7) and 5-HT1A receptor activity. J Pharmacol Exp Ther 334(1): 171–181.

Jager M, Riedel M, et al. (2010). Time course of antipsychotic treatment response in schizophrenia: results from a naturalistic study in 280 patients. Schizophr Res 118(1–3): 183–188.

Jethwa KD, Onalaja OA (2015). Antipsychotics for the management of psychosis in Parkinson's disease: systematic review and meta-analysis. BJPsych Open 1(1): 27–33.

Kane JM, Barnes TR, et al. (2010). Evaluation of akathisia in patients with schizophrenia, schizoaffective disorder, or bipolar I disorder: a post hoc analysis of pooled data from short- and long-term aripiprazole trials. J Psychopharmacol 24(7): 1019–1029.

Kane JM, Carson WH, et al. (2002). Efficacy and safety of aripiprazole and haloperidol versus placebo in patents with schizophrenia and schizoaffective disorder. J Clin Psychiatry 63: 763–771.

Kane JM, Meltzer HY, et al. (2007). Aripiprazole for treatment-resistant schizophrenia: results of a multicenter, randomized, double-blind, comparison study versus perphenazine. J Clin Psychiatry 68: 213–223.

Kane JM, Skuban A, et al. (2016). Overview of short- and long-term tolerability and safety of brexpiprazole in patients with schizophrenia. Schizophr Res 174(1–3): 93–98.

Kantrowitz JT, Citrome L (2012). Lurasidone for schizophrenia: what's different? Expert Rev Neurother 12(3): 265–273.

Karakula-Juchnowicz H, Dzikowski M, et al. (2016). The brain-gut axis dysfunctions and hypersensitivity to food antigens in the etiopathogenesis of schizophrenia. Psychiatr Pol 50(4): 747–760.

Katzman MA, Brawman-Mintzer O, et al. (2011). Extended release quetiapine fumarate (quetiapine XR) monotherapy as maintenance treatment for generalized anxiety disorder: a long-term, randomized, placebo-controlled trial. Int Clin Psychopharmacol 26(1): 11–24.

Keefe RS, Bilder RM, et al. (2007). Neurocognitive effects of antipsychotic medications in patients with chronic schizophrenia in the CATIE Trial. Arch Gen Psychiatry 64(6): 633–647.

Khan A (2008). Current evidence for aripiprazole as augmentation therapy in major depressive disorder. Expert Rev Neurother 8(10): 1435–1447.

Khan A, Joyce M, et al. (2011). A randomized, double-blind study of once-daily extended release quetiapine fumarate (quetiapine XR) monotherapy in patients with generalized anxiety disorder. J Clin Psychopharmacol 31(4): 418–428.

Kim S, Solari H, et al. (2012). Paliperidone palmitate injection for the acute and maintenance treatment of schizophrenia in adults. Patient Prefer Adherence 6: 533–545.

Kinon BJ, Volavka J, et al. (2008). Standard and higher dose of olanzapine in patients with schizophrenia or schizoaffective disorder: a randomized, double-blind, fixed-dose study. J Clin Psychopharmacol 28(4): 392–400.

Kitten AK, Hallowell SA, et al. (2018). Pimavanserin: a novel drug approved to treat Parkinson's disease psychosis. Innov Clin Neurosci 15(1–2): 16–22.

Klein L, Bangh S, Cole JB (2017). Intentional recreational abuse of quetiapine compared to other second-generation antipsychotics. West J Emerg Med 18(2): 243–250.

Komossa K, Rummel-Kluge C, et al. (2010). Olanzapine versus other atypical antipsychotics for schizophrenia. Cochrane Database Syst Rev 3: CD006654.

Komossa K, Rummel-Kluge C, et al. (2011). Risperidone versus other atypical antipsychotics for schizophrenia. Cochrane Database Syst Rev 1: CD006626.

Kontaxakis VP, Ferentinos PP, et al. (2006). Risperidone augmentation of clozapine: a critical review. Eur Arch Psychiatry Clin Neurosci 256(6): 350–355.

Kreyenbuhl J, Slade EP, et al. (2011). Time to discontinuation of first- and second-generation antipsychotic medications in the treatment of schizophrenia. Schizophr Res 131(1–3): 127–132.

Kronenfeld N, Berlin M, et al. (2017). Use of psychotropic medications in breastfeeding women. Birth Defects Res 109(12): 957–997.

Kulkarni J, Storch A, et al. (2015). Antipsychotic use in pregnancy. Expert Opin Pharmacother 16(9): 1335–1345.

Lamberti JS, Olson D, et al. (2006). Prevalence of the metabolic syndrome among patients receiving clozapine. Am J Psychiatry 163: 1273–1276.

Lee D, Baek JH, et al. (2019). Long-term response to clozapine and its clinical correlates in the treatment of tardive movement syndromes: a naturalistic observational study in patients with psychotic disorders. J Clin Psychopharmacol 39(6): 591–596.

Lehman H (1964). On acute schizophrenic patients, in Lehman H, Ban T, Eds., The Butyrophenones in Psychiatry. Montreal, QB: Psychopharmacological Research Association.

Leucht C, Heres S, et al. (2011). Oral versus depot antipsychotic drugs for schizophrenia—a critical systematic review and meta-analysis of randomised long-term trials. Schizophr Res 127(1–3): 83–92.

Leucht S, Busch R, et al. (2007). Early prediction of antipsychotic nonresponse among patients with schizophrenia. J Clin Psychiatry 68(3): 352–360.

Leucht S, Corves C, et al. (2009). Second-generation versus first-generation antipsychotic drugs for schizophrenia: a meta-analysis. Lancet 373: 31–41.

Leucht S, Komossa K, et al. (2009). A meta-analysis of head-to-head comparisons of second-generation antipsychotics in the treatment of schizophrenia. Am J Psychiatry 166(2): 152–163.

Leucht S, Tardy M, et al. (2012). Maintenance treatment with antipsychotic drugs for schizophrenia. Cochrane Database Syst Rev 5: CD008016.

Leung JG, Hasassri ME, et al. (2017). Characterization of admission types in medically hospitalized patients prescribed clozapine. Psychosomatics 58(2): 164–172.

Leweke FM, Mueller JK, et al. (2016). Therapeutic potential of cannabinoids in psychosis. Biol Psychiatry 79(7): 604–612.

Lewis SW, Barnes TR, et al. (2006). Randomized controlled trial of effect of prescription of clozapine versus other second-generation antipsychotic drugs in resistant schizophrenia. Schizophr Bull 32: 715–723.

Lexicomp (2019). https://www.wolterskluwercdi.com/lexicomp-online/

Lieb K, Vollm B, et al. (2010). Pharmacotherapy for borderline personality disorder: cochrane systematic review of randomised trials. Br J Psychiatry 196(1): 4–12.

Lieberman JA, Stroup TS (2011). The NIMH-CATIE Schizophrenia Study: what did we learn? Am J Psychiatry 168(8): 770–775.

Lieberman JA, Stroup TS, et al. (2005). Effectiveness of antipsychotic drugs in patients with chronic schizophrenia. N Engl J Med 353: 1209–1223.

Lin CH, Lin SC, et al. (2018). Early prediction of olanzapine-induced weight gain for schizophrenia patients. Psychiatry Res 263: 207–211.

Lindenmayer JP, Citrome L, et al. (2011). A randomized, double-blind, parallel-group, fixed-dose, clinical trial of quetiapine at 600 versus 1200 mg/d for patients with treatment-resistant schizophrenia or schizoaffective disorder. J Clin Psychopharmacol 31(2): 160–168.

Lipkovich I, Citrome L, et al. (2006). Early predictors of substantial weight gain in bipolar patients treated with olanzapine. J Clin Psychopharmacol 26: 316–320.

Loebel A, Cucchiaro J, et al. (2014). Lurasidone monotherapy in the treatment of bipolar I depression: a randomized, double-blind, placebo-controlled study. Am J Psychiatry 171(2): 160–168.

Lonergan E, Britton AM, et al. (2007). Antipsychotics for delirium. Cochrane Database Syst Rev 2: CD005594.

Maayan L, Vakhrusheva J, et al. (2010). Effectiveness of medications used to attenuate antipsychotic-related weight gain and metabolic abnormalities: a systematic review and meta-analysis. Neuropsychopharmacology 35(7): 1520–1530.

Mamo D, Graff A, et al. (2007). Differential effects of aripiprazole on D(2), 5-HT(2), and 5-HT(1A) receptor occupancy in patients with schizophrenia: a triple tracer PET study. Am J Psychiatry 164: 1411–1417.

Mantovani C, Labate CM, et al. (2013). Are low doses of antipsychotics effective in the management of psychomotor agitation? A randomized, rated-blind trial of 4 intramuscular interventions. J Clin Psychopharmacol 33(3): 306–312.

Marcus RN, McQuade RD, et al. (2008). The efficacy and safety of aripiprazole as adjunctive therapy in major depressive disorder: a second multicenter, randomized, double-blind, placebo-controlled study. J Clin Psychopharmacol 28(2): 156–165.

Marder SR, Sorsaburu S, et al. (2010). Case reports of postmarketing adverse event experiences with olanzapine intramuscular treatment in patients with agitation. J Clin Psychiatry 71(4): 433–441.

McCue RE, Waheed R, et al. (2006). Comparative effectiveness of second-generation antipsychotics and haloperidol in acute schizophrenia. Br J Psychiatry 189: 433–440.

McEvoy JP, Stiller RL, et al. (1986). Plasma haloperidol levels drawn at neuroleptic threshold doses: a pilot study. J Clin Psychopharmacol 6: 133–138.

McIntyre RS, Cha DS, et al. (2012). A review of published evidence reporting on the efficacy and pharmacology of lurasidone. Expert Opin Pharmacother 13(11): 1653–1659.

McKenna K, Koren G, et al. (2005). Pregnancy outcome of women using atypical antipsychotic drugs: a prospective comparative study. J Clin Psychiatry 66(4): 444–449; quiz 546.

Meltzer HY (2012). Clozapine: balancing safety with superior antipsychotic efficacy. Clin Schizophr Relat Psychoses 6(3): 134–144.

Meltzer HY, Alphs L, et. al. (2003). Clozapine treatment for suicidality in schizophrenia: International Suicide Prevention Trial (InterSePT). Arch Gen Psychiatry 60: 82–91.

Melzer-Ribeiro DL, Rigonatti SP, et al. (2017). Efficacy of electroconvulsive therapy augmentation for partial response to clozapine: a pilot randomized ECT–sham controlled trial. Arch Clin Psychiatry 44(2): 45–50.

Mercer D, Douglass AB, Links PS (2009). Meta-analyses of mood stabilizers, antidepressants and antipsychotics in the treatment of borderline personality disorder: effectiveness for depression and anger symptoms. J Pers Disord 23(2): 156–174.

Meyer JM, Simpson GM (1997). From chlorpromazine to olanzapine: a brief history of antipsychotics. Psychiatr Serv 48: 1137–1139.

Meyer JM, Stahl SM (2020). The Clozapine Handbook. Cambridge, England: Cambridge University Press.

Miceli JJ, Glue P, et al. (2007). The effect of food on the absorption of oral ziprasidone. Psychopharmacol Bull 40: 58–68.

Mohamed S, Johnson GR, et al. (2017). Effect of antidepressant switching vs augmentation on remission among patients with major depressive disorder unresponsive to antidepressant treatment: the VAST-D randomized clinical trial. JAMA 318(2): 132–145.

Mohammad OM, Osser DN (2014). The Psychopharmacology Algorithm Project at the Harvard South Shore Program: an algorithm for acute mania. Harv Rev Psychiatry 22(5): 274–294.

Morris MT, Tarpada SP (2017). Long-acting injectable paliperidone palmitate: a review of efficacy and safety. Psychopharmacol Bull 47(2): 42–52.

Nasrallah HA, Fedora R, Morton R (2019). Successful treatment of clozapine-nonresponsive refractory hallucinations and delusions with pimavanserin, a serotonin 5HT-2A receptor inverse agonist. Schizophr Res 208: 217–220.

Nelson JC, Thase ME, et al. (2012). Efficacy of adjunctive aripiprazole in patients with major depressive disorder who showed minimal response to initial antidepressant therapy. Int Clin Psychopharmacol 27(3): 125–133.

Nemani K, Hosseini Ghomi R, et al. (2015). Schizophrenia and the gut-brain axis. Prog Neuropsychopharmacol Biol Psychiatry 56: 155–160.

Nestler EJ, Hyman SE, et al. (2015). *Molecular Neuropharmacology: A Foundation for Clinical Neuroscience, 3rd Edition*. New York, NY: McGraw-Hill.

Nielsen J, Graff C, et al. (2011). Assessing QT interval prolongation and its associated risks with antipsychotics. CNS Drugs 25(6): 473–490.

Nussbaum AM, Stroup TS (2012). Paliperidone palmitate for schizophrenia. Cochrane Database Syst Rev 6: CD008296.

Nyberg S, Eriksson B, et al. (1999). Suggested minimal effective dose of risperidone based on PET-measured D2 and 5-HT2A receptor occupancy in schizophrenic patients. Am J Psychiatry 156: 869–875.

O'Brien A (2016). Comparing the risk of tardive dyskinesia in older adults with first-generation and second-generation antipsychotics: a systematic review and meta-analysis. Int J Geriatr Psychiatry 31(7): 683–693.

Oh ES, Fong TG, et al. (2017). Delirium in older persons: advances in diagnosis and treatment. JAMA 318(12): 1161–1174.

Olfson M, Marcus SC, et al. (2007). Treatment of schizophrenia with long-acting fluphenazine, haloperidol, or risperidone. Schizophr Bull 33: 1379–1387.

Ornoy A, Weinstein-Fudim L, Ergaz Z (2017). Antidepressants, antipsychotics, and mood stabilizers in pregnancy: what do we know and how should we treat pregnant women with depression. Birth Defects Res 109(12): 933–956.

Osser DN, Braun S, Fischer MA (2013). Management of the behavioral and psychological symptoms of dementia: review of current data and best practices for health care providers. Boston, MA: National Resource Center for Academic Detailing Monograph.

Osser DN, Najarian DM, Dufresne RL (1999). Olanzapine increases weight and serum triglyceride levels. J Clin Psychiatry 60: 767–770.

Osser DN, Roudsari MJ, et al. (2013). The psychopharmacology algorithm project at the Harvard South Shore Program: an update on schizophrenia. Harv Rev Psychiatry 21(1): 18–40.

Osser DN, Sigadel R (2001). Short-term inpatient pharmacotherapy of schizophrenia. Harv Rev Psychiatry 9(3): 89–104.

Ostacher M, Ng-Mak D, et al. (2018). Lurasidone compared to other atypical antipsychotic monotherapies for bipolar depression: a systematic review and network meta-analysis. World J Biol Psychiatry 19(8): 586–601.

Park Y, Hernandez-Diaz S, et al. (2018). Continuation of atypical antipsychotic medication during early pregnancy and the risk of gestational diabetes. Am J Psychiatry 175(6): 564–574.

Payne JL (2017). Psychopharmacology in pregnancy and breastfeeding. Psychiatr Clin North Am 40(2): 217–238.

PDR (2019). Prescriber's digital reference. http://www.pdr.net

Perlis RH, Welge JA, et al. (2006). Atypical antipsychotics in the treatment of mania: a meta-analysis of randomized, placebo-controlled trials. J Clin Psychiatry 67(4): 509–516.

Pi EH, Gray GE (2000). Ethnopsychopharmacology for Asians, in Ruiz P, Ed., *Ethnicity and Psychopharmacology* (Volume 19, Review of Psychiatry). Washington, DC: American Psychiatric Press, pp. 91–113.

Pigott TA, Carson WH, et al. (2003). Aripiprazole for the prevention of relapse in stabilized patients with chronic schizophrenia: a placebo-controlled 26-week study. J Clin Psychiatry 64: 1048–1056.

Pillinger T, Beck K, et al. (2017). Impaired glucose homeostasis in first-episode schizophrenia: a systematic review and meta-analysis. JAMA Psychiatry 74(3): 261–269.

Polito NB, Fellows SE (2017). Pharmacologic interventions for intractable and persistent hiccups: a systematic review. J Emerg Med 53(4): 540–549.

Potkin SG (2011). Asenapine: a clinical overview. J Clin Psychiatry 72(Suppl 1): 14–18.

Praharaj SK, Jana AK, et al. (2011). Metformin for olanzapine-induced weight gain: a systematic review and meta-analysis. Br J Clin Pharmacol 71(3): 377–382.

Quezada J, Coffman KA (2018). Current approaches and new developments in the pharmacological management of Tourette syndrome. CNS Drugs 32(1): 33–45.

Raja M (2007). Improvement or worsening of psychotic symptoms after treatment with low doses of aripiprazole. Int J Neuropsychopharmacol 10: 107–110.

Ray WA, Chung CP, et al. (2009). Atypical antipsychotic drugs and the risk of sudden cardiac death. N Engl J Med 360: 225–235.

Ray WA, Meredith S, et al. (2004). Cyclic antidepressants and the risk of sudden cardiac death. Clin Pharmacol Therap 75: 234–241.

Ray WA, Stein CM, et al. (2019). Association of antipsychotic treatment with risk of unexpected death among children and youths. JAMA Psychiatry 76(2): 162–171.

Risbood V, Lee JR, et al. (2012). Lurasidone: an atypical antipsychotic for schizophrenia. Ann Pharmacother 46(7–8): 1033–1046.

Robinson DG, Gallego JA, et al. (2015). A randomized comparison of aripiprazole and risperidone for the acute treatment of first-episode schizophrenia and related disorders: 3-month outcomes. Schizophr Bull 41(6): 1227–1236.

Robinson GE (2012). Treatment of schizophrenia in pregnancy and postpartum. J Popul Ther Clin Pharmacol 19(3): e380–e386.

Rochon PA, Normand SL, et al. (2008). Antipsychotic therapy and shortterm serious events in older adults with dementia. Arch Intern Med 168: 1090–1096.

Roffman JL, Petruzzi LJ, et al. (2018). Biochemical, physiological and clinical effects of l-methylfolate in schizophrenia: a randomized controlled trial. Mol Psychiatry 23(2): 316–322.

Sahli ZT, Tarazi FI (2018). Pimavanserin: novel pharmacotherapy for Parkinson's disease psychosis. Expert Opin Drug Discov 13(1): 103–110.

Satterthwaite TD, Wolf DH, et al. (2008). A meta-analysis of the risk of acute extrapyramidal symptoms with intramuscular antipsychotics for the treatment of agitation. J Clin Psychiatry 69: 1869–1879.

Schneider LS, Dagerman KS, et al. (2005). Risk of death with atypical antipsychotic drug treatment for dementia: meta-analysis of randomized placebo-controlled trials. JAMA 294: 1934–1943.

Schneider LS, Tariot PN, et al. (2006). Effectiveness of atypical antipsychotic drugs in patients with Alzheimer's disease. N Engl J Med 355: 1525–1538.

Schneeweiss S, Setoguchi S, et al. (2007). Risk of death associated with the use of conventional versus atypical antipsychotic drugs among elderly patients. Can Med Assoc J 176: 627–632.

Schoeler T, Petros N, et al. (2016). Effects of continuation, frequency, and type of cannabis use on relapse in the first 2 years after onset of psychosis: an observational study. Lancet Psychiatry 3(10): 947–953.

Seeman P (1992). Dopamine receptor sequences: therapeutic levels of neuroleptics occupy D2 receptors, clozapine occupies D4. Neuropsychopharmacology 7(4): 261–284.

Seeman P (2002). Atypical antipsychotics: mechanism of action. Can J Psychiatry 47(1): 27–38.

Shah RR (2005). Drug-induced QT dispersion: does it predict the risk of torsade de pointes? J Electrocardiol 38: 10–18.

Sicard MN, Zai CC, et al. (2010). Polymorphisms of the HTR2C gene and antipsychotic-induced weight gain: an update and meta-analysis. Pharmacogenomics 11(11): 1561–1571.

Sikich L, Frazier JA, et al. (2008). Double-blind comparison of first- and second-generation antipsychotics in early-onset schizophrenia and schizo-affective disorder: findings from the Treatment of Early-Onset Schizophrenia Spectrum Disorders (TEOSS) study. Am J Psychiatry 165: 1420–1431.

Sinclair DJ, Zhao S, et al. (2019). Electroconvulsive therapy for treatment-resistant schizophrenia. Cochrane Database Syst Rev 3: CD011847.

Slomski A (2019). Cannabidiol may help normalize brain function in psychosis. JAMA 321(4): 335.

Soares-Weiser K, Fernandez HH (2007). Tardive dyskinesia. Sem Neurol 27: 159–169.

Soares-Weiser K, Maayan N, et al. (2011). Vitamin E for neuroleptic-induced tardive dyskinesia. Cochrane Database Syst Rev 2: CD000209.

Solmi M, Pigato G, et al. (2018). Clinical risk factors for the development of tardive dyskinesia. J Neurol Sci 389: 21–27.

Spielmans GI, Berman MI, et al. (2013). Adjunctive atypical antipsychotic treatment for major depressive disorder: a meta-analysis of depression, quality of life, and safety outcomes. PLoS Med 10(3): e1001403.

Spina E, Scordo MG, et al. (2003). Metabolic drug interactions with new psychotropic agents. Fundam Clin Pharmacol 17: 517–538.

Stahl SM (2001). "Hit-and-run" actions at dopamine receptors, part 1: mechanism of action of atypical antipsychotics. J Clin Psychiatry 62(9): 670–671.

Stahl SM (2008). *Stahl's Essential Psychopharmacology: Neuroscientific Basis and Practical Applications*, 3rd Edition. New York, NY: Cambridge University Press.

Stoner SC, Pace HA (2012). Asenapine: a clinical review of a second-generation antipsychotic. Clin Ther 34(5): 1023–1040.

Straus SM, Bleumink GS, et al. (2004). Antipsychotics and the risk of sudden cardiac death. Arch Intern Med 164: 1293–1297.

Subeesh V, Maheswari E, et al. (2019). Novel adverse events of iloperidone: a disproportionality analysis in US Food and Drug Administration Adverse Event Reporting System (FAERS) database. Curr Drug Saf 14(1): 21–26.

Sultzer DL, Davis SM, et al. (2008). Clinical symptom responses to atypical antipsychotic medications in Alzheimer's disease: phase 1 outcomes from the CATIE-AD effectiveness trial. Am J Psychiatry 165: 844–854.

Suzuki Y, Fukui N, et al. (2012). QT prolongation of the antipsychotic risperidone is predominantly related to its 9-hydroxy metabolite paliperidone. Hum Psychopharmacol 27(1): 39–42.

Suzuki T, Uchida H, et al. (2007). How effective is it to sequentially switch among olanzapine, quetiapine and risperidone?—a randomized, open-label study of algorithm-based antipsychotic treatment to patients with symptomatic schizophrenia in the real-world clinical setting. Psychopharmacology 195: 285–295.

Swartz MS, Stroup TS, et al. (2008). What CATIE found: results from the schizophrenia trial. Psychiatr Serv 59(5): 500–506.

Tahir TA, Eeles E, et al. (2010). A randomized controlled trial of quetiapine versus placebo in the treatment of delirium. J Psychosom Res 69(5): 485–490.

Takahata K, Ito H, et al. (2012). Striatal and extrastriatal dopamine D(2) receptor occupancy by the partial agonist antipsychotic drug aripiprazole in the human brain: a positron emission tomography study with [(1)(1)C] raclopride and [(1)(1)C]FLB457. Psychopharmacology 222(1): 165–172.

Tarazi FI, Stahl SM (2012). Iloperidone, asenapine and lurasidone: a primer on their current status. Expert Opin Pharmacother 13(13): 1911–1922.

Tarsy D, Lungu C, et al. (2011). Epidemiology of tardive dyskinesia before and during the era of modern antipsychotic drugs. Handb Clin Neurol 100: 601–616.

Tiihonen J, Mittendorfer-Rutz E, et al. (2017). Real-world effectiveness of antipsychotic treatments in a nationwide cohort of 29823 patients with schizophrenia. JAMA Psychiatry 74(7): 686–693.

Tiihonen J, Taipale H, et al. (2019). Association of antipsychotic polypharmacy vs monotherapy with psychiatric rehospitalization among adults with schizophrenia. JAMA Psychiatry 76(5): 499–507.

Tiihonen J, Wahlbeck K, Kiviniemi V (2009). The efficacy of lamotrigine in clozapine-resistant schizophrenia: a systematic review and meta-analysis. Schizophr Res 109(1–3): 10–14.

Touma KTB, Scarff JR (2018). Valbenazine and deutetrabenazine for tardive dyskinesia. Innov Clin Neurosci 15(5–6): 13–16.

Trollor JN, Chen X, et al. (2009). Neuroleptic malignant syndrome associated with atypical antipsychotic drugs. CNS Drugs 23(6): 477–492.

Uguz F (2016). Second-generation antipsychotics during the lactation period: a comparative systematic review on infant safety. J Clin Psychopharmacol 36(3): 244–252.

Uguz F (2019). Antipsychotic use during pregnancy and the risk of gestational diabetes mellitus: a systematic review. J Clin Psychopharmacol 39(2): 162–167.

van Harten PN, Tenback DE (2011). Tardive dyskinesia: clinical presentation and treatment. Int Rev Neurobiol 98: 187–210.

Van Winkel R, De Hert M, et al. (2006). Screening for diabetes and other metabolic abnormalities in patients with schizophrenia and schizoaffective disorder: evaluation of incidence and screening methods. J Clin Psychiatry 67: 1493–1500.

Vayisoglu S, Anil Yagcioglu AE, et al. (2013). Lamotrigine augmentation in patients with schizophrenia who show partial response to clozapine treatment. Schizophr Res 143(1): 207–214.

Veale D, Miles S, et al. (2014). Atypical antipsychotic augmentation in SSRI treatment refractory obsessive-compulsive disorder: a systematic review and meta-analysis. BMC Psychiatry 14: 317.

Wang SM, Han C, et al. (2012). Paliperidone: a review of clinical trial data and clinical implications. Clin Drug Investig 32(8): 497–512.

Wang PS, Schneeweiss S, et al. (2005). Risk of death in elderly users of conventional vs. atypical antipsychotic medications. N Engl J Med 353: 2335–2341.

Wang G, Zheng W, et al. (2018). ECT augmentation of clozapine for clozapine-resistant schizophrenia: a meta-analysis of randomized controlled trials. J Psychiatr Res 105: 23–32.

Weiden PJ (2012). Iloperidone for the treatment of schizophrenia: an updated clinical review. Clin Schizophr Relat Psychoses 6(1): 34–44.

Weiden PJ, Manning R, et al. (2016). A randomized trial of iloperidone for prevention of relapse in schizophrenia: The REPRIEVE study. CNS Drugs 30(8): 735–747.

Weiner E, Conley RR, et al. (2010). Adjunctive risperidone for partially responsive people with schizophrenia treated with clozapine. Neuropsychopharmacology 35(11): 2274–2283.

World Health Organization (2019). World Health Organization Model List of Essential Medicines, 21st List. https://apps.who.int/iris/bitstream/handle/10665/325771/WHO-MVP-EMP-IAU-2019.06-eng.pdf?ua=1

Williams SG, Alinejad NA, et al. (2010). Statistically significant increase in weight caused by low-dose quetiapine. Pharmacotherapy 30(10): 1011–1015.

Wu RR, Zhao JP, et al. (2008). Lifestyle intervention and metformin for treatment of antipsychotic-induced weight gain: a randomized controlled trial. JAMA 299: 185–193.

Yang T, Liu Q, et al. (2017). Efficacy of olanzapine for the prophylaxis of chemotherapy-induced nausea and vomiting: a meta-analysis. Br J Clin Pharmacol 83(7): 1369–1379.

Yoodee J, Permsuwan U, Nimworapan M (2017). Efficacy and safety of olanzapine for the prevention of chemotherapy-induced nausea and vomiting: a systematic review and meta-analysis. Crit Rev Oncol Hematol 112: 113–125.

Yoon S, Jeon SW, et al. (2017). Adjunctive brexpiprazole as a novel effective strategy for treating major depressive disorder: a systematic review and meta-analysis. J Clin Psychopharmacol 37(1): 46–53.

Yury CA, Fisher JE (2007). Meta-analysis of the effectiveness of atypical antipsychotics for the treatment of behavioral problems in persons with dementia. Psychother Psychosom 76: 213–218.

Zacher JL, Roche-Desilets J (2005). Hypotension secondary to the combination of intramuscular olanzapine and intramuscular lorazepam. J Clin Psychiatry 66: 1614–1615.

Zheng W, Xiang YT, et al. (2017). Clozapine augmentation with antiepileptic drugs for treatment-resistant schizophrenia: a meta-analysis of randomized controlled trials. J Clin Psychiatry 78(5): e498–e505.

Zoccali R, Muscatello MR, et al. (2007). The effect of lamotrigine augmentation of clozapine in a sample of treatment-resistant schizophrenic patients: a double-blind, placebo-controlled study. Schizophr Res 93(1–3): 109–116.

4

Mood Stabilizers

What is a mood stabilizer? Although there is no generally accepted definition, a mood stabilizer can be defined as a medication that can treat either phase of bipolar disorder while not inducing or worsening the other phase. More conservatively, however, a mood stabilizer can be defined as an agent that has been shown to both treat *and prevent* both manic and depressive episodes. By this "two by two" definition (Bauer and Mitchner 2004), available medicines are likely only *partial* mood stabilizers at best.

Lithium and Anticonvulsants Used as Mood Stabilizers

Lithium (as a salt) has been used as a homeopathic treatment for gout and other disorders since the 1800s. Its calming effect on animals and, subsequently, on manic patients was first described in the 1940s (Cade 2000/1949). In the brain, lithium inhibits inositol phosphatases that dephosphorylate inositol phosphates that are generated by the stimulation of G proteins in neuronal membranes activated by a neurotransmitter. This inhibition may interfere with inositol regeneration and lead to its depletion in neurons, ultimately leading to decreased neuronal activity (Berridge, Downes et al. 1989; Harwood 2005; Serretti, Drago et al. 2009). Lithium also inhibits protein kinases, glycogen synthase kinase-3beta, and adenylyl cyclase (Bachmann, Schloesser et al. 2005; Lenox and Hahn 2000) and may increase the uptake of the excitatory neurotransmitter glutamate thereby reducing glutamate activity at the neuronal synapse (Shaldubina, Agam et al. 2001). It is not clear which of these (or other) mechanisms of action are responsible for lithium's clinical effects (Nestler, Hyman et al. 2015; Won and Kim 2017). Lithium also appears to have neuroprotective properties and may promote neurogenesis (Chuang 2005; Chen and Manji 2006; Bearden, Thompson et al. 2007; Nunes, Forlenza et al. 2007; Fornai, Longone et al. 2008; Moore, Cortese et al. 2009; Lyoo, Dager et al. 2010; Hajek, Bauer et al. 2012; Hajek, Kopecek et al. 2012; Won and Kim 2017).

Lithium is effective in acute manic episodes associated with bipolar disorder, as well as for long-term maintenance (Licht 2012). Lithium has not been demonstrated to have efficacy in acute bipolar depression and it does not have Food and Drug Administration (FDA) approval for this indication. Early studies provided positive data, mostly from long-term observational studies (Frances, Kahn et al. 1998; Baldessarini and Tondo 2000). However, the only large rigorously controlled study was the industry-sponsored EMBOLDEN I study, which was a randomized double-blind comparison of quetiapine (an antipsychotic), lithium, and placebo in bipolar depressed patients (62.5% bipolar I; Young et al. 2010). Lithium was not better than placebo, but quetiapine was significantly better. One caution is that the study was designed mainly to test and promote quetiapine, and industry-sponsored comparison studies find a superior result for their product over 90% of the time, presumably due usually to subtle biases in the design and conduct of the trials (Osser 2008; Heres, Davis et al. 2006).

Lithium is also the only mood stabilizer, however, with antisuicidal effects (Baldessarini, Tondo et al. 1999; Cipriani, Pretty et al. 2005; Cipriani, Hawton et al. 2013). An eight-year longitudinal study of over 50,000 patients with bipolar disorder noted that lithium (but not valproate—the most commonly used mood stabilizer in the United States, discussed later) can decrease the risk of suicide significantly (Song, Sjolander et al. 2017). This effect is distinct from lithium's mood stabilizing properties (Ahrens and Muller-Oerlinghausen 2001). This is important due to the high rate of suicide attempts of up to 32.4% in bipolar I and 36.3% in bipolar II patients (Novick, Swartz & Frank 2010; Tondo, Pompili et al. 2016). Even though lithium's antisuicidal property is not rapidly apparent, the benefits accrue over time (Young 2013). Stopping lithium increases the risk of suicide by ninefold (Tondo, Hennen & Baldessarini 2001).

Lithium also works particularly well in patients who have a strong family history of bipolar disorder (Alda 1999). It is more effective for classic acute mania than mania with mixed (depressive) features (Mohammad and Osser 2014). Genetic biomarkers for lithium response may eventually help identify bipolar patients who are likely to respond to lithium (Hou, Heilbronner et al. 2016).

Lithium has a narrow therapeutic index. A target therapeutic serum level of 0.6 to 0.75 mEq/L is recommended for maintenance treatment (Kleindienst, Severus et al. 2007; Kleindienst, Severus et al. 2005; Severus, Kleindienst et al. 2008). Serum levels of 0.75 to 1.2 mEq/L may be more effective for preventing mania, but maintaining these high levels may bring on more depressions. Serum levels higher than 1.2 mEq/L are associated with significant lithium toxicity. Long-term renal toxicity is minimized by preventing levels from exceeding 1.0 mEq/L (Kirkham, Skinner et al. 2014). Electrocardiographic changes, namely QT prolongation, may also occur more readily with serum levels greater than 1.2 mEq/L (Hsu, Liu et al. 2005). Co-administration of nonsteroidal anti-inflammatory drugs, thiazide diuretics, angiotensin-converting enzyme inhibitors, metronidazole, and tetracycline can increase lithium serum levels. Potassium-sparing diuretics and theophylline may decrease lithium serum levels (Finley, Warner & Peopody 1995).

Lithium side effects usually increase with higher serum levels, but they can occur at any dose. These may include nausea, vomiting, diarrhea, tremor, acne, psoriasis, and a benign leukocytosis. Tremor, which can begin early in treatment and become more coarse with time, can be treated by lowering the lithium dose if possible, avoiding caffeine and cigarettes, and/or adding propranolol (Gitlin 2016). Mild cognitive impairment may also occur with lithium and can be a cause of nonadherence (Wingo, Wingo et al. 2009), but often the cognitive problems are due to residual depression that has not remitted (but which could be treated more aggressively) and/or due to patients missing the creative thinking they enjoyed when manic.

Metabolic and hormonal side effects may include weight gain, nephrogenic diabetes insipidus, hypothyroidism, and hyperparathyroidism (Livingstone and Rampes 2006):

- Lithium induced weight gain may be dose-dependent but is likely to be less severe than quetiapine-, olanzapine-, or valproate-induced weight gain (McKnight, Adida et al. 2012; Bowden and Singh 2005). Lithium weight gain can come from several sources, with some easier to manage than others. Ingestion of an inorganic salt leads to increased thirst, and if caloric beverages like soda and juices are consumed, weight can increase rapidly. There can be fluid retention and abdominal bloating from ingesting lithium, and occasionally peripheral edema may develop. Use of a diuretic such as amiloride (which usually does not raise lithium levels) can help with these effects. Finally, carbohydrate cravings are reported with lithium, and these can be difficult to resist.
- Diabetes insipidus (which is a result of increased resistance to the effect of antidiuretic hormone leading to a subsequent inability to concentrate urine) can begin early in treatment and continue to affect up to 40% or more of lithium

treated patients (Grunfeld and Rossier 2009). It can cause dehydration, thirst, and polyuria (Dols, Sienaert et al. 2013). Keeping lithium doses low whenever possible and providing once-a-day dosing with the regular-release (24-hour half-life) formulation at bedtime (which gives the kidneys an opportunity to have levels drop below trough level for the second 12-hour period of the day and thus be spared exposure to high levels for the full 24 hours) may reduce these effects. Thiazides (which are otherwise best avoided with lithium due to their potential to increase lithium levels) as well as amiloride can paradoxically reduce lithium-induced polyuria (Gitlin 2016).

• Over the long run, lithium can cause hypothyroidism in up to 20% of patients (Johnston and Eagles 1999). Hypothyroidism can be treated with thyroid hormone replacement, and lithium can be continued if it has been otherwise helpful in the treatment of bipolar disorder. Some symptoms of hypothyroidism (e.g., slowed mentation, lethargy, and depressed mood) overlap with, and must be distinguished from, symptoms of worsening depression. Other symptoms include weight gain, dry skin, and cold intolerance (Gitlin 2016).

• Lithium can stimulate parathyroid hormone release and increase serum calcium (McKnight, Adida et al. 2012). Symptoms may include weakness, fatigue, and renal stones. Mild increases in calcium can be monitored without discontinuation of lithium (Gitlin 2016), but some patients who develop hyperparathyroidism may require parathyroidectomies (Meehan, Humble et al. 2015).

Worsening renal function, which can occur in 20% of patients (Lepkifker, Sverdlik et al. 2004), usually necessitates lithium discontinuation. Serious renal impairment is much less common, occurring in a placebo-corrected rate of about 0.3% (Bendz, Schon et al. 2010; McKnight, Adida et al. 2012). A recent large observation study actually found no increase in end-stage kidney disease on lithium compared with controls and no difference from patients on valproate (Kessing, Gerds et al. 2015). However, chronic kidney disease (not end-stage) was more frequent with over 20 years of lithium use (Kessing, Gerds et al. 2015; Tondo, Abramowicz et al. 2017). Kidney functions must be monitored regularly (Jefferson 2010). Because of the many complexities of lithium use, access to relevant online or textbook references is recommended.

Despite these risks, lithium has benefits that support its use over the long run. Antisuicidal and neuroprotective effects have already been mentioned. Additionally, large longitudinal studies have shown that lithium appears to improve long-term functioning. Lithium is also more likely than other treatments used for bipolar disorder to be maintained as monotherapy over time without need for additional medications (Baldessarini, Leahy et al. 2007; Kessing, Hellmund et al. 2011; Hayes, Marston et al. 2016). Finally, lithium appears to be more effective than other treatments in reducing the rates of both psychiatric and medical hospitalizations (Lahteenvuo, Tanskanen et al. 2018).

Valproate (along with carbamazepine and lamotrigine discussed later) is an anticonvulsant with putative mood-stabilizing properties. It is postulated that it exerts its effect via enhancement of gamma aminobutyric acid transmission (Johannessen 2000). It is also a use-dependent Na+ channel blocker and a calcium channel blocker. As is the case for lithium, it is not known which of valproate's neuronal actions is responsible for its therapeutic effects (Nestler, Hyman et al. 2015).

Despite more decades of clinical experience with lithium, valproate has become the most widely used mood stabilizer in the United States. This is primarily due to its wider therapeutic index, ease of use, and effective marketing by its manufacturer. It is not as popular in Europe and Asia.

Some small studies show efficacy in the treatment of bipolar depression, but most emphasis has been on use in classic manic and mixed manic episodes (Bowden, Brugger et al. 1994; Freeman, Clothier et al. 1992). However, more recent studies in acute mania failed to show differences from placebo (Wagner, Redden et al. 2009; Hirschfeld, Bowden et al. 2010), and overall valproate seems less effective than other agents for mania (Cipriani, Barbui et al. 2011). Valproate has no positive studies finding maintenance efficacy, and it is not FDA-approved for maintenance use in bipolar disorder. The large 2010 BALANCE study contributed to the evidence base for valproate's inferiority as a treatment for bipolar disorder, compared with lithium, and in combination was only slightly more effective than lithium alone (Geddes, Goodwin et al. 2010). A meta-analysis combining various studies found that valproate may have some maintenance efficacy, although the combination of lithium and valproate may be more effective in maintenance than valproate alone (Cipriani, Reid et al. 2013).

Although serum levels of 50 to 125 mcg/mL are generally considered to be within the therapeutic range (a range based on anticonvulsant usage), the best results in acute mania may occur with levels of greater than 90 mcg/mL (Allen, Hirschfeld et al. 2006).

In adults, the most troubling side effect of valproate may be weight gain, but it also causes usually benign and transient liver enzyme elevations (severe hepatotoxicity may be more common in the very young), nausea and diarrhea, hyperammonemia, and alopecia. Pancreatitis is a rare serious side effect that can be life-threatening.

Valproate may also cause possible thrombocytopenia and platelet dysfunction. Bleeding time should be measured prior to surgery even if the platelet count is normal (De Berardis, Campanella et al. 2003; Gerstner, Teich et al. 2006). Valproate is highly protein-bound: concurrent use with warfarin can displace and increase the free fraction of warfarin and increase prothrombin time. Aspirin can increase valproate levels.

Finally, valproate (like all other anticonvulsants) carries an FDA warning for suicidality.

Carbamazepine is an anticonvulsant that can enhance Na+ channel inactivation, thereby blocking action potentials and repetitive neuronal firing (Nestler, Hyman et al. 2015). It is thought to inhibit a process known as "kindling"—a process whereby repeated subthreshold electrical stimuli can lead to the development of spontaneous seizures. Hypothetically, subthreshold environmental stimuli or prior manias may similarly kindle the development and frequency of further manias (Post, Uhde et al. 1982; Post 1990).

Carbamazepine has efficacy in the treatment of acute mania and received FDA approval in 2004 (Weisler, Kalali et al. 2004; Weisler, Keck et al. 2005). It appears effective for maintenance therapy (Ceron-Litvoc, Soares et al. 2009), but probably not for acute depressive episodes associated with bipolar disorder (Ansari and Osser 2010). Serum levels of 4 to 12 mcg/mL may be therapeutic. A strong advantage of carbamazepine is its association with minimal weight gain as a side effect—which is rare among agents effective for mania. Significant side effects include dizziness, ataxia, and gastrointestinal symptoms, which all prohibit the use of loading strategies to speed response. Thrombocytopenia, leukopenia, aplastic anemia, hyponatremia, and dangerous rash may also develop with carbamazepine therapy. Like lamotrigine discussed later, carbamazepine can cause a life-threatening rash. This is found almost exclusively in patients carrying the HLA-B* 1502) gene (which is found in 10%–15% of Asians including Chinese/Taiwanese, Thai, Malaysian, and Philippinos, but not Japanese or Koreans). An FDA alert from 2007 indicated that individuals with these ethnic backgrounds should be tested for the gene if carbamazepine is to be considered (FDA 2007).

Another factor that makes treatment more difficult with carbamazepine, especially in severe mania when concurrent antipsychotics may be necessary, is its propensity to induce the activity of multiple hepatic enzymes (e.g., CYP1A2, CYP2C9, CYP2C19,

CYP3A4) that metabolize these drugs. It can therefore decrease the serum levels of other concurrently administered drugs (such as antipsychotics or benzodiazepines) and render them less effective. Carbamazepine also induces its own metabolism, with the result that over the first month the dose usually needs to be gradually increased to maintain the same level until steady state is finally reached. Notably, the antiepileptic drugs **phenobarbital, phenytoin**, and **primidone** also have similarly broad hepatic enzyme induction capacities (Perucca 2006).

Oxcarbazepine, a derivative of carbamazepine, may also have efficacy in the treatment of acute mania (Ghaemi, Berv et al. 2003; Pratoomsri, Yatham et al. 2006; Kakkar, Rehan et al. 2009). Serum levels are not routinely followed during administration, and there is less enzymatic induction with oxcarbazepine, thereby reducing the risk of drug–drug interactions. Hyponatremia, however, remains a concern and may be more likely than with carbamazepine. (Ortenzi, Paggi et al. 2008). Few studies with bipolar patients were completed before oxcarbazepine's patent protection expired and funding was then no longer available. As a result, there are insufficient efficacy data to recommend oxcarbazepine as an effective mood stabilizer, although it is still used occasionally by clinicians (Vasudev, Macritchie et al. 2011).

Lamotrigine is an anticonvulsant that may inhibit the release of the excitatory amino acid glutamate (Paraskevas, Triantafyllou et al. 2006) and may also act as a Na+ channel blocker (Nestler, Hyman et al. 2015), but its mechanism of action is not fully known. In bipolar disorder, it is often used (but not FDA-approved) for the treatment of acute bipolar depression; the effect seems to be modest. Four out of five studies failed to show separation from placebo (Calabrese, Bowden et al. 1999; Calabrese, Huffman et al. 2008), although a meta-analysis of these studies showed an overall effect size of 0.3 (considered a weak effect size) but a greater separation from placebo in more severely depressed patients (Geddes, Calabrese et al. 2009). Lamotrigine is effective and FDA-approved as maintenance therapy for depressive episodes in bipolar disorder (Bowden, Calabrese et al. 2003; Calabrese, Bowden et al. 2003; Licht, Nielsen et al. 2010).

Although lamotrigine is generally well-tolerated, there is a 0.1% to 0.3% risk of dangerous rash (i.e., toxic epidermal necrolysis—Stevens–Johnson syndrome) in adults (Calabrese, Sullivan et al. 2002; Lexicomp 2019). Gradual titration is required to decrease the risk of rash. If rash develops, lamotrigine should be discontinued and not restarted until the rash has been evaluated and found to be benign. The FDA has recently added two new warnings for aseptic meningitis and for hemophagocytic lymphohistiocytosis, an immune disorder leading to systemic inflammation and fever that can be life-threatening (FDA 2010; FDA 2018). These are expected to be rare adverse effects.

Although lamotrigine serum levels are not routinely monitored in psychiatric patients, measuring levels may be helfpul in patients who are not responding to usual maximal doses (200 mg/day). One small retrrospective study suggested that lamotrigine, like other mood stabilizers previoously noted, may have a therpaeutic window: patients who took lamotrigine for treatment of their mood disorder did better with a serum level between 5 to 11 mcg/mL (Katayama, Terao et al. 2014).

Concomitant use of lamotrigine and valproate increases lamotrigine blood levels, so lamotrigine's titration has to be at half the usual doses to reduce the risk of dangerous rash; concomitant use with carbamazepine has the opposite effect and reduces lamotrigine blood levels. The clinician should refer to the lamotrigine package insert for dosing recommendations, especially when it is combined with these other mood stabilizers. Oral contraceptives can increase lamotrigine clearance; therefore, higher doses of lamotrigine may be needed for women using both medications (although patients on lamotrigine–valproate combination may not need further adjustments in their lamotrigine dose if oral contraceptives are added; Wegner, Wilhelm et al. 2014).

Antipsychotics Used as Mood Stabilizers

Mania

All antipsychotics are expected to have efficacy in the treatment of mania (Perlis, Welge et al. 2006; Smith, Cornelius et al. 2007; Glue and Herbison 2015; Takeshima 2017). Chlorpromazine, risperidone, olanzapine, quetiapine, ziprasidone, aripiprazole, asenapine, and cariprazine are FDA-approved for the treatment of mania. These join lithium, valproate, and carbamazepine, which also have this approval.

Risperidone, olanzapine, and haloperidol may be somewhat more effective than lithium or anticonvulsants for the treatment of acute mania (Cipriani, Barbui et al. 2011; Tarr, Glue et al. 2011). Haloperidol may be the most effective (Cipriani, Barbui et al. 2011) and may have a faster onset of action than other agents (Tohen and Vieta 2009). However, it is no longer recommended for most patients with acute mania because of having the highest risk of inducing a switch to depression (Goikolea, Colom et al. 2013) and causing neuroleptic-induced dysphoria (Tohen and Zarate 1998). Improvement with antipsychotics (e.g., olanzapine and risperidone) may begin within the first week and early responders are likely to continue to improve for the duration of the period of treatment of acute symptoms (Kemp, Johnson et al. 2011). Olanzapine, however, is not an appropriate first-line treatment for mania due to its metabolic side effects (Grunze, Vieta et al. 2009; Mohammad and Osser 2014). Some second-generation antipsychotics (SGAs; e.g., quetiapine and risperidone) work better than lithium in mixed mania (Fountoulakis, Kontis et al. 2012; Swann, Lafer et al. 2013).

Bipolar Depression

For acute bipolar depression, among the SGAs, quetiapine, lurasidone, and cariprazine (at doses of 1.5 and 3 mg per day) have been shown to have clear efficacy (Calabrese, Keck et al. 2005; Thase, Macfadden et al. 2006; De Fruyt, Deschepper et al. 2012; Loebel, Cucchiaro et al. 2014; Durgam, Earley et al. 2016; Earley, Burgess et al. 2019). They have FDA approval for bipolar depression, as does olanzapine combined with fluoxetine. Although olanzapine and olanzapine–fluoxetine combination may have some efficacy (Tohen, Vieta et al. 2003), the effect may be less than quetiapine (De Fruyt, Deschepper et al. 2012), and concerns about olanzapine's adverse metabolic effects would again argue against use until most other FDA-approved and safer options have been tried. Aripiprazole, which has an FDA indication as adjunctive treatment for unipolar depression, does not appear to be efficacious for the treatment of acute bipolar depression nor for preventing depressive episodes (Keck, Calabrese et al. 2006; Thase, Jonas et al. 2008; Cruz, Sanchez-Moreno et al. 2010; De Fruyt, Deschepper et al. 2012).

Bipolar Maintenance

For maintenance therapy, FDA-approved SGA medications that have been found effective as treatments for the prevention of manic episodes consist of olanzapine, quetiapine, ziprasidone, aripiprazole, asenapine, and long-acting injectable risperidone (Tohen, Calabrese et al. 2006; Keck, Calabrese et al. 2007; Quiroz, Yatham et al. 2010). Quetiapine has one maintenance study suggesting it may prevent both manic and depressive episodes (Weisler, Nolen et al. 2011), but it did not achieve FDA approval as a maintenance monotherapy treatment for both phases of bipolar. The study was enriched with 100% acute responders to quetiapine, and despite that advantage, just as many patients did well when randomized to lithium for maintenance as to quetiapine. Nevertheless, quetiapine comes close to challenging lithium as the most broadly effective mood stabilizer with the best evidence base. In general, however, many still doubt that any SGA should be considered a mood stabilizer by the "two by two" definition (Goodwin, Whitham et al. 2011). Cariprazine did join quetiapine as one of only two SGAs that have approval for both acute bipolar mania and acute bipolar depression, but so far there are no maintenance studies with it.

There is evidence that the SGAs olanzapine, quetiapine, ziprasidone, aripiprazole, and long-acting injectable risperidone, when added to lithium or valproate, can increase maintenance efficacy for the manic phase (Tohen, Chengappa et al. 2004; Macfadden, Alphs et al. 2009; Bowden, Vieta et al. 2010; Marcus, Khan et al. 2011). In the case of quetiapine, the depressive phase was also helped (Vieta, Suppes et al. 2008; Suppes, Vieta et al. 2009).

Long-acting injectable antipsychotics in general appear to be more effective than their oral counterparts in reducing psychiatric rehospitalizations (Lahteenvuo, Tanskanen et al. 2018). Still, whether used as monotherapy or as adjunctive therapy added to a mood stabilizer, the use of antipsychotics for maintenance carries significant long-term risks and is best reserved for when lithium is unsatisfactory.

Other Anticonvulsants

Relatively newer anticonvulsants such as **topiramate, gabapentin, pregabalin, tiagabine, zonisamide,** and **levetiracetam** have had periods where they were thought to be effective for the treatment of bipolar disorder (Johannessen and Landmark 2008). However, none have placebo-controlled supportive evidence. Topiramate, for example, has four negative controlled studies in mania (Kushner, Khan et al. 2006). If used, these medications should be considered to be adjunctive treatments only (e.g., to decrease concurrent anxiety); the evidence base is insufficient to recommend their use as primary agents for the treatment of mood disorder symptoms (Anand, Bukhari et al. 2005; Grunze, Langosch et al. 2003; Grunze, Normann et al. 2001; Keck, Strawn et al. 2006; Macdonald and Young 2002; Pande, Crockatt et al. 2000; Vieta, Goikolea et al. 2003; Vieta, Manuel Goikolea et al. 2006; Vieta, Sanchez-Moreno et al. 2003; Yatham, Kusumakar et al. 2002; Young, Geddes et al. 2006; Young, Geddes et al. 2006). Older publications suggest that **clonazepam** (a benzodiazepine that has also been used as an anticonvulsant) may in addition to its sedative/hypnotic effects have mood-stabilizing effects in the treatment of mania (Sachs 1990; Sachs, Rosenbaum et al. 1990). A more recent study, however, noted that bipolar patients on long-term benzodiazepines were at a higher risk for rehospitalizations (Lahteenvuo, Tanskanen et al. 2018).

Emerging Pharmacotherapies

As discussed in the chapter on antidepressants, the phencyclidine derivative, **ketamine**, an N-methyl-D-aspartate (a glutamate receptor) antagonist, appears to show efficacy in the acute treatment of unipolar depression. This effect appears to extend to bipolar depression as well. Of note, many commonly used mood-stabilizing agents, such as lithium, valproate, and lamotrigine also appear to have some effect on the glutamatergic system, and this may point to a common therapeutic pathway (Machado-Vieira, Ibrahim et al. 2012).

Patients with depressive symptoms, who were maintained on either lithium or valproate, showed improvement in symptoms and in suicidality within 40 minutes after a single infusion of intravenous ketamine (Diazgranados, Ibrahim et al. 2010; Zarate, Brutsche et al. 2012). Manic induction was rare, and the treatment was well tolerated, the most common adverse effect being the development of transient dissociative symptoms. It is not yet known if the positive response can be sustained. Although ketamine may be superior to placebo in terms of response within the first 24 hours, it does not appear to be better than placebo for remission of bipolar depression (McCloud, Caddy et al. 2015). Also, chronic ketamine administration, if needed, may be problematic as it may be associated with increasing dissociative and perceptual disturbances.

As note earlier, esketamine, the nasally administered derivative of ketamine, has been recently received FDA approval for treatment-resistance and suicidality in patients with unipolar depression, but this approval does not yet extend to bipolar depressed patients due to lack of study in this population.

Triiodothyronine and **levothyroxine** have been studied and may be beneficial in the treatment of refractory bipolar depression (Stamm, Lewitzka et al. 2014). Supraphysiological doses of T4 may be helpful in augmenting antidepressant therapy in treatment-resistant patients (Kelly and Lieberman 2009). The antidepressant effect of thyroid hormone in a euthyroid patient has been proposed to be due to modulation of the catecholaminergic system (Chakrabarti, Giri et al. 2011).

Complementary, Alternative, and Other Pharmacotherapies

Omega-3 fatty acids continue to be considered for the treatment of bipolar depression and mania. An earlier meta-analysis suggested that adjunctive use of omega-3 fatty acids may be efficacious for bipolar depression with an effect size of 0.34, but not for bipolar mania (Sarris, Mischoulon & Schweitzer et al. 2012). Subsequent reviews have supported the use of omega-3 fatty acids as monotherapy or as adjunctive therapy in bipolar depression (Rutkofsky, Khan et al. 2017), but not as treatment that would reduce suicide risk in affective disorders (Pompili, Longo et al. 2017). On the positive side, omega-3 fatty acids are likely to be the most tolerable of all treatments studied for bipolar disorder, and they do not appear to be associated with treatment-emergent mania.

There are insufficient data to support the use of **inositol** monotherapy (Mukai, Kishi et al. 2014) or **S-adenosyl methionine** (Karas Kuzelicki 2016) for bipolar depression, and the latter may be associated with rare manic switches (Galizia, Oldani et al. 2016; Abeysundera and Gill 2018). The clinician should not assume that any "natural" supplement that may have purported antidepressant effects and is deemed safe for the treatment of unipolar depression would be safe for use in patients with bipolar depression.

Further Notes on the Clinical Use of Mood Stabilizers for Bipolar Disorder

Mood stabilization is frequently difficult to achieve in bipolar disorder. Although the goal is to use as few medications as possible and rely only on monotherapy with mood stabilizers whenever feasible, it is common that more complex psychopharmacology regimens are required. This is true for mania because the antimanic effects of lithium, valproate, and carbamazepine might not be achieved until 7 to 10 days after a therapeutic dose has been established. In the interim, sedative medications such as antipsychotics and benzodiazepines may be needed while waiting for the mood stabilizer to take effect. Once the patient is stabilized, these adjunctive medications can often be tapered, and the mood stabilizer is continued as monotherapy.

Response to lamotrigine when used for bipolar depression may take even longer: a six-week period may be needed for response. Additionally, the need for polytherapy may arise when patients do not respond (or only partially respond) to monotherapy for depression or for maintenance.

Summary of Initial Therapies for Each Phase of Bipolar Disorder

Based on the material presented in this chapter, the following general recommendations are noted:

- *Mania:* If a patient who presents with mania is taking an antidepressant, the first step is to discontinue it, or taper it over several weeks if the patient is at risk for discontinuation syndrome (Horowitz and Taylor 2019). Lithium is the first-line mood stabilizer for the treatment of acute nonmixed "classic" mania. It may be supplemented by an atypical antipsychotic (quetiapine or cariprazine may be preferred because they are also indicated for bipolar depression). Brief adjunctive treatment with a benzodiazepine should also be considered to help treat agitation, anxiety, and insomnia while more time is given for lithium to become effective. Adjunctive medications can then be tapered off, and lithium can be continued once the patient is no longer manic (Mohammad and Osser 2014). Carbamazepine is an option for adjunctive use, but its utility is limited given potential for medication interactions and slow titration.

- *Mixed mania:* SGAs are first-line (quetiapine is preferred). Valproate may be more effective than lithium for mixed episodes and may be considered for addition to the SGA. Lithium may be added as a third-line agent especially if the patient has been suicidal (Mohammad and Osser 2014).

- *Depression:* Lithium, lamotrigine, quetiapine, lurasidone, and cariprazine may be considered first-line treatments for acute bipolar depression. All are FDA-approved either for acute or at least for maintenance treatment (lithium and lamotrigine are only approved for maintenance treatment). The clinician should select the medication with the best profile of acceptability taking into account side effect vulnerabilities and patient preference. Combinations of these medications can be used if monotherapy is ineffective. Carbamazepine and valproate are not well-studied in bipolar depression, and although they might be effective in some cases, they are not preferred for initial treatment. Olanzapine and the olanzapine–fluoxetine combination may be efficacious, but the considerable potential for harm from olanzapine makes them undesirable for first-line use. Antidepressants should not be considered first-line treatments. These can be considered only in patients for whom the previously described treatments (and electroconvulsive therapy [ECT]) are ineffective or otherwise deemed unacceptable; even then, certain caveats apply (as noted later; Ansari and Osser 2010).

- *Maintenance:* Whichever mood stabilizer has been effective during the acute phase of treatment should be continued for maintenance therapy. Lithium, some SGAs, and lamotrigine (primarily for prophylaxis against depressive but not manic episodes) have efficacy as maintenance therapies. Lithium may be considered first-line given its long-term benefits—namely, suicide reduction, neuroprotective effects, improved long-term functioning, evidence of being the mood stabilizer most likely to be sufficient as monotherapy for maintenance, and possible superiority in reducing psychiatric rehospitalizations compared to other mood stabilizers. If monotherapy is ineffective, then combinations can be considered (if careful consideration is given to specific interactions and side effects). Although some SGAs have efficacy as maintenance therapies, they are primarily helpful in reducing manic rather than depressive recurrences (with the exception of quetiapine, which may protect against both, and cariprazine, which might protect against both but has not as yet been studied to delineate its maintenance properties). The larger concern with SGAs, however, is the poor long-term side effect profiles of some of them. Given that patients with bipolar disorder are likely to require lifelong maintenance treatment, long-term tolerability is a major factor in the choice of treatments. Finally, as mentioned earlier, benzodiazepines may increase the risk of rehospitalizations and are not favored for long-term maintenance therapy (Lahteenvuo, Tanskanen et al. 2018).

On the Clinical Use of Antidepressants in Bipolar Disorder

The use of antidepressants in patients with bipolar disorder remains controversial, but the evidence base indicating that they should be avoided has accumulated. Historically, antidepressants have been used to treat bipolar depression (bipolar II more than bipolar I) and older (poorly controlled) studies and algorithms did support their use. However, newer data do not support their use as first-line treatments.

The Systematic Treatment Enhancement Program—Bipolar Disorder (STEP-BD) was a publicly funded, multisite outcomes study designed to add to our understanding of how to best treat this disorder (Sachs, Thase et al. 2003; El-Mallakh, Vohringer et al. 2015). The program enrolled 4,360 bipolar patients who were being followed longitudinally at 15 sites. Some of these patients agreed to enter controlled studies of a variety of psychosocial and psychopharmacological interventions. Among the significant findings were the following:

- Psychotherapy is effective for bipolar depression, but it is a slow process. Improvement occurs in a mean of 169 days versus 279 days in the control group (Miklowitz, Otto et al. 2007).

- Antidepressants (bupropion, paroxetine) are not more effective than placebo for bipolar depression (24% for the antidepressants vs. 27% for the placebo in a six-month trial). The antidepressants, when added to a mood stabilizer, did not induce more switches to mania (10% vs. 11%), but the patients who participated in this study were probably at very low risk for switching (Sachs, Nierenberg et al. 2007).

- A group of 86 bipolar patients that had been put on an antidepressant when depressed and seemed to respond was identified. Some were rapid cyclers (four or more episodes per year). All were also on mood stabilizers such as lithium, valproate, or an SGA. These patients were randomized to stay on their antidepressants or discontinue them. The rapid-cycling patients who were continued on their antidepressant had triple the number of depressions per year compared with the nonrapid cyclers. In the patients whose antidepressant was discontinued, there was no difference in the rate of depressions between rapid and nonrapid cycling individuals. Thus, *depressive* morbidity and cycling were worsened by continuation of an antidepressant in rapid cyclers (El-Mallakh, Vohringer et al. 2015).

- A new syndrome was identified, called "ACID," for antidepressant-associated chronic irritable dysphoria (which includes a triad of irritability, dysphoria, and middle insomnia). This condition is only rarely observed in the natural course of bipolar disorder and is 10 times as likely to occur if the patient was started on an antidepressant compared with those not given one (El-Mallakh, Ghaemi et al. 2008).

- Other STEP-BD data did show that the use of antidepressants was associated with more manic symptoms. More specifically, bipolar depressed patients who had two or more associated manic symptoms, showed greater manic severity at three-month follow-up. In these cases, antidepressant use did not hasten recovery time (Goldberg, Perlis et al. 2007).

- In this patient sample 262 suicide attempts and 8 completed suicides occurred over a six-year period. Lithium seemed to offer no protective effect, contrary to data from other studies strongly suggesting that lithium helps lower suicide risk in bipolar patients. However, the patient sample clearly had a very low risk of suicidal behaviors so it was not the best population to demonstrate lithium's apparent benefit on this symptom (Marangell, Dennehy et al. 2008).
- Antidepressant continuation, in those who had responded to an antidepressant, did not confer any statistically significant longer-term benefit (Ghaemi, Ostacher et al. 2010).

Antidepressants, therefore, are considered to have limited effectiveness, and the risk of mood destabilization (both depressive and manic recurrences) continues to be a concern even if the patient is on a mood stabilizer (Pacchiarotti, Bond et al. 2013; McGirr, Vohringer et al. 2016). If a bipolar depressed patient is refractory to usual first-line treatments (i.e., lithium, lamotrigine, quetiapine, lurasidone, and cariprazine) as monotherapy and in combination and antidepressants are then being considered, the following should be taken into account (Ansari and Osser 2010):

- ECT is an effective treatment that should be considered early in the treatment algorithm for patients with urgent indications such as severe suicidality, catatonia, poor oral intake, or medical conditions (or pregnancy) that may limit the use of psychotropics.
- Patients at high risk for manic induction are not good candidates for antidepressant therapy. These include

patients with (a) a past history of antidepressant induced mania, hypomania, or mixed states; (b) a history of severe or dangerous hypomanic or manic episodes; (c) two or more concurrent manic symptoms (i.e., mixed states); (d) a history of substance abuse, and/or (e) rapid-cycling bipolar disorder (i.e., four or more episodes per year).

- If a decision is made to use antidepressants despite the previously listed concerns, bupropion, followed by selective serotonin reuptake inhibitors, may be favored as these may be less likely to cause manic switch than serotonin-norepinephrine reuptake inhibitors and tricyclic antidepressants.
- If an antidepressant is used, it should be used in combination with a mood stabilizer.
- If an antidepressant is used, it should be started at a low dose and increased gradually, and the patient should be monitored closely for signs of emerging mania.
- Consideration should be given to discontinuing antidepressant treatment after recovery from the initial depressive illness unless there is a history of sustained response with continued antidepressant use (Ghaemi, Hsu et al. 2003).

Treatment-Resistant Bipolar Disorder

Treatment-resistant bipolar disorder is not as well defined as treatment-resistant unipolar depression or treatment-resistant schizophrenia. Failing two or more treatments is rather common for bipolar patients, and by such a definition, most bipolar patients would be considered treatment-resistant. Yet there are patients who have not responded to, or have been unable to tolerate, multiple mood stabilizers and antipsychotics, alone or in combination.

Such "treatment-resistance" is more often noted in patients with bipolar depression (where fewer medication choices are available and responses are often not as robust) than in mania.

In general, ECT and clozapine are likely to be the treatments of choice for treatment-resistant bipolar disorder (Vaidya, Mahableshwarkar & Shahid 2003; Chang, Ha et al. 2006; Nielsen, Kane et al. 2012; Thirthalli, Prasad & Gangadhar 2012; Li, Tang et al. 2015; Perugi, Medda et al. 2017). Other possibly promising options could be light therapy (augmented possibly by sleep deprivation; Benedetti, Riccaboni et al. 2014; Sit, McGowan et al. 2018), pramipexole (Zarate, Payne et al. 2004; El-Mallakh, Penagaluri et al. 2010), omega-3 fatty acids (Sarris, Mischoulon et al. 2012), and triiodothyronine (Kelly and Lieberman 2009).

Clinical Use of Mood Stabilizers in Other Psychiatric Disorders

Unipolar Depression

Lithium augmentation for patients with unipolar depression was discussed briefly in the chapter for antidepressants. If an antidepressant is only partially effective in the treatment of unipolar depression, then the addition of lithium is among the most evidence-supported therapies (Dold and Kasper 2017). Lithium is likely to be effective whether it is added to a tricyclic antidepressant or to a newer antidepressant (e.g., selective serotonin reuptake inhibitor; Edwards, Hamilton et al. 2013; Nelson, Baumann et al. 2014). Lithium may also be helpful as maintenance treatment for melancholic depression (Valerio and Martino 2018). Most importantly, the antisuicidal effects of lithium may not be limited to patients with bipolar disorder: lithium may significantly decrease suicidality in patients with recurrent unipolar depression as well (Guzzetta, Tondo et al. 2007).

Aggression and Impulsivity

Valproate is often empirically used for the treatment of aggression in cognitively impaired patients with dementia or other disorders; however, clear efficacy has not been established in this regard, and potential adverse effects may outweigh benefits in some patients (Baillon, Narayana et al. 2018; Huband, Ferriter et al. 2010). Valproate may be of some benefit in reducing impulsivity and agitation in those with traumatic brain injuries (Plantier and Luaute 2016). However, clinicians seem to select valproate often as an all-purpose treatment for many patients presenting with irritability and aggression; this is not supported by the evidence base and exposes the patient to harms such as weight gain associated with this agent (Huband, Ferriter et al. 2010). For example, valproate was not effective in two placebo-controlled trials in posttraumatic stress disorder (a common cause of these symptoms), nor in one study in intermittent explosive disorder (Davis, Davidson et al. 2008; Hamner, Faldowski et al. 2009; Coccaro, Lee et al. 2015).

Dementia

Lithium potentially may help reduce the risk of dementia in the elderly, but specifics are unclear (Donix and Bauer 2016). In animal studies, lithium has been shown to interfere with the formation of neurofibrillary tangles associated with Alzheimer's disease (Leroy, Ando et al. 2010), and it appears to have some positive effects in humans with Alzheimer's disease (Forlenza, De-Paula & Diniz 2014; Forlenza, Aprahamian et al. 2016). Lithium does not appear to show any benefit in the treatment of amyotrophic lateral sclerosis (Gamez, Salvado et al. 2016; Forlenza, Aprahamian et al. 2016).

Clinical Use of Mood Stabilizers in Nonpsychiatric Disorders

Pain

Valproate is FDA-approved for migraine prophylaxis, but its use is problematic in women of childbearing age (see following discussion). Carbamazepine and oxcarbazepine are effective for the treatment or trigeminal neuralgia (Gronseth, Cruccu et al. 2008). Lamotrigine, however, does not appear to be beneficial for the treatment of neuropathic pain (Wiffen, Derry & Moore 2013).

Valproate, carbamazepine, and lamotrigine are primarily anticonvulsants. Their role in the treatment of seizure disorders is beyond the scope of this book.

Use in Women of Childbearing Potential, Pregnancy, and Breastfeeding

Pregnancy

Both treated and untreated bipolar disorders are associated with pregnancy-related complications (Boden, Lundgren et al. 2012; Scrandis 2017). Discontinuation of mood stabilizers (including discontinuation during the first trimester) is associated with an increased risk of recurrence (Viguera, Whitfield et al. 2007). Still, most mood stabilizers are known teratogens, and as with other psychiatric disorders, the risks and benefits of treatment during pregnancy should be balanced against risks of treatment discontinuation and severity of illness.

Lithium use during pregnancy is associated with cardiac anomalies including Ebstein's anomaly in the fetus, a rare congenital defect of the tricuspid valve. However, the risk is considered to be much lower than initially thought (Cohen, Friedman et al. 1994). A more recent study showed that lithium associated cardiac malformations, can occur in 2.4% of infants exposed to lithium (which includes a 0.6% prevalence of right ventricular outflow tract obstruction defects—some of which could co-occur with Ebstein's anomaly) versus 1.2% of unexposed babies (and a 0.2% prevalence of right ventricular outflow obstruction defects), an adjusted risk ratio of 1.65. The risk rises with higher doses, but is still lower than previously thought (Patorno, Huybrechts et al. 2017). It is not unreasonable to use lithium during pregnancy, although it may not always be the first choice compared to an SGA for pregnancy safety (Trixler, Gati et al. 2005; Bergink and Kushner 2014). If lithium is continued, doses may need to be increased during pregnancy to compensate for pharmacokinetic changes in the mother and then lowered shortly before or after delivery.

Valproate is associated with a high risk of teratogenic effects (i.e., neural tube defects and decreased IQ and other cognitive scores; Cohen 2007; Viguera, Koukopoulos et al. 2007; Meador, Baker et al. 2009; PDR 2019; Haskey and Galbally 2017). Because of this, a black box warning in the package insert recommends avoiding it in women of childbearing potential for all indications unless other reasonable options are not feasible. The use of folate supplementation (high doses, e.g., 5 mg/day, which some recommend) does not reduce the risk of antiepileptic-induced spina bifida or other malformations (Patel, Viguera et al. 2018; Vajda, Graham et al. 2019). Valproate may also play a role in the development of polycystic ovary syndrome (Joffe, Cohen et al. 2006; O'Donovan, Kusumakar et al. 2002).

Carbamazepine may render oral contraceptives less effective, increasing the risk of unintentional pregnancy. If pregnancy ensues, the teratogenic effects of carbamazepine are almost comparable in severity to those of valproate (Cohen 2007; Viguera, Koukopoulos et al. 2007; Vajda, Graham et al. 2019) so it also should also be avoided in women of childbearing potential.

Lamotrigine so far seems relatively safer in pregnancy than valproate and carbamazepine but may be associated with increased cleft palate (American College of Obstetricians and Gynecologists 2008; Vajda, Graham et al. 2012; Diav-Citrin, Shechtman et al. 2017; Vajda, Graham et al. 2019), although the added risk may be very small (Dolk, Wang et al. 2016). Lamotrigine is less likely than valproate to be associated with adverse effects in learning and memory in exposed children (Meador, Baker et al. 2013). However, one review noted that fetal exposure to lamotrigine (as well as to valproate or oxcarbamezapine) during pregancy may be associated with an increased risk of autism (Veroniki, Rios et al. 2017). Further studies are needed to clarify the risk.

As with lithium, an adjusted (i.e., higher) dose of lamotrigine may be needed during pregnancy—checking serum drug levels before conception and during pregnancy may help in assessing the appropriate dose. It should be kept in mind, however, that congenital malformations due to antiepilepetic drugs are possibly dose-dependent, and lamotrigine doses of 300 mg per day or less may provide the lowest relative risk compared to valproate and carbamazepine (Tomson, Battino et al. 2011).

Breastfeeding

Maternal use of mood stabilizers while breastfeeding is also problematic. Lithium and lamotrigine may be present in high levels in breast milk (Moretti, Koren et al. 2003; Newport, Pennell et al. 2008). Breastfeeding may need to be avoided while on lithium. If breastfed, the infant should be monitored for lithium toxicity and lithium serum levels (as well as other lithium-related laboratory data) should be closely monitored in both mother and infant (Moretti, Koren et al. 2003; Drug and Lactation Database 2018). Breastfeeding while taking lamotrigine apppears not to cause any severe adverse effects in infants (Dalili, Nayeri et al. 2015), although Stevens–Johnson syndrome/toxic epidermal necrolysis—albeit rarely—can occur in all age groups, including newborns and infants (Hinc-Kasprzyk, Polak-Krzeminska & Ozog-Zabolska 2015). The potential risks of lamotrigine for breastfed infants are not fully known.

Valproate and carbamazepine are not present at high levels in breast milk and are considered to be possibly safer for breast-feeding (Pacchiarotti, Leon-Caballero et al. 2016). However, their use raises the possiblity of medication-induced hepatic toxicity, which is expected to be more likely in infants and children than in adults (Dreifuss, Santilli et al. 1987). Liver function tests need to be monitored in the infant if these medications are used by the mother. However, although adverse effects in breastfed infants have been reported in the literature (Chaudron and Jefferson 2000), aggregate data appear to suggest that the prevalence of laboratory abnormalities in breastfed infants of mothers treated with the above mood stabilizers is generally low (Uguz and Sharma 2016).

Table of Mood Stabilizing Medicines

Table 4.1 summarizes the characteristics of commonly used mood-stabilizing medicines (Ansari and Osser 2015; World Health Organization 2019; Lexicomp 2019; PDR 2019). Antipsychotics with mood stabilizing efficacy were listed in Table 3.1.

TABLE 4.1 Mood-Stabilizing Medicines

Medication[a]	Adult Dosing[b]	Comments/*FDA Indication*
Lithium Carbonate (Lithobid®, Eskalith®)	For lithium carbonate: Start: 300 mg po bid-tid and check serum trough level (12 hours after last dose) after 4–5 days (after steady state) then adjust as needed. See text for serum levels. Reduce starting dose, titrate slowly, use immediate release formulation, administer all doses at bedtime, and monitor serum levels frequently in patients with mild renal impairment; avoid in patients with severe renal disease.	Check baseline chemistries, kidney function, thyroid function (TSH), ECG (in elderly and those with cardiac disease); once target dose is reached, check level, chemistries, kidney function, TSH, every 3–6 months initially, then every 6–12 months. NSAIDs, thiazide diuretics, ACE inhibitors, metronidazole, and tetracyclines can increase lithium level. On WHO Essential Medicines List for bipolar disorders. Black Box Warning: Provision and monitoring of serum lithium levels to avoid toxicity. *Mania/maintenance in bipolar disorder in patients ≥7 years old*
Divalproex Sodium, Valproic Acid, Valproate (Depakote®, Depakote ER®, Depakenc®)	For divalproex, Depakote®: Start: 250 mg po tid and check serum trough level after 4–5 days, then adjust as needed, can use loading dose of 20–30 mg/kg to hasten response. See text for serum levels. Avoid in patients with hepatic disease; monitor closely in patients with severe renal failure as uremia can increase unbound valproic acid.	Check baseline LFTs and CBC; once target dose is reached check serum level, LFTs and CBC every 3–6 months initially then yearly; can inhibit the glucuronidation of lamotrigine; can inhibit CYP2C9, CYP2C19; aspirin can increase levels; valproate is highly protein-bound so will increase free warfarin levels. On WHO Essential Medicines List for bipolar disorders. Black Box Warning: Hepatotoxicity, mitochondrial disease, pancreatitis, fetal risk *Mania/Mixed episodes associated with bipolar disorder/Migraine prophylaxis/Specific seizure disorders (see package insert)*

(continued)

TABLE 4.1 Continued

Medication[a]	Adult Dosing[b]	Comments/FDA Indication
Carbamazepine (Tegretol®, Carbatrol®, Equetro®)	For carbamazepine, Tegretol®: Start: 200 mg po bid then check serum trough level after 4–5 days. Dose requirements gradually increase over the first month due to cytochrome enzyme auto-induction. See text for serum levels. Consider reduced dose in patients with hepatic impairment; reductions in oral dose may be needed in those with severe renal impairments.	Check baseline CBC, sodium, LFTs; once target dose is reached check serum level, CBC and LFTs every 3–6 months initially, then yearly; induces CYP1A2, CYP2C9, CYP2C19, CYP3A4 and possibly others; itself is a CYP3A4 substrate. On WHO Essential Medicines List for bipolar disorders. Black Box Warning: Life-threatening rash (TEN/SJS); aplastic anemia and agranulocytosis *Acute mania and mixed episodes/ trigeminal neuralgia/specific seizure disorders (see package insert)*
Lamotrigine (Lamictal®, Lamictal XR®)	For lamotrigine, Lamictal®: Start: 25 mg po q am for first 2 weeks, then 50 mg po q am for 3rd and 4th week, then 100 mg po q am on 5th week, 200 mg po q am on 6th and 7th week, reduce these doses by 50% with concomitant valproate, and increase by 50% with concomitant carbamazepine (see package insert for full details before prescribing). Must restart at 25 mg dose if patient has not taken med for 4–5 days or longer. Dose reductions are needed in patients with moderate to severe hepatic impairments; use with caution in those with severe renal impairment.	Optimal results in bipolar depression may occur if serum level is 4–11 mcg/mL (see text); valproate and sertraline can increase levels; carbamazepine can decrease levels; monitor for rash and toxic epidermal necrolysis/Stevens-Johnson syndrome (TEN/SJS). Primarily metabolized by glucuronidation. On WHO Essential Medicines List for seizures. Black Box Warning: Life-threatening rash (TEN/SJS) *Maintenance treatment for bipolar I disorder to delay the time to occurrence of mood episodes/ Specific seizure disorders (see package insert).*

SEE PACKAGE INSERT FOR DOSING AND OTHER INFORMATION BEFORE PRESCRIBING MEDICATIONS. Dosing should be adjusted downwards ("start low, go slow" strategy) for the elderly and/or the medically compromised. Abbreviations: ACE, angiotensin-converting enzyme; bid (bis in die), twice a day; CBC, complete blood count; CYP, cytochrome P450 enzyme; ECG, electrocardiogram; kg, kilogram; LFT, liver function tests; mg, milligram; NSAIDS, nonsteroidal anti-inflammatory drugs; tid (ter in die), three times a day; TSH, thyroid-stimulating hormone; po (per os), orally; WHO, World Health Organization.

[a]Generic and U.S. brand name(s).

[b]Doses are provided for educational purposes only.

References

Abeysundera H, Gill R (2018). Possible SAMe-induced mania. BMJ Case Rep. doi:10.1136/bcr-2018-224338

Ahrens B, Muller-Oerlinghausen B (2001). Does lithium exert an independent antisuicidal effect? Pharmacopsychiatry 34(4): 132–136.

Alda M (1999). Pharmacogenetics of lithium response in bipolar disorder. J Psychiatry Neurosci 24: 154–158.

Allen MH, Hirschfeld RM, et al. (2006). Linear relationship of valproate serum concentration to response and optimal serum levels for acute mania. Am J Psychiatry 163: 272–275.

American College of Obstetricians and Gynecologists (2008). American College of Obstetricians and Gynecologists practice bulletin: clinical management guidelines for obstetrician-gynecologists, Number 92, April 2008: use of psychiatric medications during pregnancy and lactation. Obstetr Gynecol 111: 1001–1020.

Anand A, Bukhari L, et al. (2005). A preliminary open-label study of zonisamide treatment for bipolar depression in 10 patients. J Clin Psychiatry 66: 195–198.

Ansari A, Osser DN (2010). The psychopharmacology algorithm project at the Harvard South Shore Program: an update on bipolar depression. Harv Rev Psychiatry 18(1): 36–55.

Ansari A, Osser DN (2015). Psychopharmacology, A Concise Overview for Students and Clinicians, 2nd Edition. North Charleston, SC: CreateSpace.

Bachmann RF, Schloesser RJ, et al. (2005). Mood stabilizers target cellular plasticity and resilience cascades: implications for the development of novel therapeutics. Mol Neurobiol 32: 173–202.

Baillon SF, Narayana U, et al. (2018). Valproate preparations for agitation in dementia. Cochrane Database Syst Rev 10: CD003945.

Baldessarini RJ, Leahy L, et al. (2007). Patterns of psychotropic drug prescription for U.S. patients with diagnoses of bipolar disorders. Psychiatr Serv 58(1): 85–91.

Baldessarini RJ, Tondo L, et al. (1999). Effects of lithium treatment and its discontinuation on suicidal behavior in bipolar manic-depressive disorders. J Clin Psychiatry 60(Suppl 2): 77–84.

Baldessarini RJ, Tondo L (2000). Does lithium treatment still work? Evidence of stable responses over three decades. Arch Gen Psychiatry 57(2): 187–190.

Bauer MS, Mitchner L (2004). What is a "mood stabilizer"? An evidence-based response. Am J Psychiatry 161: 3–18.

Bearden CE, Thompson PM, et al. (2007). Greater cortical gray matter density in lithium-treated patients with bipolar disorder. Biol Psychiatry 62: 7–16.

Bendz H, Schon S, et al. (2010). Renal failure occurs in chronic lithium treatment but is uncommon. Kidney Int 77(3): 219–224.

Benedetti F, Riccaboni R, et al. (2014). Rapid treatment response of suicidal symptoms to lithium, sleep deprivation, and light therapy (chronotherapeutics) in drug-resistant bipolar depression. J Clin Psychiatry 75(2): 133–140.

Bergink V, Kushner SA (2014). Lithium during pregnancy. Am J Psychiatry 171(7): 712–715.

Bowden CL, Singh V (2005). Valproate in bipolar disorder: 2000 onwards. Acta Psychiatr Scand Suppl 426: 13–20.

Berridge MJ, Downes CP, et al. (1989). Neural and developmental actions of lithium: a unifying hypothesis. Cell 59(3): 411–419.

Boden R, Lundgren M, et al. (2012). Risks of adverse pregnancy and birth outcomes in women treated or not treated with mood stabilisers for bipolar disorder: population based cohort study. BMJ 345: e7085.

Bowden CL, Brugger AM, et al. (1994). Efficacy of divalproex vs. lithium and placebo in the treatment of mania. JAMA 271: 918–924.

Bowden CL, Calabrese JR, et al. (2003). A placebo-controlled 18-month trial of lamotrigine and lithium maintenance treatment in recently manic or hypomanic patients with bipolar I disorder. Arch Gen Psychiatry 60: 392–400.

Bowden CL, Singh V (2005). Valproate in bipolar disorder: 2000 onwards. Acta Psychiatr Scand Suppl 426: 13–20.

Bowden CL, Vieta E, et al. (2010). Ziprasidone plus a mood stabilizer in subjects with bipolar I disorder: a 6-month, randomized, placebo-controlled, double-blind trial. J Clin Psychiatry 71(2): 130–137.

Cade JF (2000/1949). Lithium salts in the treatment of psychotic excitement. Bull World Health Organ 78(4): 518–520.

Calabrese JR, Bowden CL, et al. (1999). A double-blind placebo-controlled study of lamotrigine monotherapy in outpatients with bipolar I depression. Lamictal 602 Study Group. J Clin Psychiatry 60: 79–88.

Calabrese JR, Bowden CL, et al. (2003). A placebo-controlled 18-month trial of lamotrigine and lithium maintenance treatment in recently depressed patients with bipolar I disorder. J Clin Psychiatry 64: 1013–1024.

Calabrese JR, Huffman RF, et al. (2008). Lamotrigine in the acute treatment of bipolar depression: results of five double-blind, placebo-controlled clinical trials. Bipolar Disord 10: 323–333.

Calabrese JR, Keck PE, et al. (2005). A randomized, double-blind, placebo-controlled trial of quetiapine in the treatment of bipolar I or II depression. Am J Psychiatry 162: 1351–1360.

Calabrese JR, Sullivan JR, et al. (2002). Rash in multicenter trials of lamotrigine in mood disorders: clinical relevance and management. J Clin Psychiatry 63(11): 1012–1019.

Ceron-Litvoc D, Soares BG, et al. (2009). Comparison of carbamazepine and lithium in treatment of bipolar disorder: a systematic review of randomized controlled trials. Hum Psychopharmacol 24(1): 19–28.

Chakrabarti I, Giri A, et al. (2011). An unusual case of thyroid papillary carcinoma with solitary cerebral metastasis presenting with neurological symptoms. Turk Patoloji Derg 27(2): 154–156.

Chang JS, Ha KS, et al. (2006). The effects of long-term clozapine add-on therapy on the rehospitalization rate and the mood polarity patterns in bipolar disorders. J Clin Psychiatry 67(3): 461–467.

Chaudron LH, Jefferson JW (2000). Mood stabilizers during breastfeeding: a review. J Clin Psychiatry 61(2): 79–90.

Chen G, Manji HK (2006). The extracellular signal-regulated kinase pathway: an emerging promising target for mood stabilizers. Curr Opin Psychiatry 19: 313–323.

Chuang DM (2005). The antiapoptotic actions of mood stabilizers: molecular mechanisms and therapeutic potentials. Ann NY Acad Sci 1053: 195–204.

Cipriani A, Barbui C, et al. (2011). Comparative efficacy and acceptability of antimanic drugs in acute mania: a multiple-treatments meta-analysis. Lancet 378(9799): 1306–1315.

Cipriani A, Hawton K, et al. (2013). Lithium in the prevention of suicide in mood disorders: updated systematic review and meta-analysis. BMJ 346: f3646.

Cipriani A, Pretty H, et al. (2005). Lithium in the prevention of suicidal behavior and all-cause mortality in patients with mood disorders: a systematic review of randomized trials. Am J Psychiatry 162: 1805–1819.

Cipriani A, Reid K, et al. (2013). Valproic acid, valproate and divalproex in the maintenance treatment of bipolar disorder. Cochrane Database Syst Rev 10: CD003196.

Coccaro EF, Lee R, et al. (2015). Inflammatory markers and chronic exposure to fluoxetine, divalproex, and placebo in intermittent explosive disorder. Psychiatry Res 229(3): 844–849.

Cohen LS (2007). Treatment of bipolar disorder during pregnancy. J Clin Psychiatry 68(Suppl 9): 4–9.

Cohen LS, Friedman JM, et al. (1994). A reevaluation of risk of in utero exposure to lithium. JAMA 271(2): 146–150.

Cruz N, Sanchez-Moreno J, et al. (2010). Efficacy of modern antipsychotics in placebo-controlled trials in bipolar depression: a meta-analysis. Int J Neuropsychopharmacol 13(1): 5–14.

Dalili H, Nayeri F, et al. (2015). Lamotrigine effects on breastfed infants. Acta Med Iran 53(7): 393–394.

Davis LL, Davidson JR, et al. (2008). Divalproex in the treatment of posttraumatic stress disorder: a randomized, double-blind, placebo-controlled trial in a veteran population. J Clin Psychopharmacol 28(1): 84–88.

De Berardis D, Campanella D, et al. (2003). Thrombocytopenia during valproic acid treatment in young patients with new-onset bipolar disorder. J Clin Psychopharmacol 23: 451–458.

De Fruyt J, Deschepper E, et al. (2012). Second generation antipsychotics in the treatment of bipolar depression: a systematic review and meta-analysis. J Psychopharmacol 26(5): 603–617.

Diav-Citrin O, Shechtman S, et al. (2017). Is it safe to use lamotrigine during pregnancy? A prospective comparative observational study. Birth Defects Res 109(15): 1196–1203.

Diazgranados N, Ibrahim L, et al. (2010). A randomized add-on trial of an N-methyl-D-aspartate antagonist in treatment-resistant bipolar depression. Arch Gen Psychiatry 67(8): 793–802.

Dold M, Kasper S (2017). Evidence-based pharmacotherapy of treatment-resistant unipolar depression. Int J Psychiatry Clin Pract 21(1): 13–23.

Dolk H, Wang H, et al. (2016). Lamotrigine use in pregnancy and risk of orofacial cleft and other congenital anomalies. Neurology 86(18): 1716–1725.

Dols A, Sienaert P, et al. (2013). The prevalence and management of side effects of lithium and anticonvulsants as mood stabilizers in bipolar disorder from a clinical perspective: a review. Int Clin Psychopharmacol 28(6): 287–296.

Donix M, Bauer M (2016). Population studies of association between lithium and risk of neurodegenerative disorders. Curr Alzheimer Res 13(8): 873–878.

Dreifuss FE, Santilli N, Langer DH, et al. (1987). Valproic acid hepatic fatalities: a retrospective review. Neurology 37(3): 379–385.

Drug and Lactation Database (2018). Lithium. https://www.ncbi.nlm.nih.gov/books/NBK501153/

Durgam S, Earley W, et al. (2016). An 8-week randomized, double-blind, placebo-controlled evaluation of the safety and efficacy of cariprazine in patients with bipolar I depression. Am J Psychiatry 173(3): 271–281.

Earley W, Burgess MV, et al. (2019). Cariprazine treatment of bipolar depression: a randomized double-blind placebo-controlled phase 3 study. Am J Psychiatry 176(6): 439–448.

Edwards SJ, Hamilton V, et al. (2013). Lithium or an atypical antipsychotic drug in the management of treatment-resistant depression: a systematic review and economic evaluation. Health Technol Assess 17(54): 1–190.

El-Mallakh RS, Ghaemi SN, et al. (2008). Antidepressant-associated chronic irritable dysphoria (ACID) in STEP-BD patients. J Affect Disord 111(2–3): 372–377.

El-Mallakh RS, Penagaluri P, et al. (2010). Long-term use of pramipexole in bipolar depression: a naturalistic retrospective chart review. Psychiatr Q 81(3): 207–213.

El-Mallakh RS, Vohringer PA, et al. (2015). Antidepressants worsen rapid-cycling course in bipolar depression: A STEP-BD randomized clinical trial. J Affect Disord 184: 318–321.

Finley PR, Warner MD, Peabody CA (1995). Clinical relevance of drug interactions with lithium. Clin Pharmacokinet 29(3): 172–191.

Food and Drug Administration (2007). Clinical Review, Adverse Events (Carbamazepine). https://www.accessdata.fda.gov/drugsatfda_docs/nda/2007/016608s098,020712s029,021710_ClinRev.pdf

Food and Drug Administration (2010). FDA Drug Safety Communication: Aseptic meningitis associated with use of Lamictal (lamotrigine). https://www.fda.gov/drugs/postmarket-drug-safety-information-patients-and-providers/fda-drug-safety-communication-aseptic-meningitis-associated-use-lamictal-lamotrigine

Food and Drug Administration (2018). FDA Drug Safety Communication: FDA warns of serious immune system reaction with seizure and mental health medicine lamotrigine. https://www.fda.gov/drugs/drug-safety-and-availability/fda-drug-safety-communication-fda-warns-serious-immune-system-reaction-seizure-and-mental-health

Forlenza OV, Aprahamian I, et al. (2016). Lithium, a therapy for AD: current evidence from clinical trials of neurodegenerative disorders. Curr Alzheimer Res 13(8): 879–886.

Forlenza OV, De-Paula VJ, Diniz BS (2014). Neuroprotective effects of lithium: implications for the treatment of Alzheimer's disease and related neurodegenerative disorders. ACS Chem Neurosci 5(6): 443–450.

Fornai F, Longone P, et al. (2008). Lithium delays progression of amyotrophic lateral sclerosis. Proc Natl Acad Sci U S A 105: 2052–2057.

Fountoulakis KN, Kontis D, et al. (2012). Treatment of mixed bipolar states. Int J Neuropsychopharmacol 15(7): 1015–1026.

Frances AJ, Kahn DA, et al. (1998). The Expert Consensus Guidelines for treating depression in bipolar disorder. J Clin Psychiatry 59(Suppl 4): 73–79.

Freeman TW, Clothier JL, et al. (1992): A double-blind comparison of valproate and lithium in the treatment of acute mania. Am J Psychiatry 149: 108–111.

Galizia I, Oldani L, et al. (2016). S-adenosyl methionine (SAMe) for depression in adults. Cochrane Database Syst Rev 10: CD011286.

Gamez J, Salvado M, et al. (2016). Lithium for treatment of amyotrophic lateral sclerosis: much ado about nothing. Neurologia 31(8): 550–561.

Geddes JR, Calabrese JR, et al. (2009). Lamotrigine for treatment of bipolar depression: independent meta-analysis and meta-regression of individual patient data from five randomised trials. Br J Psychiatry 194(1): 4–9.

Geddes JR, Goodwin GM, et al. (2010). Lithium plus valproate combination therapy versus monotherapy for relapse prevention in bipolar I disorder (BALANCE): a randomised open-label trial. Lancet 375(9712): 385–395.

Gerstner T, Teich M, et al. (2006). Valproate-associated coagulopathies are frequent and variable in children. Epilepsia 47: 1136–1143.

Ghaemi SN, Berv DA, et al. (2003). Oxcarbazepine treatment of bipolar disorder. J Clin Psychiatry 64: 943–945.

Ghaemi SN, Hsu DJ, et al. (2003). Antidepressants in bipolar disorder: the case for caution. Bipolar Disord 5(6): 421–433.

Ghaemi SN, Ostacher M, et al. (2010). Antidepressant discontinuation in bipolar depression: a Systematic Treatment Enhancement Program for Bipolar Disorder (El-Mallakh, Ghaemi, et al.) randomized clinical trial of long-term effectiveness and safety. J Clin Psychiatry 71(4): 372–380.

Gitlin M (2016). Lithium side effects and toxicity: prevalence and management strategies. Int J Bipolar Disord 4(1): 27.

Glue P, Herbison P (2015). Comparative efficacy and acceptability of combined antipsychotics and mood stabilizers versus individual drug classes for acute mania: network meta-analysis. Aust N Z J Psychiatry 49(12): 1215–1220.

Goikolea JM, Colom F, et al. (2013). Lower rate of depressive switch following antimanic treatment with second-generation antipsychotics versus haloperidol. J Affect Disord 144(3): 191–198.

Goldberg JF, Perlis RH, et al. (2007). Adjunctive antidepressant use and symptomatic recovery among bipolar depressed patients with concomitant manic symptoms: findings from the STEP-BD. Am J Psychiatry 164: 1348–1355.

Goodwin FK, Whitham EA, et al. (2011). Maintenance treatment study designs in bipolar disorder: do they demonstrate that atypical neuroleptics (antipsychotics) are mood stabilizers? CNS Drugs 25(10): 819–827.

Gronseth G, Cruccu G, et al. (2008). Practice parameter: the diagnostic evaluation and treatment of trigeminal neuralgia (an evidence-based review): report of the Quality Standards Subcommittee of the American Academy of Neurology and the European Federation of Neurological Societies. Neurology 71(15): 1183–1190.

Grunfeld JP, Rossier BC (2009). Lithium nephrotoxicity revisited. Nat Rev Nephrol 5(5): 270–276.

Grunze H, Langosch J, et al. (2003). Levetiracetam in the treatment of acute mania: an open add-on study with an on-off-on design. J Clin Psychiatry 64: 781–784.

Grunze HC, Normann C, et al. (2001). Antimanic efficacy of topiramate in 11 patients in an open trial with an on-off-on design. J Clin Psychiatry 62: 464–468.

Grunze H, Vieta E, et al. (2009). The World Federation of Societies of Biological Psychiatry (WFSBP) guidelines for the biological treatment of bipolar disorders: update 2009 on the treatment of acute mania. World J Biol Psychiatry 10(2): 85–116.

Guzzetta F, Tondo L, et al. (2007). Lithium treatment reduces suicide risk in recurrent major depressive disorder. J Clin Psychiatry 68(3): 380–383.

Hajek T, Bauer M, et al. (2012). Large positive effect of lithium on prefrontal cortex N-acetylaspartate in patients with bipolar disorder: 2-centre study. J Psychiatry Neurosci 37(3): 185–192.

Hajek T, Kopecek M, et al. (2012). Smaller hippocampal volumes in patients with bipolar disorder are masked by exposure to lithium: a meta-analysis. J Psychiatry Neurosci 37(5): 333–343.

Hamner MB, Faldowski RA, et al. (2009). A preliminary controlled trial of divalproex in posttraumatic stress disorder. Ann Clin Psychiatry 21(2): 89–94.

Harwood AJ (2005). Lithium and bipolar mood disorder: the inositol-depletion hypothesis revisited. Mol Psychiatry 10(1): 117–126.

Haskey C, Galbally M (2017). Mood stabilizers in pregnancy and child developmental outcomes: A systematic review. Aust N Z J Psychiatry 51(11): 1087–1097.

Hayes JF, Marston L, et al. (2016). Lithium vs. valproate vs. olanzapine vs. quetiapine as maintenance monotherapy for bipolar disorder: a population-based UK cohort study using electronic health records. World Psychiatry 15(1): 53–58.

Heres S, Davis J, et al. (2006). Why olanzapine beats risperidone, risperidone beats quetiapine, and quetiapine beats olanzapine: an exploratory analysis of head-to-head comparison studies of second-generation antipsychotics. Am J Psychiatry 163: 185–194.

Hinc-Kasprzyk J, Polak-Krzeminska A, Ozog-Zabolska I (2015). Toxic epidermal necrolysis. Anaesthesiol Intensive Ther 47(3): 257–262.

Hirschfeld RM, Bowden CL, et al. (2010). A randomized, placebo-controlled, multicenter study of divalproex sodium extended-release in the acute treatment of mania. J Clin Psychiatry 71(4): 426–432.

Horowitz MA, Taylor D (2019). Tapering of SSRI treatment to mitigate withdrawal symptoms. Lancet Psychiatry 6(6): 538–546.

Hou L, Heilbronner U, et al. (2016). Genetic variants associated with response to lithium treatment in bipolar disorder: a genome-wide association study. Lancet 387(10023): 1085–1093.

Hsu CH, Liu PY, et al. (2005). Electrocardiographic abnormalities as predictors for over-range lithium levels. Cardiology 103(2): 101–106.

Huband N, Ferriter M, et al. (2010). Antiepileptics for aggression and associated impulsivity. Cochrane Database Syst Rev 2: CD003499.

Jefferson JW (2010). A clinician's guide to monitoring kidney function in lithium-treated patients. J Clin Psychiatry 71(9): 1153–1157.

Joffe H, Cohen LS, et al. (2006). Valproate is associated with new-onset oligoamenorrhea with hyperandrogenism in women with bipolar disorder. Biol Psychiatry 59: 1078–1086.

Johannessen CU (2000). Mechanisms of action of valproate: a commentary. Neurochem Int 37: 103–110.

Johannessen Landmark C (2008). Antiepileptic drugs in non-epilepsy disorders: relations between mechanism of action and clinical efficacy. CNS Drugs 22: 27–47.

Johnston AM, Eagles JM (1999). Lithium-associated clinical hypothyroidism: prevalence and risk factors. Br J Psychiatry 175: 336–339.

Kakkar AK, Rehan HS, et al. (2009). Comparative efficacy and safety of oxcarbazepine versus divalproex sodium in the treatment of acute mania: a pilot study. Eur Psychiatry 24(3): 178–182.

Karas Kuzelicki N (2016). S-adenosyl methionine in the therapy of depression and other psychiatric disorders. Drug Dev Res 77(7): 346–356.

Katayama Y, Terao T, et al. (2014). Therapeutic window of lamotrigine for mood disorders: a naturalistic retrospective study. Pharmacopsychiatry 47(3): 111–114.

Keck PE Jr, Calabrese JR, et al. (2006). A randomized, double-blind, placebo-controlled 26-week trial of aripiprazole in recently manic patients with bipolar I disorder. J Clin Psychiatry 67(4): 626–637.

Keck PE Jr, Calabrese JR, et al. (2007). Aripiprazole monotherapy for maintenance therapy in bipolar I disorder: a 100-week, double-blind study versus placebo. J Clin Psychiatry 68(10): 1480–1491.

Keck PE Jr, Strawn JR, et al. (2006). Pharmacologic treatment considerations in co-occurring bipolar and anxiety disorders. J Clin Psychiatry 67(Suppl 1): 8–15.

Kelly T, Lieberman DZ (2009). The use of triiodothyronine as an augmentation agent in treatment-resistant bipolar II and bipolar disorder NOS. J Affect Disord 116(3): 222–226.

Kemp DE, Johnson E, et al. (2011). Clinical utility of early improvement to predict response or remission in acute mania: focus on olanzapine and risperidone. J Clin Psychiatry 72(9): 1236–1241.

Kessing LV, Gerds TA, et al. (2015). Use of lithium and anticonvulsants and the rate of chronic kidney disease: a nationwide population-based study. JAMA Psychiatry 72(12): 1182–1191.

Kessing LV, Hellmund G, et al. (2011). Valproate v. lithium in the treatment of bipolar disorder in clinical practice: observational nationwide register-based cohort study. Br J Psychiatry 199(1): 57–63.

Kirkham E, Skinner J, et al. (2014). One lithium level >1.0 mmol/L causes an acute decline in eGFR: findings from a retrospective analysis of a monitoring database. BMJ Open 4(11): e006020.

Kleindienst N, Severus WE, et al. (2005). Is polarity of recurrence related to serum lithium level in patients with bipolar disorder? Eur Arch Psychiatry Clin Neurosci 255: 72–74.

Kleindienst N, Severus WE, et al. (2007). Are serum lithium levels related to the polarity of recurrence in bipolar disorders? Evidence from a multicenter trial. Int Clin Psychopharmacol 22: 125–131.

Kushner SF, Khan A, et al. (2006). Topiramate monotherapy in the management of acute mania: results of four double-blind placebo-controlled trials. Bipolar Disord 8(1): 15–27.

Lahteenvuo M, Tanskanen A, et al. (2018). Real-world effectiveness of pharmacologic treatments for the prevention of rehospitalization in a Finnish nationwide cohort of patients with bipolar disorder. JAMA Psychiatry 75(4): 347–355.

Lenox RH, Hahn CG (2000). Overview of the mechanism of action of lithium in the brain: fifty-year update. J Clin Psychiatry 61(Suppl 9): 5–15.

Lepkifker E, Sverdlik A, et al. (2004). Renal insufficiency in long-term lithium treatment. J Clin Psychiatry 65: 850–856.

Leroy K, Ando K, et al. (2010). Lithium treatment arrests the development of neurofibrillary tangles in mutant tau transgenic mice with advanced neurofibrillary pathology. J Alzheimers Dis 19(2): 705–719.

Lexicomp (2019). https://www.wolterskluwercdi.com/lexicomp-online/

Li XB, Tang YL, et al. (2015). Clozapine for treatment-resistant bipolar disorder: a systematic review. Bipolar Disord 17(3): 235–247.

Licht RW (2012). Lithium: still a major option in the management of bipolar disorder. CNS Neurosci Ther 18(3): 219–226.

Licht RW, Nielsen JN, et al. (2010). Lamotrigine versus lithium as maintenance treatment in bipolar I disorder: an open, randomized effectiveness study mimicking clinical practice. The 6th trial of the Danish University Antidepressant Group (DUAG-6). Bipolar Disord 12(5): 483–493.

Livingstone C, Rampes H (2006). Lithium: a review of its metabolic adverse effects. J Psychopharmacol 20(3): 347–355.

Loebel A, Cucchiaro J, et al. (2014). Lurasidone monotherapy in the treatment of bipolar I depression: a randomized, double-blind, placebo-controlled study. Am J Psychiatry 171(2): 160–168.

Lyoo IK, Dager SR, et al. (2010). Lithium-induced gray matter volume increase as a neural correlate of treatment response in bipolar disorder: a longitudinal brain imaging study. Neuropsychopharmacology 35(8): 1743–1750.

Macdonald KJ, Young LT (2002). Newer antiepileptic drugs in bipolar disorder: rationale for use and role in therapy. CNS Drugs 16: 549–562.

Macfadden W, Alphs L, et al. (2009). A randomized, double-blind, placebo-controlled study of maintenance treatment with adjunctive risperidone long-acting therapy in patients with bipolar I disorder who relapse frequently. Bipolar Disord 11(8): 827–839.

Machado-Vieira R, Ibrahim L, et al. (2012). Novel glutamatergic agents for major depressive disorder and bipolar disorder. Pharmacol Biochem Behav 100(4): 678–687.

Marangell LB, Dennehy EB, et al. (2008): Case-control analyses of the impact of pharmacotherapy on prospectively observed suicide attempts and completed suicides in bipolar disorder: findings from STEP-BD. J Clin Psychiatry 69: 916–922.

Marcus R, Khan A, et al. (2011). Efficacy of aripiprazole adjunctive to lithium or valproate in the long-term treatment of patients with bipolar I disorder with an inadequate response to lithium or valproate monotherapy: a multicenter, double-blind, randomized study. Bipolar Disord 13(2): 133–144.

McCloud TL, Caddy C, et al. (2015). Ketamine and other glutamate receptor modulators for depression in bipolar disorder in adults. Cochrane Database Syst Rev 9: CD011611.

McGirr A, Vohringer PA, et al. (2016). Safety and efficacy of adjunctive second-generation antidepressant therapy with a mood stabiliser or an atypical antipsychotic in acute bipolar depression: a systematic review and meta-analysis of randomised placebo-controlled trials. Lancet Psychiatry 3(12): 1138–1146.

McKnight RF, Adida M, et al. (2012). Lithium toxicity profile: a systematic review and meta-analysis. Lancet 379(9817): 721–728.

Meador KJ, Baker GA, et al. (2009). Cognitive function at 3 years of age after fetal exposure to antiepileptic drugs. N Engl J Med 360(16): 1597–1605.

Meador KJ, Baker GA, et al. (2013). Fetal antiepileptic drug exposure and cognitive outcomes at age 6 years (NEAD study): a prospective observational study. Lancet Neurol 12(3): 244–252.

Meehan AD, Humble MB, et al. (2015). The prevalence of lithium-associated hyperparathyroidism in a large Swedish population attending psychiatric outpatient units. J Clin Psychopharmacol 35(3): 279–285.

Miklowitz DJ, Otto MW, et al. (2007). Psychosocial treatments for bipolar depression: a 1-year randomized trial from the Systematic Treatment Enhancement Program. Arch Gen Psychiatry 64: 419–426.

Mohammad OM, Osser DN (2014). The Psychopharmacology Algorithm Project at the Harvard South Shore Program: an algorithm for acute mania. Harv Rev Psychiatry 22(5): 274–294.

Moore GJ, Cortese BM, et al. (2009). A longitudinal study of the effects of lithium treatment on prefrontal and subgenual prefrontal gray matter volume in treatment-responsive bipolar disorder patients. J Clin Psychiatry 70(5): 699–705.

Moretti ME, Koren G, et al. (2003). Monitoring lithium in breast milk: an individualized approach for breast-feeding mothers. Ther Drug Monit 25(3): 364–366.

Mukai T, Kishi T, et al. (2014). A meta-analysis of inositol for depression and anxiety disorders. Hum Psychopharmacol 29(1): 55–63.

Nelson JC, Baumann P, et al. (2014). A systematic review and meta-analysis of lithium augmentation of tricyclic and second generation antidepressants in major depression. J Affect Disord 168: 269–275.

Nestler EJ, Hyman SE, et al. (2015). *Molecular Neuropharmacology, A Foundation for Clinical Neuroscience, 3rd Edition*. New York, NY: McGraw-Hill.

Newport DJ, Pennell PB, et al. (2008). Lamotrigine in breast milk and nursing infants: determination of exposure. Pediatrics 122(1): e223–e231.

Nielsen J, Kane JM, Correll CU (2012). Real-world effectiveness of clozapine in patients with bipolar disorder: results from a 2-year mirror-image study. Bipolar Disord 14(8): 863–869.

Novick DM, Swartz HA, Frank E (2010). Suicide attempts in bipolar I and bipolar II disorder: a review and meta-analysis of the evidence. Bipolar Disord 12(1): 1–9.

Nunes PV, Forlenza OV, et al. (2007). Lithium and risk for Alzheimer's disease in elderly patients with bipolar disorder. Br J Psychiatry 190: 359–360.

O'Donovan C, Kusumakar V, et al. (2002). Menstrual abnormalities and polycystic ovary syndrome in women taking valproate for bipolar mood disorder. J Clin Psychiatry 63: 322–330.

Ortenzi A, Paggi A, et al. (2008). Oxcarbazepine and adverse events: impact of age, dosage, metabolite serum concentrations and concomitant antiepileptic therapy. Funct Neurol 23: 97–100.

Osser DN (2008). Cleaning up evidence-based psychopharmacology. Psychopharm Rev 43(3): 19–26.

Pacchiarotti I, Bond DJ, et al. (2103). The International Society for Bipolar Disorders (ISBD) task force report on antidepressant use in bipolar disorders. Am J Psychiatry 170(11): 1249–1262.

Pacchiarotti I, Leon-Caballero J, et al. (2016). Mood stabilizers and antipsychotics during breastfeeding: focus on bipolar disorder. Eur Neuropsychopharmacol 26(10): 1562–1578.

Pande AC, Crockatt JG, et al. (2000). Gabapentin in bipolar disorder: a placebo-controlled trial of adjunctive therapy. Gabapentin Bipolar Disorder Study Group. Bipolar Disord 2: 249–255.

Paraskevas GP, Triantafyllou N, et al. (2006). Add-on lamotrigine treatment and plasma glutamate levels in epilepsy: relation to treatment response. Epilepsy Res 70(2–3): 184–189.

Patel N, Viguera AC, Baldessarini RJ (2018). Mood-stabilizing anticonvulsants, spina bifida, and folate supplementation: commentary. J Clin Psychopharmacol 38(1): 7–10.

Patorno E, Huybrechts KF, et al. (2017). Lithium use in pregnancy and the risk of cardiac malformations. N Engl J Med 376(23): 2245–2254.

PDR (2019). Precribers digital reference. http://www.pdr.net.

Perlis RH, Welge JA, et al. (2006). Atypical antipsychotics in the treatment of mania: a meta-analysis of randomized, placebo-controlled trials. J Clin Psychiatry 67(4): 509–516.

Perucca E (2006). Clinically relevant drug interactions with antiepileptic drugs. Br J Clin Pharmacol 61: 246–255.

Perugi G, Medda P, et al. (2017). The role of electroconvulsive therapy (ECT) in bipolar disorder: effectiveness in 522 patients with bipolar depression, mixed-state, mania and catatonic features. Curr Neuropharmacol 15(3): 359–371.

Plantier D, Luaute J (2016). Drugs for behavior disorders after traumatic brain injury: systematic review and expert consensus leading to French recommendations for good practice. Ann Phys Rehabil Med 59(1): 42–57.

Pompili M, Longo L, et al. (2017). Polyunsaturated fatty acids and suicide risk in mood disorders: a systematic review. Prog Neuropsychopharmacol Biol Psychiatry 74: 43–56.

Post RM (1990). Sensitization and kindling perspectives for the course of affective illness: toward a new treatment with the anticonvulsant carbamazepine. Pharmacopsychiatry 23(1): 3–17.

Post RM, Uhde TW, et al. (1982). Kindling and carbamazepine in affective illness. J Nerv Ment Dis 170(12): 717–731.

Pratoomsri W, Yatham LN, et al. (2006). Oxcarbazepine in the treatment of bipolar disorder: a review. Can J Psychiatry 51: 540–545.

Quiroz JA, Yatham LN, et al. (2010). Risperidone long-acting injectable monotherapy in the maintenance treatment of bipolar I disorder. Biol Psychiatry 68(2): 156–162.

Rutkofsky IH, Khan AS, et al. (2017). The psychoneuroimmunological role of omega-3 polyunsaturated fatty acids in major depressive disorder and bipolar disorder. Adv Mind Body Med 31(3): 8–16.

Sachs GS (1990). Use of clonazepam for bipolar affective disorder. J Clin Psychiatry 51(Suppl): 31–34; discussion 50–53.

Sachs GS, Nierenberg AA, et al. (2007). Effectiveness of adjunctive antidepressant treatment for bipolar depression. N Engl J Med 356: 1711–1722.

Sachs GS, Rosenbaum JF, et al. (1990). Adjunctive clonazepam for maintenance treatment of bipolar affective disorder. J Clin Psychopharmacol 10(1): 42–47.

Sachs GS, Thase ME, et al. (2003). Rationale, design, and methods of the systematic treatment enhancement program for bipolar disorder (STEP-BD). Biol Psychiatry 53(11): 1028–1042.

Sarris J, Mischoulon D, Schweitzer I (2012). Omega-3 for bipolar disorder: meta-analyses of use in mania and bipolar depression. J Clin Psychiatry 73(1): 81–86.

Scrandis DA (2017). Bipolar disorder in pregnancy: a review of pregnancy outcomes. J Midwifery Womens Health 62(6): 673–683.

Serretti A, Drago A, et al. (2009). Lithium pharmacodynamics and pharmacogenetics: focus on inositol mono phosphatase (IMPase), inositol poliphosphatase (IPPase) and glycogen sinthase kinase 3 beta (GSK-3 beta). Curr Med Chem 16(15): 1917–1948.

Severus WE, Kleindienst N, et al. (2008). What is the optimal serum lithium level in the long-term treatment of bipolar disorder?—a review. Bipolar Disord 10: 231–237.

Shaldubina A, Agam G, et al. (2001). The mechanism of lithium action: state of the art, ten years later. Prog Neuropsychopharmacol Biol Psych 25: 855–866.

Sit DK, McGowan J, et al. (2018). Adjunctive bright light therapy for bipolar depression: a randomized double-blind placebo-controlled trial. Am J Psychiatry 175(2): 131–139.

Smith LA, Cornelius V, et al. (2007). Pharmacological interventions for acute bipolar mania: a systematic review of randomized placebo-controlled trials. Bipolar Disord 9(6): 551–560.

Song J, Sjolander A, et al. (2017). Suicidal behavior during lithium and valproate treatment: a within-individual 8-year prospective study of 50,000 patients with bipolar disorder. Am J Psychiatry 174(8): 795–802.

Stamm TJ, Lewitzka U, et al. (2014). Supraphysiological doses of levothyroxine as adjunctive therapy in bipolar depression: a randomized, double-blind, placebo-controlled study. J Clin Psychiatry 75(2): 162–68.

Suppes T, Vieta E, et al. (2009). Maintenance treatment for patients with bipolar I disorder: results from a North American study of quetiapine in combination with lithium or divalproex (trial 127). Am J Psychiatry 166(4): 476–488.

Swann AC, Lafer B, et al. (2013). Bipolar mixed states: an International Society for Bipolar Disorders task force report of symptom structure, course of illness, and diagnosis. Am J Psychiatry 170(1): 31–42.

Takeshima M (2017). Treating mixed mania/hypomania: a review and synthesis of the evidence. CNS Spectr 22(2): 177–185.

Tarr GP, Glue P, et al. (2011). Comparative efficacy and acceptability of mood stabilizer and second generation antipsychotic monotherapy for acute mania—a systematic review and meta-analysis. J Affect Disord 134(1–3): 14–19.

Thase ME, Jonas A, et al. (2008). Aripiprazole monotherapy in nonpsychotic bipolar I depression: results of 2 randomized, placebo-controlled studies. J Clin Psychopharmacol 28(1): 13–20.

Thase ME, Macfadden W, et al. (2006). Efficacy of quetiapine monotherapy in bipolar I and II depression: a double-blind, placebo-controlled study (the BOLDER II study). J Clin Psychopharmacol 26: 600–609.

Thirthalli J, Prasad MK, Gangadhar BN (2012). Electroconvulsive therapy (ECT) in bipolar disorder: a narrative review of literature. Asian J Psychiatr 5(1): 11–17.

Tohen M, Calabrese JR, et al. (2006). Randomized, placebo-controlled trial of olanzapine as maintenance therapy in patients with bipolar I disorder responding to acute treatment with olanzapine. Am J Psychiatry 163(2): 247–256.

Tohen M, Chengappa KN, et al. (2004). Relapse prevention in bipolar I disorder: 18-month comparison of olanzapine plus mood stabiliser v. mood stabiliser alone. Br J Psychiatry 184: 337–345.

Tohen M, Vieta E (2009). Antipsychotic agents in the treatment of bipolar mania. Bipolar Disord 11(Suppl 2): 45–54.

Tohen M, Vieta E, et al. (2003). Efficacy of olanzapine and olanzapine-fluoxetine combination in the treatment of bipolar I depression. Arch Gen Psychiatry 60(11): 1079–1088.

Tohen M, Zarate CA Jr (1998). Antipsychotic agents and bipolar disorder. J Clin Psychiatry 59(Suppl 1): 38–48; discussion 49.

Tomson T, Battino D, et al. (2011). Dose-dependent risk of malformations with antiepileptic drugs: an analysis of data from the EURAP epilepsy and pregnancy registry. Lancet Neurol 10(7): 609–617.

Tondo L, Abramowicz M, et al. (2017). Long-term lithium treatment in bipolar disorder: effects on glomerular filtration rate and other metabolic parameters. Int J Bipolar Disord 5(1): 27.

Tondo L, Hennen J, Baldessarini RJ (2001). Lower suicide risk with long-term lithium treatment in major affective illness: a meta-analysis. Acta Psychiatr Scand 104(3): 163–172.

Tondo L, Pompili M, et al. (2016). Suicide attempts in bipolar disorders: comprehensive review of 101 reports. Acta Psychiatr Scand 133(3): 174–186.

Trixler M, Gati A, et al. (2005). Use of antipsychotics in the management of schizophrenia during pregnancy. Drugs 65(9): 1193–1206.

Uguz F, Sharma V (2016). Mood stabilizers during breastfeeding: a systematic review of the recent literature. Bipolar Disord 18(4): 325–333.

Vaidya NA, Mahableshwarkar AR, Shahid R (2003). Continuation and maintenance ECT in treatment-resistant bipolar disorder. J ECT 19(1): 10–16.

Vajda FJ, Graham JE, et al. (2012). Teratogenicity of the newer antiepileptic drugs—the Australian experience. J Clin Neurosci 19(1): 57–59.

Vajda FJ, Graham JE, et al. (2019). Antiepileptic drugs and foetal malformation: analysis of 20 years of data in a pregnancy register. Seizure 65: 6–11.

Valerio MP, Martino DJ (2018). Differential response to lithium between melancholic and non-melancholic unipolar depression. Psychiatry Res 269: 183–184.

Vasudev A, Macritchie K, et al. (2011). Oxcarbazepine for acute affective episodes in bipolar disorder. Cochrane Database Syst Rev 12: CD004857.

Veroniki AA, Rios P, et al. (2017). Comparative safety of antiepileptic drugs for neurological development in children exposed during pregnancy and breast feeding: a systematic review and network meta-analysis. BMJ Open 7(7): e017248.

Vieta E, Goikolea JM, et al. (2003). 1-year follow-up of patients treated with risperidone and topiramate for a manic episode. J Clin Psychiatry 64: 834–839.

Vieta E, Manuel Goikolea, J, et al. (2006). A double-blind, randomized, placebo-controlled, prophylaxis study of adjunctive gabapentin for bipolar disorder. J Clin Psychiatry 67: 473–477.

Vieta E, Sanchez-Moreno J, et al. (2003). Adjunctive topiramate in bipolar II disorder. World J Biol Psychiatry 4: 172–176.

Vieta E, Suppes T, et al. (2008). Efficacy and safety of quetiapine in combination with lithium or divalproex for maintenance of patients with bipolar I disorder (international trial 126). J Affect Disord 109(3): 251–263.

Viguera AC, Koukopoulos A, et al. (2007). Teratogenicity and anticonvulsants: lessons from neurology to psychiatry. J Clin Psychiatry 68(Suppl 9): 29–33.

Viguera AC, Whitfield T, et al. (2007). Risk of recurrence in women with bipolar disorder during pregnancy: prospective study of mood stabilizer discontinuation. Am J Psychiatry 164(12): 1817–1824; quiz 1923.

Wagner KD, Redden L, et al. (2009). A double-blind, randomized, placebo-controlled trial of divalproex extended-release in the treatment of bipolar disorder in children and adolescents. J Am Acad Child Adolesc Psychiatry 48(5): 519–532.

Wegner I, Wilhelm AJ, et al. (2014). Effect of oral contraceptives on lamotrigine levels depends on comedication. Acta Neurol Scand 129(6): 393–398.

Weisler RH, Kalali AH, et al. (2004). A multicenter, randomized, double-blind, placebo-controlled trial of extended-release carbamazepine capsules as monotherapy for bipolar disorder patients with manic or mixed episodes. J Clin Psychiatry 65: 478–484.

Weisler RH, Keck PE, et al. (2005). Extended-release carbamazepine capsules as monotherapy for acute mania in bipolar disorder: a multicenter, randomized, double-blind, placebo-controlled trial. J Clin Psychiatry 66: 323–330.

Weisler RH, Nolen WA, et al. (2011). Continuation of quetiapine versus switching to placebo or lithium for maintenance treatment of bipolar I disorder (Trial 144: a randomized controlled study). J Clin Psychiatry 72(11): 1452–1464.

230 | PSYCHOPHARMACOLOGY

Wiffen PJ, Derry S, Moore RA (2013). Lamotrigine for chronic neuro-pathic pain and fibromyalgia in adults. Cochrane Database Syst Rev 12: CD006044.

Wingo AP, Wingo TS, et al. (2009). Effects of lithium on cognitive performance: a meta-analysis. J Clin Psychiatry 70(11): 1588–1597.

Won E, Kim YK (2017). An oldie but goodie: lithium in the treatment of bipolar disorder through neuroprotective and neurotrophic mechanisms. Int J Mol Sci 18(12).

World Health Organization (2019). World Health Organization model list of essential medicines, 21st list. https://apps.who.int/iris/bitstream/handle/10665/325771/WHO-MVP-EMP-IAU-2019.06-eng.pdf?ua=1

Yatham LN, Kusumakar V, et al. (2002). Third generation anticonvulsants in bipolar disorder: a review of efficacy and summary of clinical recommendations. J Clin Psychiatry 63: 275–283.

Young AH (2013). Review: lithium reduces the risk of suicide compared with placebo in people with depression and bipolar disorder. Evid Based Ment Health 16(4): 112.

Young AH, Geddes JR, et al. (2006). Tiagabine in the maintenance treatment of bipolar disorders. Cochrane Database Syst Rev: CD005173.

Young AH, Geddes JR, et al. (2006). Tiagabine in the treatment of acute affective episodes in bipolar disorder: efficacy and acceptability. Cochrane Database Syst Rev: CD004694.

Young AH, McElroy SL, et al. (2010). A double-blind, placebo-controlled study of quetiapine and lithium monotherapy in adults in the acute phase of bipolar depression (EMBOLDEN I). J Clin Psychiatry 71(2): 150–162.

Zarate CA Jr, Brutsche NE, et al. (2012). Replication of ketamine's antidepressant efficacy in bipolar depression: a randomized controlled add-on trial. Biol Psychiatry 71(11): 939–946.

Zarate CA, Payne JL, et al. (2004). Pramipexole for bipolar II depression: a placebo-controlled proof of concept study. Biol Psychiatry 56(1): 54–60.

5

Stimulants and Other ADHD Medicines

There have been significant increases in stimulant prescriptions for adults with attention-deficit/hyperactivity (ADHD) in recent years (Safer 2016) as the evidence base has been growing (Cortese, Adamo et al. 2018). Most ADHD medications have been prescribed by nonpsychiatric physicians (Olfson, Blanco et al. 2013).

The diagnosis of ADHD in adults is sometimes problematic, but the American Psychiatric Association (APA) added anchor details to the criteria in DSM-5 (APA 2013) that are relevant for adults, and European guidelines have been developed (Canadian Attention Deficit Hyperactivity Disorder Resource Alliance 2011; Kooij, Bijlenga et al. 2019) to aid the process. DSM-5 also reduced the required number of symptoms required for the diagnosis in adults, from six to five out of nine for both the hyperactive and inattention subtypes. Diagnosis currently requires evidence that at least several (but not all five) symptoms were present prior to age 12 (APA 2013). This is often difficult to establish retrospectively and relying on a patient's self-report of childhood ADHD symptoms is likely to be inaccurate in most patients (Mannuzza, Klein et al. 2002; Modesto-Lowe, Chaplin et al. 2015). Getting consultation from a parent or other close observer of the person in childhood is strongly advised. When earlier ADHD symptoms are suspected, it is difficult to rule out other etiologies for these symptoms (e.g., family stressors, childhood depression, learning disorders, etc.).

Nevertheless, there are adults with undiagnosed ADHD, many of whom have other comorbid psychiatric illnesses, who continue to suffer chronic symptoms through adulthood and may benefit from treatment. Others may have had a clear history and diagnosis of ADHD in childhood and as adults may need to have pharmacological treatments considered or resumed. ADHD patients have poorer long-term social and functional outcomes than those without ADHD (e.g., motor vehicle accidents, arrests and convictions for criminal behavior, divorces, accidents and injuries, work attendance and performance, cigarette smoking, and early pregnancies), and yet these can be significantly improved with treatment (Shaw, Hodgkins et al. 2012). Pharmacotherapy can help improve both the primary symptoms of attention deficit, hyperactivity and impulsivity, as well as improve social, functional, and executive functioning in adults with ADHD (Bitter, Angyalosi et al. 2012). Many believe that functional improvement is more strongly related to the acquisition of new skills and behaviors that have to be taught via behavioral therapies. Medications can help patients be more receptive to and able to utilize psychotherapeutic approaches. Unfortunately, many adult patients do not adhere to pharmacotherapy over the long term, which reduces their potential impact (Edvinsson and Ekselius 2018).

Medications available for the treatment of ADHD in adults are discussed next. The use of psychotropics for the treatment of ADHD in children and adolescents is beyond the scope of this chapter. Medication trials in children are discussed here only to help with discussions relevant to adult pharmacotherapy.

Stimulants

Stimulants (or more specifically psychostimulants) are the most effective and usual first-line treatments for nonsubstance-abusing patients with ADHD. **Methylphenidate, dextroamphetamine,** mixed **amphetamine salts**, and **lisdexamfetamine** (a pro-drug converted slowly in the bloodstream to dextroamphetamine) are examples of stimulants used in the treatment of ADHD.

Methylphenidate and amphetamines enhance norepinephrinergic and dopaminergic transmission in the brain. Methylphenidate may primarily disrupt the presynaptic reuptake of these neurotransmitters, whereas amphetamines may do the same while additionally enhancing their intracellular and extracellular release. These effects may occur in the ascending reticular activating system as well as in the regulation of "top–down" cortical-thalamic-striatal circuits (Nestler, Hyman & Malenka 2015). Amphetamines seem to be more potent in their effects than methylphenidate in adults (Cortese, Adamo et al. 2018). Stimulants in general appear to be more efficacious than nonstimulants for ADHD (Cunill, Castells et al. 2016).

Assuming correct diagnosis and adequate dose, stimulants' beneficial effects on attentional symptoms, impulsivity, and hyperactivity are immediate and subside with medication clearance. Emotional dysregulation and oppositional-defiant symptoms may also improve with treatment if they are associated with ADHD (Marchant, Reimherr et al. 2011). Other improvements, such as a reduction in automobile accidents, may also be seen (Cox, Davis et al. 2012). There is recent concern about a possible increase in suicide risk in adults with ADHD (Stickley, Tachimori et al. 2018); results from one longitudinal study suggest that long-term methylphenidate may reduce this risk (Huang, Wei et al. 2018), but more studies are needed to confirm this protective effect.

Short half-life formulations need to be administered multiple times during the day, but not near bedtime. In recent years multiple formulations, such as extended-release, longer-acting, and transdermal medications, have been developed to decrease dosing variations and pharmacokinetic fluctuations and to provide continuous drug effect throughout the day (Ermer, Adeyi & Pucci 2010). It is not clear, however, if differences in drug release formulations improve overall efficacy and outcome in adults (Castells, Ramos-Quiroga et al. 2011). In regard to adequate dosing of stimulants in adults, daily dosing based on body weight (i.e., doses up to 1–1.3 mg/kg/day for methylpenidate and 0.5–0.65 mg/kg/day for amphetamine salts) may provide better results if lower doses are not effective (Spencer, Biederman et al. 2005; Sachdev and Trollor 2000; Biederman, Mick et al. 2006). However, in terms of dosing stimulants, there is significant variablity in pharmacokinetics and response; therefore, starting a stimulant at a low dose and titrating it gradaully allows for better ongoing assessments of effectiveness and tolerability and better individualization of treatment (Ermer, Adeyi & Pucci 2010; Wilens, Morrison & Prince 2011).

Stimulant side effects include decreased appetite, insomnia, and anxiety, necessitating gradual dose titration to improve tolerability. Decreased libido and sweating can also occur (Edvinsson and Ekselius 2018). Blood pressure and heart rate can also increase with stimulant administration so patients with significant cardiac disease may not be good candidates for these medications. When used in healthy adults, however, the short- and long-term cardiac effects of stimulants appear to be mild, and these medicines are generally well tolerated (Bejerot, Ryden et al. 2010; Cooper, Habel et al. 2011; Habel, Cooper et al. 2011; Hammerness, Surman et al. 2011; Edvinsson and Ekselius 2018; Mosholder, Taylor et al. 2018). A Food and Drug Administration (FDA) advisory notes that adults treated with ADHD medications (including atomoxetine, discussed later) do not appear to show an increased risk of serious cardiovascular events, although these medications should be avoided in those with "serious heart problems" (FDA 2011). Possible growth retardation and the development of transient tics, although of concern in children, are not likely to be problematic in adults. In addition to severe cardiovascular abnormalities, the presence of angle-closure glaucoma (which is much more prevalent in patients of Asian descent; Congdon, Wang & Tielsch 1992) and pheochromocytoma are contraindications to stimulant therapy.

Chronic stimulant use (or overuse) can lead to psychosis in susceptible individuals (e.g., patients with schizophrenia or at high risk for schizophrenia), but increased psychosis can also be seen after just one dose (Curran, Byrappa et al. 2004) or otherwise early in treatment. The risk may be greater with amphetamines than with methylphenidate (Moran, Ongur et al. 2019). Given the difficulties in reliably identifying susceptible individuals, all treated patients should be monitored carefully for the emergence of psychosis (Kraemer, Uekermann et al. 2010). Fortunately, most cases of treatment-emergent psychosis resolve completely within days of stimulant discontinuation (Ross 2006). Psychosis is a rare outcome when psychiatrists prescribe stimulants for ADHD compared with when primary care clinicians prescribe them (Moran, Ongur et al. 2019), which may be due to their greater experience and capacity to diagnose persons at risk for psychotic disorders.

Lastly, medication interactions of note include the possible emergence of a hypertensive crisis if stimulants are combined with monoamine oxidase inhibitors. Also, to avoid additive adverse effects, prescription stimulants should not be combined with illicit stimulants such as cocaine, 3,4-methylenedioxymethamphetamine, or methamphetamine. Caffeine taken concurrently with stimulants may increase the risk of tachycardia, and a hyperadrenergic reaction may be seen in patients using over-the-counter ephedra/ephedrine-related compounds such as pseudoephedrine.

The major concern regarding the use of stimulants in adults, however, is the risk of misuse (Compton, Han et al. 2018). This seems related to the stimulants' ability to increase dopaminergic effects in the reward and reinforcement circuitry in the nucleus accumbens. Euphoria, tolerance, and addictive behaviors may develop in susceptible individuals. In the United States, stimulants are highly regulated; they are Schedule II drugs—which indicates that the Drug Enforcement Administration designates them as being in the highest risk category for controlled substances that have an established therapeutic use. Misusers of stimulants are more likely than nonusers to have ADHD, conduct disorder, or substance use disorders (Wilens, Zulauf et al. 2016).

Of note, most misuse of prescribed stimulants occurs with immediate-release formulations. Immediate-release formulations may be four times as likely to be misused than extended-release ones (Dupont, Coleman et al. 2008). Sudden dopamine increases in the nucleus accumbens are thought to be associated with reinforcing effects that might facilitate stimulant abuse. Minimum effective doses or slow-release formulations may therefore serve to decrease the risk of medication abuse. A larger dose of an extended-release stimulant may be *less* reinforcing that a smaller dose of an immediate-release stimulant (Volkow 2006).

The risks of addiction and misuse have led some clinicians to be wary of using stimulants even when treatment with these medications is otherwise medically indicated. However, if the diagnosis of ADHD is accurate, these medications need not be avoided in patients who do not have a history of substance abuse. A clear risk and benefit assessment is necessary. If they do have such a history, then stimulants should probably be avoided in most cases. However, appropriate monitoring and supervision may decrease the risk of abuse. Data suggest no increase in risk of subsequent abuse of stimulants when children and adolescents with ADHD are treated with stimulants (Biederman, Monuteaux et al. 2008). However, this may depend on the developmental stage at which treatment is provided: starting prescription stimulants during high school and college may actually increase the subsequent risk of drug abuse (McCabe, Teter & Boyd 2006; Kollins 2008).

The question arises as to whether stimulant therapy might sometimes decrease the risk of stimulant abuse in some adults. Agonist therapy has been successful in treating some individuals with opioid and tobacco use disorders, and it has been proposed that cocaine and amphetamine use disorders may sometimes respond to a similar strategy. ADHD is considered to be a risk factor for substance abuse. Older data regarding treatment of ADHD as a way to decrease the risk of substance abuse were mixed (Wilens 2004; Wilens, Faraone et al. 2003). More recently, however, there has been some evidence to show that extended-release amphetamine salts (at high doses of 60 and 80 mg daily) may help decrease cocaine use and ADHD symptoms in patients with both disorders (Levin, Mariani et al. 2015) and (combined with topiramate) may reduce cocaine use in patients without ADHD (Mariani, Pavlicova et al. 2012). Levin and colleagues also showed in their high-dose amphetamine salts trial that when improvement in ADHD occurred in the first two weeks, abstinence from cocaine became more likely (Levin, Choi et al. 2018). Extended-release methylphenidate use may decrease methamphetamine use and cravings in methamphetamine users (Rezaei, Emami et al. 2015). In another study of 54 men who resided in a medium security prison in Sweden and who had co-diagnoses of amphetamine dependence and ADHD, extended-release methylphenidate at doses up to 180 mg daily or placebo was initiated 14 days before their release from prison (Konstenius, Jayaram-Lindstrom et al. 2014). They were followed for 24 weeks. The methylphenidate group had significantly more improvement in ADHD and were significantly more likely to have negative amphetamine urines and to be retained in treatment.

Lastly, students and clinicians should be aware that **pemoline** (previously marketed as Cylert®), a central nervous system "stimulant" with an unclear mechanism of action, was used for many years and was deemed to be effective for the treatment of ADHD. Evidence about a significant increase in the risk of hepatotoxicity and hepatic failure (Shevell 1997) led to an FDA boxed warning about these risks in 1999, and the FDA subsequently concluded that these risks outweighed potential benefits (Stein 2005). Pemoline is no longer marketed or sold in the United States or Europe but is still available in Japan where no cases of hepatotoxicity have apparently been reported (Shader 2017).

Nonstimulant Medicines for ADHD

Atomoxetine, a selective norepinephrine reuptake inhibitor (Bymaster, Katner et al. 2002; Yu, Li & Markowitz 2016), has shown efficacy in, and has been primarily marketed for, the treatment of ADHD (Michelson, Adler et al. 2003; Young, Sarkis et al. 2011; Durell, Adler et al. 2013; Ravishankar, Chowdappa et al. 2016). As might be expected by its mechanism of action, it may also have antidepressant effects, but there are no published data to support its use as monotherapy in the treatment of major depression.

Unlike stimulants, which can rapidly improve ADHD symptoms, atomoxetine requires several weeks of treatment before initial response occurs. In children, response in one month may predict greater response later (Savill, Buitelaar et al. 2015). Atomoxetine's efficacy versus placebo in six weeks may be only slightly less than that of methylphenidate (Newcorn, Kratochvil et al. 2008). A meta-analysis of atomoxetine and long-acting (osmotic release) methylphenidate for ADHD found that efficacy against placebo was not significantly different for the two medications in studies up to three months duration (Bushe, Day et al. 2016). Response may increase over the first six months and become comparable to that of methylphenidate (Clemow and Bushe 2015). Because response to atomoxetine is gradual, it may not be felt as robustly as when taking stimulants. In adults, atomoxetine may have greater efficacy in improving symptoms of inattention than those of hyperactivity and impulsivity (Ravishankar, Chowdappa et al. 2016). A practical difficulty in using atomoxetine in patients with ADHD is that it takes so long to work and requires the patient to take the medication with good adherence while waiting for this benefit. This is difficult for many individuals with severe ADHD to remember to do, especially when they are not noticing any benefit. Separation from placebo may not begin to occur for three to five weeks in some studies.

There have been no studies showing that atomoxetine can work in adult patients who have failed to respond to initial trials with stimulants such as methylphenidate. However, there is one study in children and adolescents showing that 43% can respond to atomoxetine after failing a six-week trial of methylphenidate (Newcorn, Kratochvil et al. 2008).

Atomoxetine has been studied in patients with ADHD recently obtaining abstinence from an alcohol use disorder (Wilens, Adler et al. 2008). ADHD symptoms significantly improved, and heavy drinking days were reduced by 23% over 12 weeks compared with placebo, although the time to relapse of heavy drinking did not differ. It seemed reasonably well-tolerated, and discontinuation rates were low.

Atomoxetine may cause increases in blood pressure and heart rate (Stiefel and Besag 2010; Liang, Lim et al. 2018), nausea, dry mouth, insomnia, fatigue, and decreased appetite (Walker, Mason et al. 2015). Insomnia may be more significant in poor metabolizers of this drug (Wynchank, Bijlenga et al. 2017). Rare hepatic injury has also been reported (Reed, Buitelaar et al. 2016). Atomoxetine is not associated with abuse or dependence (Upadhyaya, Desaiah et al. 2013).

Extended-release formulations of **clonidine** and **guanfacine** (alpha-2 adrenergic agonists that act on inhibitory autoreceptors and may modulate the effects of norepinephrine) have been shown to have efficacy in treating ADHD symptoms in children and adolescents but not in adults (Connor, Fletcher et al. 1999; Biederman, Melmed et al. 2008; Daviss, Patel et al. 2008; Palumbo, Sallee et al. 2008; Sallee and Eaton 2010; Croxtall 2011; Bukstein and Head 2012; Wilens, Bukstein et al. 2012). They have been used as monotherapy or as adjuncts to stimulants (Childress and Sallee 2012). Mild decreases in blood pressure and heart rate can be seen in both. If they do not work as well in adults, it could be because the symptoms that these agents improve the most in youths, such as hyperactivity and impulsivity, can diminish in adulthood. Nearly

40% of patients taking clonidine and nearly 60% of patients taking guanfacine may experience drowsiness sometime during treatment (Lexicomp 2019), which, if persistent, may suggest limited utility in adult patients with primarily attentional symptoms. However, clonidine and guanfacine have been reported to improve aggression in a prison population (Mattes 2016). Although these medicines have not been specifically studied in adults with ADHD, it may be reasonable to consider them when alternatives to stimulants are needed.

In adults, antidepressants with noradrenergic and/or dopaminergic effects may be helpful in the treatment of ADHD symptoms, although again response is generally weaker than that expected from stimulants (Meszaros, Czobor et al. 2007). These include **bupropion** (Wilens, Spencer et al. 2001; Maneeton, Maneeton et al. 2011; Verbeeck, Bekkering et al. 2017), **tricyclic antidepressants** (especially the more noradrenergic **desipramine** and **nortriptyline**; Higgins 1999; Prince, Wilens et al. 2000; Wilens, Biederman et al. 1996; Ghanizadeh 2013), and the serotonin-norepinephrine reuptake inhibitors **venlafaxine** and **duloxetine** (Popper 1997; Mahmoudi-Gharaei, Dodangi et al. 2011; Amiri, Farhang et al. 2012; Bilodeau, Simon et al. 2014). These antidepressants may be helpful for ADHD patients with comorbid unipolar depression, but they should be avoided for most patients with comorbid bipolar disorder.

Despite uncertainities about the mechanism of action of **modafinil** (and its newer R-enantiomer armodafinil), it has been proposed that these drugs may have potential efficacy for ADHD given that they may act as dopamine reuptake inhibitors (Loland, Mereu et al. 2012). Studies in children have shown potential promise for modafinil (Biederman, Swanson et al. 2006; Wang, Han et al. 2017). In adults, however, recent reviews suggest a lack of efficacy for modafinil in the treatment of ADHD (Taylor and Russo 2000; Cortese, Adamo et al. 2018; Stuhec, Lukic & Locatelli 2019). It has been disappointing also as a cognitive enhancer other than in the context of improving wakefulness in people with narcolepsy and related disorders (Kredlow, Keshishian et al. 2019).

Complementary, Alternative, and Other Pharmacotherapies

Although various herbal preparations have been studied as cognition-enhancers in adults, there are very few agents that have been studied specifically for adult ADHD. Even in child and adolescent populations where herbal therapies (e.g., *Melissa officinalis*, *Valeriana officinalis*, *Passiflora incarnate*, **pine bark extract**, and **Gingko biloba**) have been studied, there are insufficient data to allow any clear conclusions to be drawn (Anheyer, Lauche et al. 2017).

There is interest in the role of **omega-3** supplementation in adults with ADHD. Children with ADHD may have reduced omega-3 levels, and supplementation may provide modest benefits (Hawkey and Nigg 2014). Additionally, lower omega-3 levels in the blood appeared to correlate with increased ADHD symptoms (and aggression) in a sample of male prisoners (Meyer, Byrne et al. 2015). Still, there are no controlled studies assessing the efficacy of omega-3 supplementation for ADHD symptoms in adults.

Melatonin has been studied in children and adolescents with ADHD and sleep onset insomnia (Weiss, Wasdell et al. 2006; Van der Heijden, Smits et al. 2007; Bendz and Scates 2010). It appears to be helpful with sleep onset but not with cognitive symptoms.

Further Notes on the Clinical Use of Medicines for Adult ADHD

The greatest initial challenge in providing effective treatment of ADHD is in arriving at an accurate diagnosis. Although some investigators have raised the possibility of adult-onset ADHD as a disorder that might be distinct from childhood-onset ADHD (Moffitt, Houts et al. 2015; Agnew-Blais, Polanczyk et al. 2016; Caye, Rocha et al. 2016), the question has not yet been settled. Until it is, the clinician should make every effort to screen for childhood symptoms whenever this is possible and to adhere to the DSM's (already liberalized) criteria and symptom checklist. Neuropsychological testing may be helpful in supporting the diagnosis, especially if there is suspicion that other cognitive deficits are present, but it is not usually required for diagnosis. Pharmacotherapy has been studied in patients meeting DSM criteria for ADHD; psychological testing has not been used to establish diagnosis in these studies, and testing results have not been associated with or found to predict medication response.

Clinicians should keep in mind that many ADHD symptoms are nonspecific and may be due to other conditions such as depression, anxiety, or substance use. Therefore, a comprehensive psychiatric evaluation is needed to rule out other etiologies for ADHD symptoms and to uncover medical (e.g., cardiac) or psychiatric comorbidities that may need to be addressed before diagnosis and treatment. This evaluation should also include questions regarding family histories of ADHD and cardiac disease.

Starting Pharmacotherapy in Adults

Once the patient is accurately diagnosed and other psychiatric and medical concerns have been addressed, patients with adult ADHD are likely to benefit from available pharmacotherapy. Because stimulants have generally been found to be more efficacious than nonstimulants, they are usual first-line treatments for ADHD in patients who are not at high risk for substance use disorders. There are two basic classes of stimulant products: methylphenidate products and amphetamine products. Most experts consider them equally effective, although they have not been subjected to head-to-head comparisons. Methylphenidate products have had more study, and in some countries, amphetamine products are not available for prescription. Many clinicians in the United States and around the world start with a methylphenidate product, although a recent meta-analysis cited earlier found, based on a relatively small number of studies, that outcome among adults was somewhat better with amphetamine products (Cortese, Adamo et al. 2018).

Immediate-release formulations (for methylphenidate and amphetamines) are often started at a low dose and titrated gradually to arrive at the dose that is effective in improving targeted symptoms for the three to five hours following each administration. This dose can then be repeated twice per day. Once the minimum effective dose has been established, the patient could be switched to an extended release formulation of the same drug (for ease of use and possible decreased risk of misuse). The medication can be then continued on a daily basis.

Alternatively, some clinicians initiate treatment with an extended release formulation of methylphenidate or amphetamine salts and titrate it gradually as needed and tolerated. Lisdexamfetamine is only available in a long-acting once-a-day formulation and is slower acting than others and possibly less likely to be misused. Lisdexamfetamine is likely to be more expensive than other available stimulants.

In patients for whom stimulants' potential risks are concerning, atomoxetine is often considered. If it is used, the patient should be made aware that response to atomoxetine is likely to be gradual and may need a period of three to six months (Clemow and Bushe 2015). Atomoxetine, as previously mentioned, may be more helpful for inattention than for hyperactivity or impulsivity (Ravishankar, Chowdappa et al. 2016). Clonidine and guanfacine might be considered for adult patients with prominent hyperactivity symptoms.

Drug Holidays

Drug holidays—that is, intentionally pausing stimulant therapy for days or weeks—may be useful for some patients who are not likely to incur severe consequences (e.g., motor vehicle accidents) on days in which they do not use their stimulant. Taking drug holidays is a way to diminish the stimulant's adverse effects on sleep and appetite (and growth in children), to decrease the risk of medication tolerance, and to help assess the need for stimulants in an ongoing manner (Ibrahim and Donyai 2015; Kolar, Keller et al. 2008). As needed (prn) use, rather than everyday use, may also serve to decrease drug exposure and adverse effects and may be appropriate for some adult patients. On the other hand, for patients who drive or have severe ADHD, consistent daily adherence may be needed to decrease the risks of problematic sequelae of ADHD (Bikic and Dalsgaard 2018).

Long-Term Use

Since many adults with ADHD begin treatment as children, stimulants (or nonstimulants) are often prescribed over many years. Published reviews do not show any adverse effects in patients who have continued stimulants for one to four years (Fredriksen, Halmoy et al. 2013; Fredriksen and Peleikis 2016). In clinical practice, therapeutic use of amphetamines appears well tolerated over the long run. However, supratherapeutic doses may adversely affect memory and executive functioning (Nestler, Hyman et al. 2015)—these are adverse effects that are shared with chronic use of methamphetamine (Rusyniak 2013). Since stimulant therapy may continue for decades, further studies are needed to clarify longer-term risks.

ADHD and Sleep

There is new interest in the interplay between sleep and ADHD. Insomnia is highly prevalent in patients with ADHD. In some patients, however, insomnia is secondary to pharmacological treatments (Wynchank, Bijlenga et al. 2017). Avoiding stimulant use too close to bedtime can minimize insomnia. Baseline insomnia can be treated by the addition of a sleep medication without abuse potential.

Treatment of ADHD in College Students

As previously noted, uncertainties regarding accurate diagnosis and treatment-emergent risks can influence the decision of whether or not to treat adult ADHD patients with stimulants. In a challenging subgroup of adults—namely, college students—the processes of first identifying those with true ADHD and then performing an appropriate treatment risk/benefit analysis can be particularly difficult. Given growing concerns about the potential misuse of prescription stimulants on college campuses (Benson, Flory et al. 2015; Compton, Han et al. 2018), clinicians should be aware of the following caveats when considering the diagnosis and treatment of college students with ADHD:

(1) The prevalence of ADHD is estimated to be 5.9% to 7.1% in children and adolescents and 2% to 8% in college students (DuPaul, Weyandt et al. 2009; Green and Rabiner 2012; Willcutt 2012). These college student estimates, however, are mostly based on self-report measures and not based on comprehensive evaluations of representative samples. It is reasonable to assume that the prevalence would be lower if strict diagnostic criteria are applied (e.g., presence of sufficient symptomatology, early onset of symptoms, impairment in multiple domains) and if the assessment involves third-party corroboration and the ruling out of other contributing disorders. It is important to keep in mind that self-reporting of symptoms alone may not

be sufficient for a diagnosis of ADHD (McGough and Barkley 2004; DuPaul, Weyandt et al. 2009; Green and Rabiner 2012).

(2) The self-report of subjective improvements in cognitive functioning with past stimulant use also does not, by itself, confirm the presence of ADHD. Healthy adults given stimulants may perceive and report subjective cognitive enhancements even when these perceived improvements are not confirmed by objective measures (Ilieva, Boland et al. 2013).

(3) Even though a subgroup of cocaine users may have ADHD, the self-reported experience of a paradoxical "calming" effect from past cocaine use is *not* pathognomonic of ADHD. There is no published evidence suggesting a correlation between this paradoxical reaction to cocaine and the diagnosis of ADHD.

(4) Malingering to obtain prescriptions for stimulants (e.g., by feigning or exaggerating symptoms) is not uncommon among college students and may occur in up to 50% of students presenting with ADHD symptoms (Green and Rabiner 2012). Also, it is difficult to identify which of the students seeking care are malingerers.

(5) There is a dearth of double-blind, placebo-controlled studies investigating the efficacy of stimulants in college students with ADHD. The one available small study is of short duration and does not assess academic outcomes (which are often the ostensible reasons for students asking for stimulants in the first place; Dupaul, Weyandt et al. 2012; Green and Rabiner 2012). On the other hand, there are several (albeit some small) randomized controlled trials that indicate that that mindfullness-based cognitive therapy, neurofeedbak training, dialectic behavioral group skills training, and working memory training can be effective in this specific

population (Gropper, Gotlieb et al. 2014; Fleming, McMahon et al. 2015; Ryoo and Son 2015; Gu, Xu & Zhu 2018).

(6) The percentage of ADHD diagnosed students who have diverted (shared or sold) their ADHD medications at least once in their lifetime may be above 60% (Garnier, Arria et al. 2010). In one large survey, the number of students who reported illicit use of prescription stimulants was greater than those who reported medical use of these medications (McCabe, Teter et al. 2006). The vast majority of college students who misuse stimulants obtain them from a friend (Wilens, Zulauf et al. 2016).

(7) Students with ADHD have a higher risk of alcohol-related problems (Rooney, Chronis-Tuscano et al. 2015), and inattention in college students with ADHD may be partly due to alcohol use (Mesman 2015).

(8) Whereas children who begin stimulant therapy during elementary school do not appear to be at an elevated risk of stimulant or other drug use during college compared to those who have never been prescribed stimulants, students who began treatment in high school or college may have significantly higher rates of reporting stimulant misuse compared to those who have never been prescribed stimulants (McCabe, Teter et al. 2006).

In summary, caution should be used when considering stimulants for college students with ADHD. As for all patients, a comprehensive assessment should be performed before treatment is initiated. In addition to relying on direct observation, clinicians should attempt to elicit DSM-supported criteria and symptomatology, clarify past history of symptoms, corroborate present and past history with parents or others close to the patient, and obtain objective functional records or other cognitive testing when indicated and available. Although corroboration of history by significant others is not always possible or practical when evaluating adults with ADHD, it may be of significant value for arriving at an appropriate diagnosis (especially if the patient's reliability as an informant is in question).

During treatment, clinicians should make every effort to reduce the risk of medication misuse before prescribing stimulants. The establishment of a therapeutic alliance with the patient and, more concretely, the use of treatment contracts and close monitoring may be helpful in this regard—here again, enlisting the alliance of a family member could be invaluable. To reduce risks, nonstimulant medicines can be considered as alternatives to stimulants when necessary (even though the nonstimulants may take much longer to work and in the end be slightly less effective). Finally, nonpharmacological treatments, such as cognitive-behavior therapy, should be considered for treating adult ADHD (although cognitive-behavior therapy may be more effective in combination with medications; Mongia and Hechtman 2012).

Treatment-Resistant ADHD

In patients who do not respond to stimulants, dose optimization (by basing dose on weight) may be helpful. If stimulants are ineffective or intolerable, then atomoxetine is often tried, although there is actually no evidence available in adults showing that atomoxetine can work after adequate trials of simulants (e.g., methylphenidate and an amphetamine product) have failed.

Patients who do not respond to monotherapy with stimulants or atomoxetine are frequently considered for combinations of these medications. This combination is not studied in adults, but one review noted that, despite variable response, the combination of a stimulant and atomoxetine appeared well tolerated in children and adolescents (Treuer, Gau et al. 2013). Stimulant combinations with clonidine or guanfacine may also be tried (Childress and Sallee

2014), although there is insufficient evidence to confirm improved efficacy for any combined therapies in adults. Finally, monotherapy with bupropion, desipramine, or a serotonin-norepinephrine reuptake inhibitor can also be tried, although again there is no evidence suggesting that after failure on two stimulants and atomoxetine one of these could be effective.

Clinical Use of Stimulants in Other Psychiatric Disorders

Unipolar Depression

Stimulants have been historically used in the treatment of anergic, medically ill, mildly depressed, often elderly patients. In these elderly and/or terminally ill patients, fatigue and apathy may improve with stimulant therapy (Hardy 2009). Response can often be noted in a matter of days. Although stimulants can improve certain symptoms of depression, there is still insufficient evidence to claim that they can be generally effective antidepressants in other patients with major depression (Satel and Nelson 1989; Malhi, Byrow et al. 2016; McIntyre, Lee et al. 2017).

Although stimulants may not fully treat acute depression, it has been proposed that they may have a role to play in facilitating "cognitive remission" after remission from a major depressive disorder (Bortolato, Miskowiak et al. 2016). Modafinil (not a stimulant) may improve memory in patients who have persistent cognitive dysfunction related to major depression after remission from their depressive episode (Kaser, Deakin et al. 2017), and lisdexamfetamine may improve executive dysfunction in similar patients (Madhoo, Keefe et al. 2014). There is still insufficient evidence to recommend routine use of these medications in this context.

Bipolar Depression

Stimulants are sometimes considered for treatment-resistant bipolar depression when mood stabilizers and antipsychotics are ineffective or intolerable. They are also sometimes considered for the treatment of ADHD in patients with comorbid bipolar disorder. There is controversy regarding the efficacy and safety of stimulants in these patients. A retrospective chart review of 137 adults with bipolar disorder treated with various stimulants found that 40% developed stimulant-associated mania or hypomania, suggesting a fairly high risk to this intervention; 25% improved (Wingo and Ghaemi 2008). A more recent and much larger study confirmed a sevenfold risk of treatment-emergent mania with stimulant monotherapy in patients with bipolar disorder, but there was no increased risk if the patient was also treated concurrently with a mood stabilizer (Viktorin, Ryden et al. 2017). Viktorin and colleagues actually found a protective effect of stimulant use on mania induction as reflected by a hazard ratio of 0.6 compared to bipolar patients not treated with a stimulant.

Binge-Eating Disorder

Lisdexamfetamine has efficacy and FDA approval for treatment of patients with binge-eating disorder and can help reduce weight in these patients (Brownley, Berkman et al. 2016). Doses at the higher end of the usual therapeutic range may be necessary (Citrome 2015). Methylphenidate may also reduce binge episodes (Quilty, Allen et al. 2019). It is reasonable to assume that all stimulants would have similar effects (as they all share appetite- and weight-reducing effects in patients without eating disorders), but none have been as extensively studied as lisdexamfetamine for binge-eating disorder.

Clinical Use of Stimulants in Nonpsychiatric Disorders

Fatigue

Stimulants have been studied and deemed potentially helpful for moderate to severe cancer-related fatigue (Yennurajalingam and Bruera 2014), chronic fatigue syndrome (Blockmans and Persoons 2016), and postconcussive "mental fatigue" (Johansson, Wentzel et al. 2017), but there is insufficient evidence to suggest their routine use in these or similar medical conditions.

The neurological use of methylphenidate, dextroamphetamine, and mixed-amphetamine salts for the treatment of narcolepsy is beyond the scope of this chapter.

Use in Women of Childbearing Potential, Pregnancy, and Breastfeeding

Pregnancy

There are relatively little data regarding the use of ADHD medications during pregnancy, but what are available suggest that exposure to methylphenidate does not appear to increase the risk of major congenital malformations (Pottegard, Hallas et al. 2014; Diav-Citrin, Shechtman et al. 2016), with the exception of a recent study that found a small increase in the risk of cardiac malformations in infants exposed to methylphenidate (but not to amphetamines) in utero (Huybrechts, Broms et al. 2018). There may be an increased risk of spontaneous abortions in patients taking methylphenidate, but the increase may be partly due to the underlying ADHD (Bro, Kjaersgaard et al. 2015; Diav-Citrin, Shechtman et al. 2016). Maternal methylphenidate and amphetamine–dextroamphetamine use may be associated with very small increases in the risk of preeclampsia and preterm births (Cohen, Hernandez-Diaz et al. 2017) and use of stimulants in late pregnancy may adversely affect fetal growth (Freeman 2014). All these associations may be due to confounding by indication.

In many cases, if ADHD is not severe, women are likely to be advised to discontinue pharmacotherapy during pregnancy. If ADHD is severe or places the mother at risk (e.g., from severe functional impairments or motor vehicle accidents) then nonpharmacological accommodations can first be considered before less frequent prn use of stimulants is considered (Freeman 2014).

There are insufficient data to support the use of nonstimulant pharmacotherapies for ADHD during pregnancy.

Breastfeeding

There are even less data to support the use of methylphenidate or amphetamines while breastfeeding. Impaired sleep and appetite and growth retardation are areas of concern for the infant if stimulants are ingested through breast milk.

Table of ADHD Medicines

Table 5.1 summarizes the characteristics of selected ADHD medicines (Ansari and Osser 2015; PDR 2019; Lexicomp 2019). Antidepressants used in the treatment of ADHD are listed in Table 1.1.

TABLE 5.1 ADHD Medicines

Medication[a]	Adult Dosing[b]	Comments/FDA Indications
Methylphenidate (Stimulant) (Ritalin®, Ritalin LA®, Ritalin SR®, Concerta®, Aptensio XR®, Cotempla XR-ODT®, Daytrana®, Metadate CD®, Metadate ER®, Methylin®, JORNAY PM®, QuilliChew ER ®, Quillivant XR®) And Dexmethylphenidate (Focalin®, Focalin XR®)	For Ritalin®: Start: 5 mg po bid (morning and afternoon) and increase weekly by 10 mg/day, divide bid or tid with last dose not after 6 pm, maximum 60 mg/day with bid-tid dosing. (See package insert for other formulations). Doses should be individualized: some studies found doses up to 1.0–1.3 mg/kg/day may be needed. No hepatic or renal dose adjustments provided by manufacturer for Ritalin®.	Carries risk of abuse; may decrease appetite and cause insomnia, may cause psychosis. Avoid if significant cardiac problems are present. Monitor blood pressure and heart rate. Does not appear to be metabolized by hepatic CYP450 enzymes. Black Box Warning: Abuse and dependence *Treatment of ADHD and narcolepsy (for some formulations)*
Amphetamine salts (Stimulant) (Adderall®, Adderall XR®, Mydayis®)	For Adderall®: Start: 5 mg po q AM or AM and midday, and increase weekly by 5 mg/day, maximum 60 mg/day with bid dosing (morning and afternoon). (See package insert for XR formulation). Doses should be individualized: some have suggested doses of 0.5–0.65 mg/kg/day. Use with caution in patients with hepatic or renal impairments.	Carries risk of abuse; may decrease appetite and cause insomnia, may cause psychosis. Avoid if significant cardiovascular disease is present. Monitor blood pressure and heart rate. Metabolized by CYP2D6. Black Box Warning: Abuse and dependence; cardiovascular risk. *Treatment of ADHD and narcolepsy (for immediate release only)*

(continued)

TABLE 5.1 Continued

Medication[a]	Adult Dosing[b]	Comments/FDA Indications
Dextroamphetamine (Stimulant) (Dexedrine®, DextroStat®, Procentra®, Zenzedi®)	For Dexedrine®: Start: 5 mg po q AM or morning and midday and increase weekly by 5 mg/ day, maximum 40 mg/day with bid dosing (morning and afternoon). (See package insert for other formulations). Use with caution in patients with hepatic or renal impairments.	Carries risk of abuse; may decrease appetite and cause insomnia, may cause psychosis. Avoid if significant cardiovascular disease is present. Monitor blood pressure and heart rate. Black Box Warning: Abuse and dependence; cardiovascular risk. *Treatment of ADHD and narcolepsy*
Lisdexamfetamine dimesylate (Stimulant) (Vyvanse®)	Start: 10–30 mg po q AM. May adjust in 10 mg/ day increments at weekly intervals. Max 70 mg/day. Use with caution in patients with hepatic impairment. Max dose is lower in patients with renal impairment.	Pro-drug, converted to dextroamphetamine in the bloodstream. Carries risk of abuse; may decrease appetite and cause insomnia, may cause psychosis. Less likely to be snorted than other stimulant formulations. Slow onset and slow offset of effect. Avoid if significant cardiovascular disease is present. Monitor blood pressure and heart rate. Black Box Warning: Abuse and dependence *Treatment of ADHD and moderate to severe binge-eating disorder in adults*
Atomoxetine (Selective Norepinephrine Reuptake Inhibitor) (Strattera®)	Start: 40 mg po q AM or divided bid (morning and afternoon), after 3 days increase to 80 mg po q AM or divided bid, maximum 100 mg/day. Reduce dosing in patients with hepatic impairment.	No risk of abuse; much slower response than with stimulants; CYP2D6 substrate. Monitor for treatment-emergent suicidality. Black Box Warning: Suicidality *Treatment of ADHD*

TABLE 5.1 Continued

Medication[a]	Adult Dosing[b]	Comments/FDA Indications
Clonidine Extended Release (Alpha 2 agonist) (Kapvay®)	Adult dosing unclear. However, may start at 0.1 mg po qhs then increase to 0.1 mg po bid. Uptitrate weekly if needed. Max dose 0.4 mg/day in divided doses. Taper when discontinuing to avoid rebound hypertension. May need lower doses and increased monitoring in patients with hepatic or renal impairments.	Extended release formulation. Nonextended release tablets and extended release transdermal patch indicated for the treatment of hypertension. Monitor for low blood pressure and heart rate. May potentiate other sedating medications. *Treatment of ADHD as monotherapy, or as an adjunct to a stimulant, in pediatric patients*
Guanfacine Extended Release (Alpha 2A agonist) (Intuniv®)	Adult dosing unclear. However, may start at 1 mg po q AM or qhs. Adjust by 1 mg/day in weekly intervals. Max dose is 4 mg/day. If 2 or more doses are missed, then retitrate starting at 1 mg per day. (See package insert for weight-based dosing). Taper when discontinuing to avoid rebound hypertension. Dose reductions may be necessary in patients with hepatic or renal impairments.	Extended release. Nonextended release given for hypertension. Monitor for low blood pressure and heart rate. May potentiate other sedating medications. CYP3A4 substrate. *Treatment of ADHD as monotherapy and as adjunct to a stimulant*

SEE PACKAGE INSERT FOR DOSING AND OTHER INFORMATION BEFORE PRESCRIBING MEDICATIONS. All doses listed here are for use in adults, not for children. Dosing should be adjusted downwards ("start low, go slow" strategy) for the elderly and/or the medically compromised. Abbreviations: ADHD, attention-deficit/hyperactivity disorder; bid (bis in die), twice a day; CYP, cytochrome P450 enzyme; mg, milligram; po (per os), orally; tid (ter in die), three times a day; q (quaque), every; qhs (quaque hora somni), every bedtime.

[a]Generic and U.S. brand name(s).

[b]Doses are provided for educational purposes only.

References

Agnew-Blais JC, Polanczyk GV, et al. (2016). Evaluation of the persistence, remission, and emergence of attention-deficit/hyperactivity disorder in young adulthood. JAMA Psychiatry 73(7): 713–720.

American Psychiatric Association (2013). *DSM 5. Diagnostic and Statistical Manual of Mental Disorders, 5th Edition.* Arlington, VA: American Psychiatric Publishing.

Amiri S, Farhang S, et al. (2012). Double-blind controlled trial of venlafaxine for treatment of adults with attention deficit/hyperactivity disorder. Hum Psychopharmacol 27(1): 76–81.

Anheyer D, Lauche R, et al. (2017). Herbal medicines in children with attention deficit hyperactivity disorder (ADHD): a systematic review. Complement Ther Med 30: 14–23.

Ansari A, Osser DN (2015). *Psychopharmacology, A Concise Overview for Students and Clinicians, 2nd Edition.* North Charleston, SC: CreateSpace.

Bejerot S, Ryden EM, et al. (2010). Two-year outcome of treatment with central stimulant medication in adult attention-deficit/hyperactivity disorder: a prospective study. J Clin Psychiatry 71(12): 1590–1597.

Bendz LM, Scates AC (2010). Melatonin treatment for insomnia in pediatric patients with attention-deficit/hyperactivity disorder. Ann Pharmacother 44(1): 185–191.

Benson K, Flory K, et al. (2015). Misuse of stimulant medication among college students: a comprehensive review and meta-analysis. Clin Child Fam Psychol Rev 18(1): 50–76.

Biederman J, Melmed RD, et al. (2008). A randomized, double-blind, placebo-controlled study of guanfacine extended release in children and adolescents with attention-deficit/hyperactivity disorder. Pediatrics 121(1): e73–e84.

Biederman J, Mick E, et al. (2006). A randomized, placebo-controlled trial of OROS methylphenidate in adults with attention-deficit/hyperactivity disorder. Biol Psychiatry 59(9): 829–835.

Biederman J, Monteaux MC, et al. (2008). Stimulant therapy and risk for subsequent substance use disorders in male adults with ADHD: a naturalistic controlled 10-year follow-up study. Am J Psychiatry 165: 597–603.

Biederman J, Swanson JM, et al. (2006). A comparison of once-daily and divided doses of modafinil in children with attention-deficit/hyperactivity disorder: a randomized, double-blind, and placebo-controlled study. J Clin Psychiatry 67: 727–735.

Bikic A, Dalsgaard S (2018). Pharmacological treatment reduces the risk of motor vehicle crashes among men and women with ADHD. Evid Based Ment Health 21(2): 79.

Bilodeau M, Simon T, et al. (2014). Duloxetine in adults with ADHD: a randomized, placebo-controlled pilot study. J Atten Disord 18(2): 169–175.

Bitter I, Angyalosi A, et al. (2012). Pharmacological treatment of adult ADHD. Curr Opin Psychiatry 25(6): 529–534.

Blockmans D, Persoons P (2016). Long-term methylphenidate intake in chronic fatigue syndrome. Acta Clin Belg 71(6): 407–414.

Bortolato B, Miskowiak KW, et al. (2016). Cognitive remission: a novel objective for the treatment of major depression? BMC Med 14: 9.

Bro SP, Kjaersgaard MI, et al. (2015). Adverse pregnancy outcomes after exposure to methylphenidate or atomoxetine during pregnancy. Clin Epidemiol 7: 139–147.

Brownley KA, Berkman ND, et al. (2016). Binge-eating disorder in adults: a systematic review and meta-analysis. Ann Intern Med 165(6): 409–420.

Bukstein OG, Head J (2012). Guanfacine ER for the treatment of adolescent attention-deficit/hyperactivity disorder. Expert Opin Pharmacother 13(15): 2207–2213.

Bushe C, Day K, et al. (2016). A network meta-analysis of atomoxetine and osmotic release oral system methylphenidate in the treatment of attention-deficit/hyperactivity disorder in adult patients. J Psychopharmacol 30(5): 444–458.

Bymaster FP, Katner JS, et al. (2002). Atomoxetine increases extracellular levels of norepinephrine and dopamine in prefrontal cortex of rat: a potential mechanism for efficacy in attention deficit/hyperactivity disorder. Neuropsychopharmacology 27: 699–711.

Canadian Attention Deficit Hyperactivity Disorder Resource Alliance (2011). Canadian ADHD Practice Guidelines, 3rd Edition. Toronto, ON: Author.

Castells X, Ramos-Quiroga JA, et al. (2011). Amphetamines for attention deficit hyperactivity disorder (ADHD) in adults. Cochrane Database Syst Rev 6: CD007813.

Caye A, Rocha TB, et al. (2016). Attention-deficit/hyperactivity disorder trajectories from childhood to young adulthood: evidence from a birth cohort supporting a late-onset syndrome. JAMA Psychiatry 73(7): 705–712.

Childress AC, Sallee FR (2012). Revisiting clonidine: an innovative add-on option for attention-deficit/hyperactivity disorder. Drugs Today 48(3): 207–217.

Childress AC, Sallee FR (2014). Attention-deficit/hyperactivity disorder with inadequate response to stimulants: approaches to management. CNS Drugs 28(2): 121–129.

Citrome L (2015). Lisdexamfetamine for binge eating disorder in adults: a systematic review of the efficacy and safety profile for this newly approved indication—what is the number needed to treat, number needed to harm and likelihood to be helped or harmed? Int J Clin Pract 69(4): 410–421.

Clemow DB, Bushe CJ (2015). Atomoxetine in patients with ADHD: a clinical and pharmacological review of the onset, trajectory, duration of response and implications for patients. J Psychopharmacol 29(12): 1221–1230.

Cohen JM, Hernandez-Diaz S, et al. (2017). Placental complications associated with psychostimulant use in pregnancy. Obstet Gynecol 130(6): 1192–1201.

Compton WM, Han B, et al. (2018). Prevalence and correlates of prescription stimulant use, misuse, use disorders, and motivations for misuse among adults in the United States. Am J Psychiatry 175(8): 741–755.

Congdon N, Wang F, Tielsch JM (1992). Issues in the epidemiology and population-based screening of primary angle-closure glaucoma. Surv Ophthalmol 36(6): 411–423.

Connor DF, Fletcher KE, et al. (1999). A meta-analysis of clonidine for symptoms of attention-deficit hyperactivity disorder. J Am Acad Child Adoles Psychiatry 38: 1551–1559.

Cooper WO, Habel LA, et al. (2011). ADHD drugs and serious cardiovascular events in children and young adults. N Engl J Med 365(20): 1896–1904.

Cortese S, Adamo N, et al. (2018). Comparative efficacy and tolerability of medications for attention-deficit hyperactivity disorder in children, adolescents, and adults: a systematic review and network meta-analysis. Lancet Psychiatry 5(9): 727–738.

Cox DJ, Davis JM, et al. (2012). Long-acting methylphenidate reduces collision rates of young adult drivers with attention-deficit/hyperactivity disorder. J Clin Psychopharmacol 32(2): 225–230.

Croxtall JD (2011). Clonidine extended-release: in attention-deficit hyperactivity disorder. Paediatr Drugs 13(5): 329–336.

Cunill R, Castells S, et al. (2016). Efficacy, safety and variability in pharmacotherapy for adults with attention deficit hyperactivity disorder: a meta-analysis and meta-regression in over 9000 patients. Psychopharmacology 233(2): 187–197.

Curran C, Byrappa N, et al. (2004). Stimulant psychosis: systematic review. Br J Psychiatry 185: 196–204.

Daviss WB, Patel NC, et al. (2008). Clonidine for attention-deficit/hyperactivity disorder: II. ECG changes and adverse events analysis. J Am Acad Child Adolesc Psychiatry 47(2): 189–198.

Diav-Citrin O, Shechtman S, et al. (2016). Methylphenidate in pregnancy: a multicenter, prospective, comparative, observational study. J Clin Psychiatry 77(9): 1176–1181.

DuPaul GJ, Weyandt LL, et al. (2009). College students with ADHD: current status and future directions. J Atten Disord 13(3): 234–250.

Dupaul GJ, Weyandt LL, et al. (2012). Double-blind, placebo-controlled, crossover study of the efficacy and safety of lisdexamfetamine dimesylate in college students with ADHD. J Atten Disord 16(3): 202–220.

Dupont RL, Coleman JJ, et al. (2008). Characteristics and motives of college students who engage in nonmedical use of methylphenidate. Am J Addict 17(3): 167–171.

Durell TM, Adler LA, et al. (2013). Atomoxetine treatment of attention-deficit/hyperactivity disorder in young adults with assessment of functional outcomes: a randomized, double-blind, placebo-controlled clinical trial. J Clin Psychopharmacol 33(1): 45–54.

Edvinsson D, Ekselius L (2018). Long-term tolerability and safety of pharmacological treatment of adult attention-deficit/hyperactivity disorder: a 6-year prospective naturalistic study. J Clin Psychopharmacol 38(4): 370–375.

Ermer JC, Adeyi BA, Pucci ML (2010). Pharmacokinetic variability of long-acting stimulants in the treatment of children and adults with attention-deficit hyperactivity disorder. CNS Drugs 24(12): 1009–1025.

Fleming AP, McMahon RJ, et al. (2015). Pilot randomized controlled trial of dialectical behavior therapy group skills training for ADHD among college students. J Atten Disord 19(3): 260–271.

Food and Drug Administration (2011). FDA Drug Safety Communication: Safety review update of medications used to treat attention-deficit/hyperactivity disorder (ADHD) in children and young adults: https://www.fda.gov/drugs/drug-safety-and-availability/fda-drug-safety-communication-safety-review-update-medications-used-treat-attention

Fredriksen M, Halmoy A, et al. (2013). Long-term efficacy and safety of treatment with stimulants and atomoxetine in adult ADHD: a review of controlled and naturalistic studies. Eur Neuropsychopharmacol 23(6): 508–527.

Fredriksen M, Peleikis DE (2016). Long-term pharmacotherapy of adults with attention deficit hyperactivity disorder: a literature review and clinical study. Basic Clin Pharmacol Toxicol 118(1): 23–31.

Freeman MP (2014). ADHD and pregnancy. Am J Psychiatry 171(7): 723–728.

Garnier LM, Arria AM, et al. (2010). Sharing and selling of prescription medications in a college student sample. J Clin Psychiatry 71(3): 262–269.

Ghanizadeh A (2013). A systematic review of the efficacy and safety of desipramine for treating ADHD. Curr Drug Saf 8(3): 169–174.

Green AL, Rabiner DL (2012). What do we really know about ADHD in college students? Neurotherapeutics 9(3): 559–568.

Gropper RJ, Gotlieb H, et al. (2014). Working memory training in college students with ADHD or LD. J Atten Disord 18(4): 331–345.

Gu Y, Xu G, Zhu Y (2018). A randomized controlled trial of mindfulness-based cognitive therapy for college students With ADHD. J Atten Disord 22(4): 388–399.

Habel LA, Cooper WO, et al. (2011). ADHD medications and risk of serious cardiovascular events in young and middle-aged adults. JAMA 306(24): 2673–2683.

Hammerness PG, Surman CB, et al. (2011). Adult attention-deficit/hyperactivity disorder treatment and cardiovascular implications. Curr Psychiatry Rep 13(5): 357–363.

Hardy SE (2009). Methylphenidate for the treatment of depressive symptoms, including fatigue and apathy, in medically ill older adults and terminally ill adults. Am J Geriatr Pharmacother 7(1): 34–59.

Hawkey E, Nigg JT (2014). Omega-3 fatty acid and ADHD: blood level analysis and meta-analytic extension of supplementation trials. Clin Psychol Rev 34(6): 496–505.

Higgins ES (1999). A comparative analysis of antidepressants and stimulants for the treatment of adults with attention-deficit hyperactivity disorder. J Fam Pract 48: 15–20.

Huang KL, Wei HT, et al. (2018). Risk of suicide attempts in adolescents and young adults with attention-deficit hyperactivity disorder: a nationwide longitudinal study. Br J Psychiatry 212(4): 234–238.

Huybrechts KF, Broms G, et al. (2018). Association between methylphenidate and amphetamine use in pregnancy and risk of congenital malformations: a cohort study from the International Pregnancy Safety Study Consortium. JAMA Psychiatry 75(2): 167–175.

Ibrahim K, Donyai P (2015). Drug holidays from ADHD medication: international experience over the past four decades. J Atten Disord 19(7): 551–568.

Ilieva I, Boland J, et al. (2013). Objective and subjective cognitive enhancing effects of mixed amphetamine salts in healthy people. Neuropharmacology 64: 496–505.

Johansson B, Wentzel AP, et al. (2017). Long-term treatment with methylphenidate for fatigue after traumatic brain injury. Acta Neurol Scand 135(1): 100–107.

Kaser M, Deakin JB, et al. (2017). Modafinil improves episodic memory and working memory cognition in patients with remitted depression: a double-blind, randomized, placebo-controlled study. Biol Psychiatry Cogn Neurosci Neuroimaging 2(2): 115–122.

Kolar D, Keller A, et al. (2008). Treatment of adults with attention-deficit/hyperactivity disorder. Neuropsychiatr Dis Treat 4(2): 389–403.

Kollins SH (2008). ADHD, substance use disorders, and psychostimulant treatment: current literature and treatment guidelines. J Atten Disord 12(2): 115–125.

Konstenius M, Jayaram-Lindstrom N, et al. (2014). Methylphenidate for attention deficit hyperactivity disorder and drug relapse in criminal offenders with substance dependence: a 24-week randomized placebo-controlled trial. Addiction 109(3): 440–449.

Kooij JJS, Bijlenga D, et al. (2019). Updated European Consensus Statement on diagnosis and treatment of adult ADHD. Eur Psychiatry 56: 14–34.

Kraemer M, Uekermann J, et al. (2010). Methylphenidate-induced psychosis in adult attention-deficit/hyperactivity disorder: report of 3 new cases and review of the literature. Clin Neuropharmacol 33(4): 204–206.

Kredlow MA, Keshishian A, et al. (2019). The efficacy of modafinil as a cognitive enhancer: a systematic review and meta-analysis. J Clin Psychopharmacol 39(5): 455–461.

Levin FR, Choi CJ, et al. (2018). How treatment improvement in ADHD and cocaine dependence are related to one another: a secondary analysis. Drug Alcohol Depend 188: 135–140.

Levin FR, Mariani JJ, et al. (2015). Extended-release mixed amphetamine salts vs placebo for comorbid adult attention-deficit/hyperactivity disorder and cocaine use disorder: a randomized clinical trial. JAMA Psychiatry 72(6): 593–602.

Lexicomp (2019). https://www.wolterskluwercdi.com/lexicomp-online/

Liang EF, Lim SZ, et al. (2018). The effect of methylphenidate and atomoxetine on heart rate and systolic blood pressure in young people and adults with attention-deficit hyperactivity disorder (ADHD): systematic review, meta-analysis, and meta-regression. Int J Environ Res Public Health 15(8): E1789s.

Loland CJ, Mereu M, et al. (2012). R-modafinil (armodafinil): a unique dopamine uptake inhibitor and potential medication for psychostimulant abuse. Biol Psychiatry 72(5): 405–413.

Madhoo M, Keefe RS, et al. (2014). Lisdexamfetamine dimesylate augmentation in adults with persistent executive dysfunction after partial or full remission of major depressive disorder. Neuropsychopharmacology 39(6): 1388–1398.

Mahmoudi-Gharaei J, Dodangi N, et al. (2011). Duloxetine in the treatment of adolescents with attention deficit/hyperactivity disorder: an open-label study. Hum Psychopharmacol 26(2): 155–160.

Malhi GS, Byrow Y, et al. (2016). Stimulants for depression: on the up and up? Aust N Z J Psychiatry 50(3): 203–207.

Maneeton N, Maneeton B, et al. (2011). Bupropion for adults with attention-deficit hyperactivity disorder: meta-analysis of randomized, placebo-controlled trials. Psychiatry Clin Neurosci 65(7): 611–617.

Mannuzza S, Klein RG, et al. (2002). Accuracy of adult recall of childhood attention deficit hyperactivity disorder. Am J Psychiatry 159(11): 1882–1888.

Marchant BK, Reimherr FW, et al. (2011). Methylphenidate transdermal system in adult ADHD and impact on emotional and oppositional symptoms. J Atten Disord 15(4): 295–304.

Mariani JJ, Pavlicova M, et al. (2012). Extended-release mixed amphetamine salts and topiramate for cocaine dependence: a randomized controlled trial. Biol Psychiatry 72(11): 950–956.

Mattes JA (2016). Treating ADHD in prison: focus on alpha-2 agonists (clonidine and guanfacine). J Am Acad Psychiatry Law 44(2): 151–157.

McCabe SE, Teter CJ, Boyd CJ (2006). Medical use, illicit use and diversion of prescription stimulant medication. J Psychoactive Drugs 38(1): 43–56.

McGough JJ, Barkley RA (2004). Diagnostic controversies in adult attention deficit hyperactivity disorder. Am J Psychiatry 161(11): 1948–1956.

McIntyre RS, Lee Y, et al. (2017). The efficacy of psychostimulants in major depressive episodes: a systematic review and meta-analysis. J Clin Psychopharmacol 37(4): 412–418.

Mesman GR (2015). The relation between ADHD symptoms and alcohol use in college students. J Atten Disord 19(8): 694–702.

Meszaros A, Czobor P, et al. (2007). Pharmacotherapy of adult attention deficit/hyperactivity disorder (ADHD): a systematic review. Psychiatria Hungarica 22: 259–270.

Meyer BJ, Byrne MK, et al. (2015). Baseline omega-3 index correlates with aggressive and attention deficit disorder behaviours in adult prisoners. PLoS One 10(3): e0120220.

Michelson D, Adler L, et al. (2003). Atomoxetine in adults with ADHD: two randomized, placebo-controlled studies. Biol Psychiatry 53: 112–120.

Modesto-Lowe V, Chaplin M, et al. (2015). Universal precautions to reduce stimulant misuse in treating adult ADHD. Cleve Clin J Med 82(8): 506–512.

Moffitt TE, Houts R, et al. (2015). Is adult ADHD a childhood-onset neurodevelopmental disorder? evidence from a four-decade longitudinal cohort study. Am J Psychiatry 172(10): 967–977.

Mongia M, Hechtman L (2012). Cognitive behavior therapy for adults with attention-deficit/hyperactivity disorder: a review of recent randomized controlled trials. Curr Psychiatry Rep 14(5): 561–567.

Moran LV, Ongur D, et al. (2019). Psychosis with methylphenidate or amphetamine in patients with ADHD. N Engl J Med 380(12): 1128–1138.

Mosholder AD, Taylor L, et al. (2018). Incidence of heart failure and cardiomyopathy following initiation of medications for attention-deficit/hyperactivity disorder: a descriptive study. J Clin Psychopharmacol 38(5): 505–508.

Nestler EJ, Hyman SE, Malenka RC (2015). *Molecular Neuropharmacology: A Foundation for Clinical Neuroscience, 3rd Edition*. New York, NY: McGraw-Hill.

Newcorn JH, Kratochvil CJ, et al. (2008). Atomoxetine and osmotically released methylphenidate for the treatment of attention deficit hyperactivity disorder: acute comparison and differential response. Am J Psychiatry 165(6): 721–730.

Olfson M, Blanco C, et al. (2013). Trends in office-based treatment of adults with stimulants in the United States. J Clin Psychiatry 74(1): 43–50.

Palumbo DR, Sallee FR, et al. (2008). Clonidine for attention-deficit/hyperactivity disorder: I. Efficacy and tolerability outcomes. J Am Acad Child Adolesc Psychiatry 47(2): 180–188.

PDR (2019). Prescriber's digital reference. http://www.pdr.net.

Popper CW (1997). Antidepressants in the treatment of attention-deficit/ hyperactivity disorder. J Clin Psychiatry 58(Suppl 14): 14–29.

Pottegard A, Hallas J, et al. (2014). First-trimester exposure to methylphenidate: a population-based cohort study. J Clin Psychiatry 75(1): e88–e93.

Prince JB, Wilens TE, et al. (2000). A controlled study of nortriptyline in children and adolescents with attention deficit hyperactivity disorder. J Child Adolesc Psychopharmacol 10: 193–204.

Quilty LC, Allen TA, et al. (2019). A randomized comparison of long acting methylphenidate and cognitive behavioral therapy in the treatment of binge eating disorder. Psychiatry Res 273: 467–474.

Ravishankar V, Chowdappa SV, et al. (2016). The efficacy of atomoxetine in treating adult attention deficit hyperactivity disorder (ADHD): a meta-analysis of controlled trials. Asian J Psychiatr 24: 53–58.

Reed VA, Buitelaar JK, et al. (2016). The safety of atomoxetine for the treatment of children and adolescents with attention-deficit/hyperactivity disorder: a comprehensive review of over a decade of research. CNS Drugs 30(7): 603–628.

Rezaei F, Emami M, et al. (2015). Sustained-release methylphenidate in methamphetamine dependence treatment: a double-blind and placebo-controlled trial. Daru 23: 2.

Rooney M, Chronis-Tuscano AM, Huggins S (2015). Disinhibition mediates the relationship between ADHD and problematic alcohol use in college students. J Atten Disord 19(4): 313–327.

Ross RG (2006). Psychotic and manic-like symptoms during stimulant treatment of attention deficit hyperactivity disorder. Am J Psychiatry 163(7): 1149–1152.

Rusyniak DE (2013). Neurologic manifestations of chronic methamphetamine abuse. Psychiatr Clin North Am 36(2): 261–275.

Ryoo M, Son C (2015). Effects of Neurofeekback training on EEG, continuous performance task (CPT), and ADHD symptoms in ADHD-prone college students. J Korean Acad Nurs 45(6): 928–938.

Sachdev PS, Trollor JN (2000). How high a dose of stimulant medication in adult attention deficit hyperactivity disorder? Aust N Z J Psychiatry 34(4): 645–650.

Safer DJ (2016). Recent trends in stimulant usage. J Atten Disord 20(6): 471–477.

Sallee FR, Eaton K (2010). Guanfacine extended-release for attention-deficit/hyperactivity disorder (ADHD). Expert Opin Pharmacother 11(15): 2549–2556.

Satel SL, Nelson JC (1989). Stimulants in the treatment of depression: a critical overview. J Clin Psychiatry 50: 241–249.

Savill NC, Buitelaar JK, et al. (2015). The efficacy of atomoxetine for the treatment of children and adolescents with attention-deficit/hyperactivity disorder: a comprehensive review of over a decade of clinical research. CNS Drugs 29(2): 131–151.

Shader RI (2017). Risk evaluation and mitigation strategies (REMS), pemoline, and what is a signal? Clin Ther 39(4): 665–669.

Shaw M, Hodgkins P, et al. (2012). A systematic review and analysis of long-term outcomes in attention deficit hyperactivity disorder: effects of treatment and non-treatment. BMC Med 10: 99.

Shevell M (1997). Pemoline associated hepatic failure: a critical analysis of the literature. Pediatr Neurol 16(4): 353.

Spencer T, Biederman J, et al. (2005). A large, double-blind, randomized clinical trial of methylphenidate in the treatment of adults with attention-deficit/hyperactivity disorder. Biol Psychiatry 57(5): 456–463.

Stein J (2005, December 9). FDA Alert: Pemoline market withdrawal. New England Journal of Medicine, Journal Watch. https://www.jwatch.org/pa200512090000003/2005/12/09/fda-alert-pemoline-market-withdrawal

Stickley A, Tachimori H, et al. (2018). Attention-deficit/hyperactivity disorder symptoms and suicidal behavior in adult psychiatric outpatients. Psychiatry Clin Neurosci 72(9): 713–722.

Stiefel G, Besag FM (2010). Cardiovascular effects of methylphenidate, amphetamines and atomoxetine in the treatment of attention-deficit hyperactivity disorder. Drug Saf 33(10): 821–842.

Stuhec M, Lukic P, Locatelli I (2019). Efficacy, acceptability, and tolerability of lisdexamfetamine, mixed amphetamine salts, methylphenidate, and modafinil in the treatment of attention-deficit hyperactivity disorder in adults: a systematic review and meta-analysis. Ann Pharmacother 53(2): 121–133.

Taylor FB, Russo J (2000). Efficacy of modafinil compared to dextroamphetamine for the treatment of attention deficit hyperactivity disorder in adults. J Child Adolesc Psychopharmacol 10(4): 311–320.

Treuer T, Gau SS, et al. (2013). A systematic review of combination therapy with stimulants and atomoxetine for attention-deficit/hyperactivity disorder, including patient characteristics, treatment strategies, effectiveness, and tolerability. J Child Adolesc Psychopharmacol 23(3): 179–193.

Upadhyaya HP, Desaiah D, et al. (2013). A review of the abuse potential assessment of atomoxetine: a nonstimulant medication for attention-deficit/hyperactivity disorder. Psychopharmacology 226(2): 189–200.

Van der Heijden KB, Smits MG, et al. (2007). Effect of melatonin on sleep, behavior, and cognition in ADHD and chronic sleep-onset insomnia. J Am Acad Child Adolesc Psychiatry 46(2): 233–241.

Verbeeck W, Bekkering GE, et al. (2017). Bupropion for attention deficit hyperactivity disorder (ADHD) in adults. Cochrane Database Syst Rev 10: CD009504.

Viktorin A, Ryden E, et al. (2017). The risk of treatment-emergent mania with methylphenidate in bipolar disorder. Am J Psychiatry 174(4): 341–348.

Volkow ND (2006). Stimulant medications: how to minimize their reinforcing effects? Am J Psychiatry 163(3): 359–361.

Walker DJ, Mason O, et al. (2015). Atomoxetine treatment in adults with attention-deficit/hyperactivity disorder. Postgrad Med 127(7): 686–701.

Wang SM, Han C, et al. (2017). Modafinil for the treatment of attention-deficit/hyperactivity disorder: a meta-analysis. J Psychiatr Res 84: 292–300.

Weiss MD, Wasdell MB, et al. (2006). Sleep hygiene and melatonin treatment for children and adolescents with ADHD and initial insomnia. J Am Acad Child Adolesc Psychiatry 45(5): 512–519.

Wilens TE (2004). Impact of ADHD and its treatment on substance abuse in adults. J Clin Psychiatry 65(Suppl 3): 38–45.

Wilens TE, Adler LA, et al. (2008). Atomoxetine treatment of adults with ADHD and comorbid alcohol use disorders. Drug Alcohol Depend 96(1–2): 145–154.

Wilens TE, Biederman J, et al. (1996). Six-week, double-blind, placebo-controlled study of desipramine for adult attention deficit hyperactivity disorder. Am J Psychiatry 153: 1147–1153.

Wilens TE, Bukstein O, et al. (2012). A controlled trial of extended-release guanfacine and psychostimulants for attention-deficit/hyperactivity disorder. J Am Acad Child Adolesc Psychiatry 51(1): 74–85 e72.

Wilens TE, Faraone SV, et al. (2003). Does stimulant therapy of attention-deficit/hyperactivity disorder beget later substance abuse? A meta-analytic review of the literature. Pediatrics 111: 179–185.

Wilens TE, Morrison NR, Prince J (2011). An update on the pharmacotherapy of attention-deficit/hyperactivity disorder in adults. Expert Rev Neurother 11(10): 1443–1465.

Wilens TE, Spencer TJ, et al. (2001). A controlled clinical trial of bupropion for attention deficit hyperactivity disorder in adults. Am J Psychiatry 158(2): 282–288.

Wilens T, Zulauf C, et al. (2016). Nonmedical stimulant use in college students: association with attention-deficit/hyperactivity disorder and other disorders. J Clin Psychiatry 77(7): 940–947.

Willcutt EG (2012). The prevalence of DSM-IV attention-deficit/hyperactivity disorder: a meta-analytic review. Neurotherapeutics 9(3): 490–499.

Wingo AP, Ghaemi SN (2008). Frequency of stimulant treatment and of stimulant-associated mania/hypomania in bipolar disorder patients. Psychopharmacol Bull 41(4): 37–47.

Wynchank D, Bijlenga D, et al. (2017). Adult attention-deficit/hyperactivity disorder (ADHD) and insomnia: an update of the literature. Curr Psychiatry Rep 19(12): 98.

Yennurajalingam S, Bruera E (2014). Review of clinical trials of pharmacologic interventions for cancer-related fatigue: focus on psychostimulants and steroids. Cancer J 20(5): 319–324.

Young JL, Sarkis E, et al. (2011). Once-daily treatment with atomoxetine in adults with attention-deficit/hyperactivity disorder: a 24-week, randomized, double-blind, placebo-controlled trial. Clin Neuropharmacol 34(2): 51–60.

Yu G, Li GF, Markowitz JS (2016). Atomoxetine: a review of its pharmacokinetics and pharmacogenomics relative to drug disposition. J Child Adolesc Psychopharmacol 26(4): 314–326.

6

Treatments for Substance Use Disorders

The past few decades have seen a dramatic increase in the number of pharmacological options available for the treatment of substance use disorders. Pharmacotherapeutic treatments are now available for the treatment of opioid, alcohol, and tobacco use disorders. Other medications are under investigation, but none are approved yet for treating individuals with other substances use disorders.

Clinicians should consider the use of available pharmacotherapies if a patient has been unable to maintain sobriety on his or her own. However, in treating patients with substance use, the beneficial effects of psychosocial interventions should not be overlooked (Dutra, Stathopoulou et al. 2008; Hartmann-Boyce, Stead et al. 2014; Dugosh, Abraham et al. 2016; Khan, Tansel et al. 2016). In fact, pharmacological interventions should be considered as only one part of a multifaceted treatment plan for the treatment of substance use disorders.

Pharmacological treatments include agonist or antagonist medications used to replace or block the effects of the specific substance used or medications that may act to otherwise reduce the likelihood of use (e.g., by decreasing cravings), providing aversive reactions if the substance is used, or affecting limbic reward systems. The medical treatment of withdrawal states that emerge upon substance discontinuation are outside the scope of this chapter but have been reviewed elsewhere (Miller, Fiellin et al. 2019; Kranzler, Ciraulo, Zindel 2014).

Medicines for Opioid Use Disorder

Methadone, a synthetic opioid mu-receptor agonist first introduced in 1964, is a long-acting analgesic that has shown efficacy in maintenance treatment (also referred to as "methadone maintenance treatment" or "medication-assisted treatment") for patients with a history of opioid dependence. When compared to nonopioid replacement therapies, methadone is significantly more effective in reducing heroin use and maintaining patients in treatment (Mattick, Breen et al. 2009). Methadone maintenance treatment (along with other opioid dependence treatments discussed later) may also reduce the secondary problems associated with opioid use, such as criminality, infectious diseases (e.g., HIV), and death (Gowing, Farrell et al. 2006; Gibson, Degenhardt et al. 2008; Sordo, Barrio et al. 2017; Evans, Zhu et al. 2019).

Although methadone (at relatively low doses; e.g., 5 mg twice a day) can be prescribed as an analgesic by individual physicians in the United States, methadone for the treatment of heroin dependence can only be dispensed by centers registered and authorized to do so by regulatory agencies. The initial daily methadone dose is low, but it is gradually increased over many months in patients attending these centers until a high dose (of usually 90–120 mg/day or higher) is reached that stops cravings for illicit opioids and reduces incentives for drug-seeking behaviors (Faggiano, Vigna-Taglianti et al. 2003). For each patient, the dose is individualized until the desired anticraving effect is reached; some patients may require higher doses, while others may do well with lower doses (Fareed, Casarella et al. 2010). However, doses higher than 60 mg/day are likely to retain more patients in treatment than those under 60 mg/day (Bao, Liu et al. 2009).

Methadone can cause respiratory depression (especially in patients who are not tolerant to opioids) as well as adverse central nervous system (CNS) effects, especially if it is used concurrently with other sedatives (Food and Drug Administration [FDA] 2016a). The concomitant use of methadone and benzodiazepines (or alcohol) increases the concern for potentially fatal respiratory depression (Caplehorn and Drummer 2002; Saber-Tehrani, Bruce & Altice 2011). Despite the risks of concomitant use, an FDA advisory from 2017 suggests that opioid addiction medicines such as methadone (and buprenorphine, discussed later) should not be withheld or immediately stopped in patients who use benzodiazepines, since the risks of untreated opioid addiction may outweigh the risk of respiratory depression from this combination (FDA 2017). Instead attempts should be made to minimize (or taper off) benzodiazepine use, even though this may not always succeed.

Methadone can also cause dose-dependent QT prolongation (Ehret, Voide et al. 2006). Methadone-treated patients who have other reasons for QT prolongation may benefit from electrocardiographic monitoring, especially when the daily methadone dose is greater than 100 mg per day (Medicines and Healthcare Products Regulatory Agency & Commission on Human Medicines 2006). The risk of QT prolongation increases if a patient on methadone maintenance is treated with other QT prolongers (e.g., antipsychotics, tricyclic antidepressants, citalopram, trazodone). Caution should also be used when combining methadone with hepatic CYP3A4 inhibitors (e.g., ketoconazole, erythromycin, fluoxetine, fluvoxamine, and grapefruit juice), CYP2D6 inhibitors (e.g., fluoxetine, paroxetine, and bupropion) or other CYP450 inhibitors as these can increase methadone serum levels (Kapur, Hutson et al. 2011) and the risk of respiratory and cardiac effects. CYP450 inducers (e.g., carbamazepine), on the other hand, may decrease methadone levels by metabolizing it to its inactive metabolite, thereby placing the patient at risk for opioid withdrawal (Saber-Tehrani, Bruce et al. 2011). Many antiretroviral drugs can inhibit and/or induce different hepatic enzymes and can therefore affect methadone levels; patients on these medication combinations should be monitored more carefully (Taylor, Paton & Kapur 2015, pp. 601–604).

Finally, other adverse effects of methadone may include severe constipation, dry mouth, nausea, vomiting, increased sweating, weight gain, edema, and sexual dysfunction.

Buprenorphine is an opioid mu-receptor partial agonist (with very high affinity for this receptor) and an opioid kappa-receptor antagonist that is used as an alternative to methadone for maintenance therapy in opioid dependence (Fudala, Bridge et al. 2003; Soyka 2017). Like methadone, buprenorphine is used to diminish cravings for other opioids. It is more effective than placebo in decreasing illicit opioid use, but its relative efficacy compared to methadone may depend on the doses used: fixed medium to high buprenorphine doses are more likely to have similar efficacy to methadone (Mattick, Kimber et al. 2008; Mattick, Breen et al. 2014). Long-term outcomes appear to be similar to those of methadone (Hser, Evans et al. 2016).

Buprenorphine treatment has the benefit of "normalizing" patients' lives and decreasing stigma. In the United States, buprenorphine can be prescribed in an office-based setting, for example, with weekly counseling and weekly dispensing, without requiring daily administration in a methadone center (Fiellin, Pantalon et al. 2006). Buprenorphine is less dangerous than methadone in overdose; it has a lower risk of respiratory depression given its partial opioid agonist properties and ceiling effect at high doses (Walsh, Preston et al. 1994). Early treatment with buprenorphine may be associated with lower overall mortality than treatment with methadone (Bell, Trinh et al. 2009).

However, like methadone, concurrent use of buprenorphine with benzodiazepines (or alcohol) significantly increases the risk of death from respiratory depression (Megarbane, Hreiche et al. 2006; Kintz 2001; Tracqui, Kintz & Ludes 1998). The use of buprenorphine maintenance in patients with a history of polydrug (e.g., concurrent benzodiazepine or alcohol) use, therefore, carries added risk. The severe medical risks from the nonmedical concurrent use of benzodiazepines and buprenorphine, however, are likely to be less than those from nonmedical use of benzodiazepines and methadone (Lee, Klein-Schwartz et al. 2014).

In addition to medication interactions with benzodiazepines and alcohol, buprenorphine may have pharmacokinetic interactions with other medications as well. Most notably, medications that inhibit the CYP3A4 hepatic enzyme (e.g., ritonavir and other medicines listed earlier) can increase the serum level of buprenorphine, leading to CNS effects such as sedation.

When used in outpatient treatment, buprenorphine is combined with the opioid antagonist **naloxone** and administered sublingually. In sublingual form the buprenorphine is absorbed while the naloxone is not. When swallowed and absorbed through the gastrointestinal (GI) tract, naloxone undergoes extensive first-pass liver metabolism, decreasing its systemic availability. Buprenorphine is combined with naloxone to discourage intravenous abuse of this medication: if this combination is misused intravenously, the naloxone effect predominates and blocks opioid effects such as euphoria and instead may precipitate opioid withdrawal.

Buprenorphine used for opioid dependence is available in other formulations as well. A buprenorphine/naloxone sublingual film formulation was developed to further decrease the risk of diversion and/or accidental overdose. The risk of misusing the film by injection appears to be lower than that of tablets (Butler, Black et al. 2018). Sublingual buprenorphine without naloxone is also available; its use, however, is best limited to inpatient settings where its administration can be supervised.

The FDA has recently approved a once-monthly injectable buprenorphine as well as a six-month subdermal buprenorphine implant with similar effectiveness to sublingual buprenorphine (Rosenthal, Lofwall et al. 2016; Haight, Learned et al. 2019). These may be very helpful for patients who have difficulty adhering to daily doses and for those who may be at risk of diversion of their prescribed medication.

Buprenorphine may also be beneficial in chronic pain patients who are at risk of opioid dependence. Because it is only a partial agonist, higher doses may be needed when buprenorphine is used as an analgesic. Methadone may be better for patients with opioid use disorder and severe ongoing pain, but either may be helpful in patients previously taking morphine, oxycodone, or fentanyl for pain and/or for those who have developed opioid-induced hyperalgesia (Daitch, Frey et al. 2012). It should be noted that transdermal buprenorphine, marketed for the treatment of chronic pain, is not approved for outpatient maintenance treatment for opioid use disorders.

Naltrexone is a nonselective opioid antagonist that blocks the effects of illicit opioids. Naltrexone has FDA approval in a monthly injectable formulation for relapse prevention in opioid dependence following opioid detoxification (Krupitsky, Nunes et al. 2011; PDR 2019; Kunoe, Lobmaier et al. 2014). It also appears to decrease the rate of relapse for opioid-using adults in the criminal justice system (Lee, Friedmann et al. 2016). Prior to the availability of the injectable formulation, oral naltrexone had been available and used occasionally for opioid-dependent patients who had significant external supports and motivation to ensure adherence to this medication (Kirchmayer, Davoli et al. 2003). Highly motivated addicted physicians and other professionals sometimes benefited from oral naltrexone treatment for opioid dependence (Ling and Wesson 1984; Washton, Gold et al. 1984). In others, it was not effective. The need for daily adherence to oral medication is avoided with long-acting injectable naltrexone, although monthly adherence is still required, and injection-site pain is sometimes problematic. Injectable naltrexone may be more efficacious than oral naltrexone, especially when the former is combined with psychosocial interventions (Brooks, Comer et al. 2010). It may be twice as likely to maintain patients with opioid use disorders in treatment over a six-month period compared to oral naltrexone (Sullivan, Bisaga et al. 2019). Finally, the effectiveness of injectable naltrexone in the first three months of abstinence appears to be comparable to that of daily buprenorphine/naloxone therapy (Tanum, Solli et al. 2017).

Subcutaneous slow-release naltrexone implants have recently been investigated for long-term use in opioid use disorders and the preliminary evidence is promising (Kunoe, Lobmaier et al. 2009; Hulse, Ngo et al. 2010; Kunoe, Lobmaier et al. 2010; Krupitsky, Zvartau et al. 2012). One study also found that it may have efficacy in the treatment of polydrug (heroin and cocaine) dependence (Tiihonen, Krupitsky et al. 2012). However, this formulation has not yet been approved by the FDA for use in the United States.

Clinicians should be aware that the risk of death from opioid overdose is still present for patients taking long-acting naltrexone. A relapsing patient may intentionally use an extremely high amount of an opioid to achieve euphoria by overcoming the blockade effect of naltrexone. This increases the risk of respiratory depression and death. Patients need to be educated about this risk before beginning treatment.

Naloxone is a nonselective opioid antagonist used to reverse respiratory depression in patients who have overdosed on an opioid. Although the medical treatment of drug overdose is generally outside the scope of this book, all clinicians should become familiar with the use of intranasal naloxone. In the hospital emergency department, naloxone is administered intravenously. Outside the hospital, the newly available nasal spray formulation allows for naloxone's administration in the community setting. Due to the significantly increased use of illicit and prescription opioids, any clinician may come across an individual in the community who has become increasingly sedated and somnolent and who has slow or shallow respirations due to an opioid overdose. The rapid administration of naloxone may save that individual's life.

The effects of naloxone in reversing respiratory depression are rapid but brief in duration. One dose is sufficient for reversal in two thirds of patients, two doses are needed for nearly another third, and a small minority may yet require more (FDA 2016b). Repeated doses may need to be administered if somnolence and respiratory depression recur. The effect of naloxone may be reduced if the patient's respiratory depression is due to an overdose of buprenorphine (PDR 2019).

Upon naloxone administration, patients can become quickly alert and, in some cases, can become belligerent. Patients who are opioid dependent may go into severe withdrawal due to the rapid blockade of their opioid receptors. Those with pre-existing cardiovascular disease may exhibit adverse cardiovascular effects. All patients will need to be monitored medically afterward, and emergency medical services are still needed to arrive at the scene.

Naloxone nasal spray can be prescribed to opioid-dependent patients so that it can be available to their families or cohabitants in case of overdose. However, despite increased awareness and benefits of naloxone, only a very small number of patients receive a prescription for this medication (Follman, Arora et al. 2019). To increase access, the FDA has recently approved a generic version of the naloxone nasal spray (FDA 2019a), and over-the-counter naloxone may not be far behind (FDA 2019b).

Medicines for Alcohol Use Disorder

Disulfiram, one of the earliest treatments developed for substance use disorders, acts by producing disturbing physical effects if alcohol is concurrently consumed. It disrupts ethanol metabolism by irreversibly inhibiting aldehyde dehydrogenase, thereby leading to a significant accumulation of the ethanol metabolite acetaldehyde, which is associated with severely unpleasant adverse effects (and cardiac stress). Anticipation of expected adverse effects from drinking helps disulfiram's effectiveness (Mutschler, Grosshans et al. 2016). Although there is no evidence that it helps maintain abstinence over the long run, it may be useful as a disincentive to ethanol use in the short term (Suh, Pettinati et al. 2006). It retains its effect on aldehyde dehydrogenase for up to two weeks, so even if the patient stops taking disulfiram and plans to drink, there may be time to reconsider and enlist other supportive mechanisms to maintain sobriety before it loses effectiveness. Supervised treatment (i.e., ensuring medication adherence) plays a major role in disulfiram's short-term effectiveness (Jorgensen, Pedersen et al. 2011; Petrov, Krogh et al. 2011). Ultimately, however, most patients who wish to drink do so by discontinuing disulfiram, and many drink while still on it, placing themselves at severe risk. Therefore, like all pharmacotherapies for ethanol dependence, external supports (such as family supervision of medication adherence) and nonpharmacological therapies (such as ongoing counseling and behavioral therapies) are needed for continued effectiveness (Hughes and Cook 1997; Lingford-Hughes, Welch et al. 2004). Notably, a randomized comparison of disulfiram versus naltrexone and acamprosate (discussed later) in 243 patients, all of whom received brief cognitive-behavioral psychotherapy, showed disulfiram to be more advantageous than the other agents (Laaksonen, Koski-Jannes et al. 2008). Another retrospective comparative study of 353 patients found supervised disulfiram to be more effective than acamprosate, especially in patients with longer duration of alcohol use (Diehl, Ulmer et al. 2010).

Patients who are beginning disulfiram treatment should be informed of possible medication interactions and the need for avoidance of alcohol in foods (e.g., sauces), topical preparations (e.g., perfumes), and mouthwashes. Disulfiram is not recommended for patients with cardiac disease, significant liver disease, peripheral neuropathy, or psychosis. In patients with cardiac disease, the disulfiram reaction may precipitate a cardiac event by acutely increasing stress on the heart. Deaths from cardiovascular events have occurred, but avoidance of treating patients with cardiac disease may have lessened this incidence over time (Chick 1999).

Acamprosate may increase the number of abstinence days and decrease overall alcohol consumption long term in alcohol-dependent patients (Sass, Soyka et al. 1996; Whitworth, Fischer et al. 1996; Kranzler and Van Kirk 2001; Mann, Lehert et al. 2004; Boothby and Doering 2005). Although acamprosate may reduce drinking, its overall clinical effect is relatively modest (Rosner, Hackl-Herrwerth et al. 2010). Its mechanism of action is unclear although it is thought to involve the enhancement of gamma aminobutyric acid (GABA) transmission and possibly the antagonism or reduction of the excitatory neurotransmitter glutamate (Littleton and Zieglgansberger 2003). It is generally well-tolerated, with mild GI symptoms (e.g., diarrhea) as the most commonly seen adverse effects. It is renally excreted and therefore patients who are renally impaired will need dose adjustments, and those with severe renal impairment should not take it at all. Acamprosate may be administered, however, to patients with liver disease.

Evidence from a large multicenter study has shed doubt on the effectiveness of acamprosate (Anton, O'Malley et al. 2006)—see following discussion. Researchers have observed that acamprosate appears to do better in European studies that in U.S. studies, although the reasons for this are unclear.

Acamprosate is administered in large 333 mg tablets and the usual dose is two tablets (666 mg) three times daily. Many patients have difficulty adhering to this regimen, which reduces effectiveness. However, others who are committed to abstinence find the three daily doses to be an important reminder of the lurking presence of their alcohol use disorder and do not mind the inconvenience.

Naltrexone, as noted in the discussion on opioid use disorders, is an opioid receptor antagonist. Alcohol can increase the release of endogenous opioids in the brain, which may contribute to its euphoric effects. Naltrexone may reduce the opioid-mediated dopamine-dependent aspect of alcohol's reinforcing properties (possibly in the nucleus accumbens and the ventral tegmental area of the brain) and modestly reduce alcohol use in dependent patients (Gonzalez and Weiss 1998; Srisurapanont and Jarusuraisin 2005;

Soyka and Rosner 2008; Anton 2008). It appears to be most beneficial in severe alcoholics (Pettinati, O'Brien et al. 2006), in alcoholics who smoke (Fucito, Park et al. 2012), and possibly in alcoholics
with a history of childhood adversity (Savulich, Riccelli et al. 2017).
As noted, a long-acting (i.e., every four weeks) injectable preparation is available (Garbutt, Kranzler et al. 2005; O'Malley, Garbutt
et al. 2007) and, like oral naltrexone, appears to be efficacious in
severe alcoholics (Pettinati, Silverman et al. 2011). Both can be
helpful in abstinent and nonabstinent patients (who do not require
medical withdrawal from alcohol). Naltrexone may cause mild GI
symptoms and infrequent transaminitis that requires monitoring.
Patients on naltrexone must not be given opioids for pain management: they will either be ineffective, or, as noted, overdose
and death may result if high opioid doses are administered in an
attempt to override the effect of naltrexone.

Some studies have suggested superior efficacy of naltrexone
as compared to acamprosate (Rubio, Jimenez-Arriero et al. 2001;
Anton, O'Malley et al. 2006; Morley, Teesson et al. 2006). The
U.S. government-sponsored COMBINE study, which compared
naltrexone, acamprosate, and the combination of the two, all combined with medical management (i.e., brief meetings with a healthcare provider in a primary care setting), found naltrexone to be
more effective than acamprosate. It also found that the meetings
with a healthcare provider increased the likelihood of abstinence
(Anton, O'Malley et al. 2006). It should be noted that the dose of
naltrexone used in this study was twice the usual dose (100 mg/day
vs. 50 mg/day).

Although this is a subject meriting greater discussion, naltrexone's disruption of alcohol's reinforcing effects may lead clinically
into an overall decrease in "cravings" for alcohol (Helstrom, Blow
et al. 2016; Ray, Green et al. 2019). Although not proven by any
well-designed studies, there is a strong suspicion by clinicians and
researchers that naltrexone (and probably acamprosate as well)
are not particularly effective for preventing relapse in alcohol

use disorder patients who drink intentionally to "self-medicate" intense distress or dysphoria or to fall asleep when there are no other effective means available. The craving that naltrexone may prevent is the kind that is associated with the pleasure of ingesting the beverage, the kind that is stimulated by seeing a commercial or encountering others drinking socially or by the odor of the beverage. Often, when experiencing such cravings, the patient will reason that maybe they could just have one drink, enjoy it, and not continue to drink. However, that first drink will then stimulate extreme additional cravings to have a second drink, and relapse will be inevitable. O'Malley and colleagues found that after one drink, the relapse rate on placebo was 81% whereas it was 50% if the patient was on naltrexone (O'Malley, Jaffe et al. 1996). Although 50% is still a high rate and taking one drink is not advised, the potential for public health benefits from the use of naltrexone seems to be considerable.

Finally, individuals with a specific polymorphism of the mu-opioid receptor gene (OPRM1; i.e., individuals with an Asp40 allele—coding for a receptor with increased beta-endorphin binding and activity; Bond, LaForge et al. 1998) may be more likely to respond to naltrexone (Anton, Oroszi et al. 2008). However, a recent study did not confirm differential response to naltrexone in heavy drinkers based on this polymorphism (Oslin, Leong et al. 2015)

Other Potentially Effective Medicines for Alcohol Use Disorder

Other medications have been studied for the treatment of alcohol use disorders. Although none of these medications are FDA-approved for this indication, they may be considered as adjuncts or as secondary treatments when primary treatments are either contraindicated or ineffective.

There is evidence to support the use of the anticonvulsant **topiramate** for the treatment of alcohol dependence, but doses up to 300 mg/day may be needed (Johnson, Ait-Daoud et al. 2003; Johnson, Rosenthal et al. 2007; De Sousa 2010; Guglielmo, Martinotti et al. 2015). It is likely to be more efficacious than placebo in increasing the number of abstinence days and in decreasing the percentage of heavy drinking days (Arbaizar, Diersen-Sotos et al. 2010). Also, topiramate (at mean doses of 200 mg/day or higher) may be more efficacious than naltrexone (50 mg/day; Baltieri, Daro et al. 2008; Florez, Saiz et al. 2011). It is hypothesized that it helps reduce alcohol use by facilitating GABA inhibition, antagonizing excitatory glutamate receptors, and suppressing alcohol-induced dopamine release from the nucleus accumbens, thereby diminishing the reinforcing effects of alcohol (Olmsted and Kockler 2008; De Sousa 2010). Topiramate may also regulate alcohol use by affecting behavioral impulsivity (Rubio, Martinez-Gras et al. 2009).

Topiramate has several important side effects, probably more so than those of FDA-approved options for treating alcohol use disorder. Symptomatic kidney stones develop in 2.1% of patient (and additional patients have asymptomatic ones; Dell'Orto, Belotti et al. 2014). Cognitive impairment, paresthesias in the limbs, hyperchloremic metabolic acidosis, and glaucoma are other significant problem areas. It also frequently causes weight loss, although, of course, many patients would find that to be a benefit.

Pregabalin, an anticonvulsant (and as discussed earlier, a potential anxiolytic), has also shown possible efficacy in the treatment of alcohol dependence (Martinotti, Di Nicola et al. 2010; Oulis and Konstantakopoulos 2012) at doses of 150 to 450 mg/day and especially in those with comorbid generalized anxiety disorder (Guglielmo, Martinotti et al. 2012). Similarly, **gabapentin**, at doses of 900 mg twice daily, was found effective in a placebo-controlled randomized trial of 150 patients (Mason, Quello et al. 2014). Gabapentin has similar structure and pharmacodynamics to pregabalin while currently costing much less because of its generic status. Both gabapentin and pregabalin can be abused and may be misused in combination with alcohol, benzodiazepines, and opioids. Furthermore, patients with a history of alcohol or substance use may be at higher risk of misuse (Smith, Havens & Walsh 2016; Bonnet and Scherbaum 2017; Evoy, Covvey et al. 2019). Therefore, the use of pregabalin or gabapentin in patients with alcoholism (or other substance abuse) may be problematic.

A small number of studies have indicated a possible role for other anticonvulsants such as **carbamazepine, oxcarbazepine**, and **divalproex** in the treatment of alcohol dependence (Mueller, Stout et al. 1997; Longo, Campbell et al. 2002; Martinotti, Di Nicola et al. 2007), but there is insufficient evidence to recommend their use as primary treatments for reducing alcohol use. It should not be assumed that all anticonvulsants will be helpful in alcohol use disorders: in a small open-label study, **levetiracetam** treatment actually increased alcohol consumption in half of the patients studied (Mitchell, Grossman et al. 2012), and another study showed no effect in relapse prevention (Richter, Effenberger et al. 2012).

Ondansetron, an antiemetic with 5-HT3 receptor antagonist activity, has emerged as an agent with possible efficacy for this indication (Johnson, Ait-Daoud et al. 2000; Johnson, Roache et al. 2000; Correa Filho and Baltieri 2013). The antidepressant **mirtazapine** is also a 5-HT3 antagonist but has not been studied for this indication *per se*. However, mirtazapine had been shown in earlier studies to reduce alcohol cravings and drinking in alcoholic patients with comorbid depression (Yoon, Pae et al. 2006; Cornelius, Douaihy et al. 2012). In a subsequent study, however, mirtazapine failed to show an improvement in alcohol consumption, despite improvements in depression (Cornelius, Chung et al. 2016a), and a concurrent review of other published data by the same authors reached the same conclusion (Cornelius, Chung et al. 2016b).

Baclofen, a GABA-B receptor agonist, has been studied for both alcohol withdrawal and for ongoing treatment (Addolorato and Leggio 2010; Lyon, Khan et al. 2011). However, in both contexts, despite some evidence of beneficial response, no conclusions can be reached regarding its overall efficacy given mixed results from studies with different outcomes and different sample populations (Muzyk, Rivelli et al. 2012; Liu and Wang 2013). Findings from a more recent review did not change this impression (Minozzi, Saulle et al. 2018).

Prazosin, an alpha-1 adrenergic antagonist modulating noradrenergic effects (previously discussed for PTSD symptoms), has had a few very small pilot studies showing possible effects on alcohol consumption (Simpson, Saxon et al. 2009; Fox, Anderson et al. 2012; Simpson, Malte et al. 2015). Its use may decrease anxiety associated with alcohol deprivation in animal models (Rasmussen, Kincaid & Froehlich 2017), and a more recent controlled study noted efficacy in decreasing alcohol consumption in humans when prazosin was used at high doses (Simpson, Saxon et al. 2018). Further studies are needed.

Sertraline, a selective serotonin reuptake inhibitor (SSRI), has been studied for the treatment of alcoholism. Interestingly, the effect of this medication on reducing the number of drinking days may be dependent on the alcoholism subtype. Patients who are Type A (later onset, lower vulnerability) alcoholics may respond positively to sertraline whereas Type B (early onset/higher severity) alcoholics may exhibit poorer outcomes than placebo (Pettinati, Volpicelli et al. 2000; Dundon, Lynch et al. 2004; Kranzler, Armeli et al. 2011; Kranzler, Armeli et al. 2012). Similar adverse outcomes had been noted earlier with **fluoxetine** (Kranzler, Burleson et al. 1996). The relationship between age of onset and response to sertraline may depend on the serotonin transporter genotype (Kranzler, Armeli et al. 2011). In one study, a combination of sertraline and naltrexone improved drinking outcomes and depression compared to either treatment alone (Pettinati, Oslin et al. 2010). One might conclude that clinicians should be aware that ongoing SSRI treatment could be harmful for some patients with alcohol use disorders, while being possibly beneficial for some others. As regards the utility of antidepressants in general for coexisting depression and alcohol dependence, the quality of aggregate evidence is poor, and if there are any improvements in both disorders, the "clinical relevance may be modest" (Agabio, Trogu & Pani 2018).

Medicines for Tobacco Use Disorder

Nicotine replacement therapy (NRT) is used to decrease withdrawal symptoms during smoking tapering and cessation and can double the odds of quitting (Silagy, Lancaster et al. 2004). NRT can be delivered transdermally via a patch or transmucosally by gum, inhaler, nasal spray, or dissolving lozenge. Given significant first-pass metabolism by the liver, nicotine is minimally effective if ingested orally. All other available modes of delivery are likely to be effective (Silagy, Lancaster et al. 2004) and may increase the rate of quitting by 50% to 70% (Stead, Perera et al. 2012). A more recent large study confirmed the efficacy of the nicotine patch over placebo (Anthenelli, Benowitz et al. 2016). Combining two forms of nicotine delivery, such as a patch and a rapid delivery form of nicotine as needed at key times (e.g., a patch plus gum or lozenge), may increase the odds of smoking cessation (Piper, Smith et al. 2009; Heydari, Marashian et al. 2012; Stead, Perera et al. 2012). Actual dosing and duration of treatment vary slightly for each formulation, although all nicotine replacement treatments involve setting a target date for smoking cessation followed by a gradual taper of the nicotine replacement over two to three months. In a review of 88 trials, success rates on 6- to 12-month follow-up averaged 16% versus 10% on placebo (Silagy, Mant et al. 2000). The number needed to treat (NNT) was 17; that is, 17 patients need to be treated before 1 will be successful who would not have quit on placebo. These are not very good odds; therefore, patients should be encouraged to make repeated efforts to quit. Caution should be used in patients with a history of cardiac disease, especially when using the nicotine patch (while avoiding the patch if there is a history of serious arrhythmias, angina, or immediately post-myocardial infarction), although an extensive review of available trials found no evidence that NRT increases the risk of heart attacks (Stead, Perera et al. 2012). Patients should not smoke at all while wearing the transdermal nicotine patch, although often this advice is not heeded. Nausea and headaches can occur frequently with NRT. Insomnia and nightmares may occur with the patch, and many patients prefer to have it removed at bedtime. However, strong cravings the next morning may make it very difficult to resist smoking before putting on the next day's patch.

In terms of medication interactions, it is important to note that if patients who are smoking cigarettes (which induces CYP450 enzymes, such as CYP1A2) replace smoking with NRTs (which do not induce these enzymes), adjustments may be needed to the doses of their concurrent medications (e.g., clozapine) whose serum levels may rise with the discontinuation of cigarette use.

Electronic cigarettes (e-cigarettes), which provide inhaled nicotine through a smokeless device, were initially heralded as a promising aid for smoking cessation or, at least, for conversion to a less harmful form of nicotine. A large number of products (vaping devices) rapidly became available (Breland, Spindle et al. 2014). Nicotine concentrations in these devices are variable, and the long-term risks of inhaled compounds that are added to aerosolize the nicotine are not known. More recently there have been reports of seizures following the use of vaping devices; these may be due to high-dose nicotine toxicity or due to the presence of adulterants (FDA 2019c).

Data from the Centers for Disease Control and Prevention's 2011–2018 National Youth Tobacco Survey showed that among middle school students e-cigarette use increased 8-fold from 2011 to 2018, and among high school students the increase was nearly 14-fold. From 2017 to 2018, "current" e-cigarette use increased by nearly 50% in middle school students and nearly 80% in high school students (Cullen, Ambrose et al. 2018). The FDA has banned their sale to those who are less than 18 years old, and some states have restricted them to those who are 21 or older.

More recently, as of this writing, there have been reports of over 1,000 cases of a peculiar lung ailment in persons using vaping devices; 20 people have died. Intensive investigation is underway to determine the cause of these ailments. In the United States, Massachusetts has instituted a four-month halt on all sales of vaping materials pending the outcome of these investigations, and many other areas have imposed partial bans.

Evidence is also accumulating that e-cigarettes are initiating many people into nicotine use disorders (Dutra and Glantz 2014). High-nicotine concentration e-cigarette use in adolescents has been shown to increase the risk of smoking cigarettes (Goldenson, Leventhal et al. 2017). Patterns of use have suggested that their use may actually decrease the chance of smoking cessation, and, as such, e-cigarettes should not be considered nicotine replacement "therapies" (Kalkhoran and Glantz 2016). E-cigarettes cannot be recommended for smoking cessation, given the availability of other safer NRTs.

Bupropion, an antidepressant with dopaminergic effects at the nucleus accumbens (also see section on antidepressants) is also efficacious for smoking cessation (Jorenby, Leischow et al. 1999; Johnson 2010; Hughes, Stead et al. 2014; Anthenelli, Benowitz et al. 2016). An additional mechanism, noted anecdotally, may be that it gives a very unpleasant taste to the cigarette smoke. However, it does not seem to have that effect on chewing tobacco users, and it seems to have no efficacy for patients who want to quit "dipping" (Ebbert, Elrashidi & Stead 2015). Bupropion should be started for two weeks and reach a dose of 150 mg twice daily before the target stop date, and then it is continued for at least three months. The addition of NRT to bupropion can increase the chances of abstinence compared to the use of either drug alone (Jorenby, Leischow et al. 1999). Bupropion should be avoided in patients with histories of seizures or eating disorders.

Another antidepressant, **nortriptyline**, may also increase long-term smoking cessation rates (Hughes, Stead et al. 2014), but its side effect profile is problematic, and it is not FDA-approved for this indication. The effects on smoking cessation from bupropion and nortriptyline are independent of their effects on depressive symptoms. SSRIs do not seem to be similarly effective (Hughes, Stead et al. 2014). **Clonidine** may also have some effectiveness for smoking cessation (Cahill, Stevens et al. 2013).

Varenicline is an alpha-4 beta-2 nicotinic acetylcholine receptor partial agonist, with higher affinity than nicotine for this receptor. It is the latest advance in nicotine addiction treatment and the most expensive of all available treatments. It may have effectiveness that is comparable to, or greater than that of, bupropion and NRT for smoking cessation (Gonzales, Rennard et al. 2006; Jorenby, Hays et al. 2006; Tonstad, Tonnesen et al. 2006; Bolliger, Issa et al. 2011; Mills, Wu et al. 2012; Cahill, Stevens et al. 2013; Anthenelli, Benowitz et al. 2016; Baker, Piper et al. 2016).

Although varenicline appears to be generally well-tolerated, treatment-emergent mood changes and psychosis had been reported earlier in susceptible patients (Freedman 2007; Kohen and Kremen 2007; Ahmed, Ali et al. 2013). Higher rates of suicidality had been associated with varenicline treatment than with other treatments used for smoking cessation (Moore, Furberg et al. 2011). However, in a reanalysis of 17 placebo-controlled trials plus a new Department of Defense data set, no evidence of adverse neuropsychiatric events was found (Gibbons and Mann 2013). These results were further supported by the large multicenter Evaluating Adverse Events in a Global Smoking Cessations Study (EAGLES) trial (Anthenelli, Benowitz et al. 2016). This study enrolled 8,000 smokers, 4,000 of whom had a comorbid significant mental illness (e.g., depression, bipolar, schizophrenia, anxiety disorders) along with tobacco use disorder. Subjects were randomized to varenicline, bupropion, nicotine patch, or placebo. The study found varenicline more effective than the other three treatments, and there was no difference from placebo in major neuropsychiatric side effects such as suicidal thoughts or behaviors, aggressive behaviors, mood episodes, or anxiety symptoms. As a result, the FDA removed the warning box on these problems from the package insert in 2017. There were more of these adverse effects in subjects with comorbid mental illness, as expected, but again there was no difference from placebo. The investigators concluded, and the new package insert states, that these problems can occur when one tries to quit smoking, but they come from the nicotine withdrawal and not from varenicline, bupropion, or NRT. Another more recent study showed that all three medications were effective for patients with pre-existing psychiatric disease (Evins, Benowitz et al. 2019) The FDA also recommended, however, that patients taking varenicline (or bupropion) stop these medications if they develop "any side effects on mood, behavior or thinking" (FDA 2018). The primary adverse effect from varenicline appears to be nausea. Insomnia is also common, and nightmares may occur especially in patients with nightmares from pre-existing conditions like posttraumatic stress disorder.

Historically, there were mixed findings regarding a possible increased risk of cardiovascular events associated with varenicline treatment (Singh, Loke et al. 2011; Prochaska and Hilton 2012; Svanstrom, Pasternak et al. 2012). More recent findings, again from the large EAGLES study, found that varenicline (as well as bupropion and NRT) did not increase cardiovascular risks in patients without unstable cardiovascular conditions (e.g., recent myocardial infarction or uncontrolled hypertension; Benowitz, Pipe et al. 2018). In the vast majority of patients, the benefits of smoking cessation were likely to outweigh cardiac risks.

Medicines for Other Substance Use Disorders

There are no FDA-approved medications for the treatment of substance use disorders other than those approved for opioid, alcohol, and tobacco use disorders. However, some treatments have been studied for cocaine, cannabis, and amphetamine use disorders.

Cocaine Use Disorder

Two double-blind, randomized, placebo-controlled, 12-week studies have shown that **topiramate** (discussed previously) may have some efficacy in reducing cocaine use. The first study used doses up to 300 mg per day and noted robust response in terms of urinary cocaine-free weeks (Johnson, Ait-Daoud et al. 2013). The second study used doses up to 200 mg per day and noted reductions in crack cocaine use in the first four weeks of treatment but not in the subsequent two months (Baldacara, Cogo-Moreira et al. 2016). Nevertheless, topiramate may be a potential first-line consideration for treating cocaine use disorders. **Disulfiram** (which may work through a mechanism different from that in alcohol use disorders) has been studied in a placebo-controlled study and shown to have some efficacy in reducing cocaine use (Carroll, Fenton et al. 2004), but its reputation as aversive therapy for alcohol use disorders may be problematic for many patients. Tolerability, however, appeared to be similar to that of placebo. Finally, **modafinil** showed some efficacy and was well tolerated, but the results were not very impressive (Dackis, Kampman et al. 2005). Modafinil could be considered perhaps for more severe addicts who have had more severe cocaine withdrawal and have not been abstinent very long.

Cannabis Use Disorder

Dronabinol, a synthetic delta-9-THC, has been studied for the treatment of cannabis use disorder. A placebo-controlled study found no difference in the reduction of marijuana use with dronabinol as compared to placebo, although treatment retention and withdrawal symptoms were improved with the former (Levin, Mariani et al. 2011). Subsequent trials for dronabinol are lacking. Another study showed that **naltrexone** maintenance reduced cannabis use compared to placebo, possibly by decreasing positive reinforcing effects of cannabis in subjects who used marijuana daily and were not seeking treatment for their use (Haney, Ramesh et al. 2015).

Amphetamine Use Disorder

Finally, a review of pharmacotherapy studies for the treatment of methamphetamine or amphetamine-type stimulant use disorders did not find significant efficacy for any medication, despite the finding that some medications such as **naltrexone** and **methylphenidate** were helpful in subgroups of patients (Brensilver, Heinzerling & Shoptaw 2013). Subsequent placebo-controlled studies support the possible efficacy of sustained-release methylphenidate for the treatment of methamphetamine abuse (Ling, Chang et al. 2014; Rezaei, Emami et al. 2015).

Complementary, Alternative, and Other Pharmacotherapies

Opioid Use Disorders

Proponents of "medical marijuana" argue that **cannabis** is a safe and "natural" herbal treatment for chronic pain and that its use could decrease widespread opioid use. One recent review, however, found that the quality of evidence supporting the use of cannabis-based medicines for chronic neuropathic pain is poor, the analgesic effects are not robust, and the potential harms may outweigh the benefits (Mucke, Phillips et al. 2018).

It has also been observed that some states that have medical cannabis laws have lower opioid overdose mortality rates (Bachhuber, Saloner et al. 2014). However, it is difficult to establish a direct causation relationship between the two. Additionally, the putative benefits in terms of reducing opioid-related mortality would have to be weighed against any adverse individual or societal effects that may arise from the increased use of cannabis (e.g., the risk of psychosis, motor vehicle accidents, etc.). There are no controlled trials that show that prescribing cannabinoids to patients with opioid use disorder actually decreases opioid use or the risk of overdose. **Cannabidiol**, however, may decrease cravings in abstinent patients with heroin use disorder (Hurd, Spriggs et al. 2019).

Alcohol Use Disorder

Past studies suggested a possible reduction of alcohol misuse from a single dose of lysergic acid diethylamide (LSD; Krebs and Johansen 2012). More recently, researchers have studied the effect of the hallucinogen **psilocybin** on alcohol use. A few small pilot studies suggest possible response for patients with tobacco and alcohol dependence (Johnson, Garcia-Romeu et al. 2014; Bogenschutz, Forcehimes et al. 2015). The reported transformative experiences of those who ingest psilocybin during supportive therapy are quite varied: they are described by some authors as "experiences of catharsis, forgiveness, self-compassion, and love," which may help the individual reduce or discontinue alcohol use (Bogenschutz, Podrebarac et al. 2018). However, given the distinctly personal effects of this drug, it is difficult to generalize the purported effects to the general population without larger longitudinal studies. Psilocybin is a schedule I drug with high potential for abuse.

Tobacco Use Disorder

A 2014 review found no benefits from **St. John's wort** or **S-adenosyl methionine** for smoking cessation (Hughes, Stead et al. 2014).

Further Notes on the Clinical Use of Medicines for Substance Use Disorders

Several medication options have been discussed in this chapter for the treatment of opioid, alcohol, and tobacco use disorders. However, for any of these to be successful, patient motivation is essential; without it, adherence to treatment is not likely. Furthermore, these treatments are unlikely to succeed without psychosocial supports or non-pharmacological therapies. "Favorable external circumstances" (including external supports) and patient motivation are likely to increase the chance that a patient will remain in treatment (Ali, Green et al. 2017).

Initiating and Continuing Treatment

Opioid Use Disorders

As discussed, both methadone and buprenorphine/naloxone combination at optimized doses and injectable naltrexone are efficacious for the treatment of opioid use disorders. The buprenorphine/naloxone combination, however, is increasingly considered first-line therapy compared to methadone, because of its effect in "normalizing" treatment and its more favorable safety profile.

Patients who are actively using illicit opioids (e.g., heroin) need to discontinue use (for 6–24 hours) and be in at least moderate opioid withdrawal before taking their first sublingual dose of buprenorphine/naloxone. Because of buprenorphine's high affinity for opioid mu-receptors, starting it sooner may displace the pre-existing opioid and lead to rapid opioid withdrawal. If a patient is using a long-acting opioid, then the longer-acting opioid should be gradually tapered and preferably discontinued until the patient is in moderate opioid withdrawal; a longer period of time since discontinuation (up to 48 hours) and possibly inpatient treatment may be needed before initiating buprenorphine.

Once an adequate fixed dose (e.g., 8–16 mg per day) of buprenorphine is achieved, that dose may be continued. Doses should be individualized, and higher doses are sometimes considered for those with severe opioid dependence (Maremmani, Rolland et al. 2016). Buprenorphine alone (without naloxone) is not recommended for ongoing outpatient use, given its greater risk of diversion and misuse (if the buprenorphine is injected intravenously). Longer-acting buprenorphine formulations (monthly injections or implants) are not combined with naloxone, and patients who have tolerated sublingual buprenorphine/naloxone may be changed to these longer-acting options. However, there is still minimal clinical experience with these formulations.

Methadone can be used as an alternative to buprenorphine for patients with severe or long-standing opioid dependence who may benefit from the increased daily structure of attending a methadone clinic. As previously discussed, dosing is started at a low dose at a methadone clinic and gradually titrated to higher doses over many months. During early treatment, before anticraving doses are reached, patients are still at risk of relapse and therefore intensifying psychological and other supportive therapies would be beneficial. Once the patient is stable on higher doses, ongoing treatment reduces relapse.

Clinicians should be aware that patients maintained on high-dose methadone who are admitted to the medical/surgical units of hospitals for unrelated medical care are likely to need to continue their daily dose of methadone. However, high doses should never be administered without independent confirmation with the methadone center administering this drug to confirm the actual dose that the patient has been receiving prior to admission. Even three to four days of methadone discontinuation may significantly reduce a patient's tolerance to the respiratory depressant effects of this drug. To decrease the risk of death from respiratory depression, a single dose of methadone should never exceed 20 mg when independent confirmation of higher doses is still pending. Subsequent dose increments can then be added as necessary and as tolerated.

Methadone or buprenorphine can be continued long term, or indefinitely, if tolerated. If a patient requests discontinuation, then a gradual taper would be necessary to decrease the risks of opioid withdrawal. The risks of destabilization and relapse are likely to be high for most patients who discontinue medical treatment regardless of the medication used. Mortality risk may increase in the months following buprenorphine or methadone discontinuation (Bell, Trinh et al. 2009). Therefore, patients should have a sustained period of stability as well as increased psychosocial supports in place before treatment discontinuation is considered.

Monthly injectable naltrexone is a viable alternative to opioid replacement therapy; however, it frequently is not available. It requires opioid discontinuation and resolution of opioid withdrawal symptoms prior to initiation, which may complicate treatment for some patients and increase the risk of early relapse. However, after this initial phase, treatment results may be comparable to those of buprenorphine (Lee, Nunes et al. 2018). Naltrexone does not replace opioids and therefore may be less favored by some opioid dependent patients. Oral naltrexone is not an effective first-line treatment for opioid use disorders unless the patient is supervised daily to ensure strict adherence to the medication; otherwise, treatment retention is low (Minozzi, Amato et al. 2011).

Alcohol Use Disorder

Pharmacotherapy is often offered to patients with moderate to severe alcohol use, but regardless of severity, counseling and/or use of group therapies should always be recommended for patients with an alcohol use disorder. If the patient is agreeable to pharmacotherapy, either oral naltrexone or acamprosate could be considered (Jonas, Amick et al. 2014). There can be a slight edge toward naltrexone as first-line treatment in the United States, given acamprosate's poorer efficacy in U.S. studies and its need for three-times-a day-dosing. Both medications may be more efficacious if their use is preceded by a brief period of abstinence (Maisel, Blodgett et al. 2013).

Alcoholic patients starting naltrexone would benefit from measuring baseline liver transaminases given that this medication can increase these values further (although significant liver toxicity is uncommon at usual therapeutic doses). If the patient has pre-existing liver disease, then acamprosate can be considered preferentially. Acamprosate, on the other hand, is not favored if the patient is renally impaired.

If adherence to oral naltrexone is poor, then supervised dosing or a switch to long-acting injectable may be considered. As previously noted, oral or injectable naltrexone should not be administered to a patient who is taking opioids concurrently.

Disulfiram is usually not an appropriate first-line medication for patients with alcohol use disorders given the acute medical risks if a patient drinks while taking this medication. There may be an exception to this, however, in patients who may be at risk of behavior that may result in imminent death with each alcohol relapse (e.g., in an otherwise relatively stable patient who attempts suicide only when he or she is intoxicated). Even then, the patient's motivation for treatment should be assessed before it is initiated. Disulfiram is much more likely to be efficacious if dose administration is supervised (e.g., by a spouse or a parent).

Tobacco Use Disorder

All three FDA-approved medications for smoking cessation are appropriate as first-line therapies for this indication. NRT, especially the combination of a patch and lozenge or gum, is affordable and easily accessible as an over-the-counter treatment. Due to the large EAGLES study results that varenicline may be more effective than bupropion or the nicotine patch and has comparable safety, it may be chosen as first-line (Anthenelli, Benowitz et al. 2016). However, a smaller study suggested that it may not be more effective than combination NRT formulations (Cahill, Stevens et al. 2013).

The usual dose of varenicline is 1 mg twice daily. After a week on this dose, patients can set a quit date. If they fail it, they can continue it for two more weeks and try to quit again. It may take several trials before there can be success with quitting, but it may help to examine the circumstances maintaining the usage of the few remaining cigarettes and to apply cognitive or behavioral strategies to eliminate these (e.g., the one that goes with coffee in the morning—maybe skip the coffee). If the patient has reduced cigarette use by at least 50% but has not quit, one study shows that it can be beneficial to increase the varenicline dose to 1.5 mg twice daily (Karam-Hage, Kypriotakis et al. 2019). This did not work, however, if the patient had failed to achieve a 50% reduction.

Bupropion may be appropriate for patients who have comorbid unipolar depression and/or attention-deficit/hyperactivity disorder and/or those who are concerned about weight gain after smoking cessation (although those with past seizures or eating disorders cannot take this medication). All treatments should be continued for several months (or longer if needed) after smoking cessation. This should be stressed at the beginning when patients commence these therapies.

Increasing behavioral supports for patients treated with medication for smoking cessation is likely to increase the chances of smoking cessation regardless of which medication is used (Stead, Koilpillai et al. 2015).

Treatment-Resistant Substance Use Disorders

Substance abuse treatments often fail due to reasons that are not related to the pharmacological effects of the therapies used. Possible nonadherence to treatment, diversion of therapeutic medications (in the case of buprenorphine), concurrent psychiatric disorders, poor social supports, or unsuspected polysubstance use should be addressed to increase treatment response.

Opioid Use Disorder

Patients who relapse on buprenorphine/naloxone or methadone may benefit from increased psychosocial supports and increased doses to help control cravings. Switching from opioid maintenance treatments to injectable naltrexone (or vice versa) may also be considered.

Those who relapse on maximum daily doses of buprenorphine may be tried on methadone. Those who divert sublingual buprenorphine may be tried on monthly injectable buprenorphine or oral methadone. Those who were initially started on methadone but have been unable to tolerate this medication can be switched to buprenorphine (once methadone is tapered off and the patient is in moderate opioid withdrawal).

It is important to keep in mind that medication-assisted therapy is likely to be more effective with the addition of psychotherapy (McLellan, Arndt et al. 1993). Both buprenorphine and methadone are FDA-approved for use *in conjunction* with psychosocial therapies (even if these were to be only marginally helpful). Therefore, pharmacotherapy without psychosocial therapies may be considered *partial* treatment. Failure of such treatment therefore does not necessarily constitute "treatment resistance."

Alcohol Use Disorder

Patients who fail treatment with either naltrexone (oral and injectable) or acamprosate may try the other. Even though complete abstinence is preferred, for both agents treatment response may be defined as a significant reduction of alcohol use, and the lack of abstinence, therefore, is not necessarily grounds for discontinuation of either medication. If both medications are insufficiently helpful in monotherapy, then they may be combined if tolerated, although there is not much evidence supporting this combination (Anton, O'Malley et al. 2006). If combination therapy is still not helpful then disulfiram monotherapy may be considered in patients who are not at high risk of adverse cardiovascular events or this medication's other potential adverse effects. Supervised disulfiram administration may be more effective than naltrexone or acamprosate (Laaksonen, Koski-Jannes et al. 2008).

Ondansetron, prazosin, or the anticonvulsants reviewed previously may also be considered in patients who do not respond to FDA-approved treatments, as long as their potential benefits appear to outweigh their risks. At every step, psychosocial supports should also be increased.

Tobacco Use Disorder

If varenicline, bupropion, and NRT monotherapies are not helpful in smoking cessation, combination treatments may be considered. The combination of NRT and bupropion may be more effective than bupropion or NRT alone (Jorenby, Leischow et al. 1999; Stead, Perera et al. 2012). However, adding bupropion to NRT may not improve the chances for long-term cessation (Hughes, Stead et al. 2014).

The combination of varenicline and NRT would be expected to have questionable pharmacodynamic value, given that they overlap in their effects on nicotine receptors. However, a randomized trial in 446 smokers found that varenicline worked better when a nicotine patch was added two weeks prior to the quit date, compared to varenicline alone (Koegelenberg, Noor et al. 2014). Fifty-five percent were able to quit for three months on the combination versus 41% on just varenicline (odds ratio = 1.85). Side effects varied in both groups. It might be that the NRT blunts the withdrawal symptoms, which, as the EAGLES study showed, are not reduced by varenicline. The patient is able to use the anticraving effects of the varenicline to convert to NRT monotherapy and then can taper this off gradually.

Finally, the addition of bupropion to varenicline may be of modest benefit over varenicline alone (Ebbert, Hatsukami et al. 2014).

Use in Women of Childbearing Potential, Pregnancy, and Breastfeeding

Pregnancy

Opioid Use Disorder

Illicit opioid use during pregnancy is associated with multiple risks to the fetus, including the risk of maternal death from overdose. Maternal opioid use may also lead to more preterm births, fetal death, growth restriction, and acquisition of infectious diseases if illicit opioids are used intravenously. For opioids in general, the risks of congenital malformations are not fully known. One review found that it was difficult to reach definitive conclusions about the teratogenicity of opioids, although oral cleft, cardiac septal defects, and clubfoot were more commonly reported in the reviewed studies (Lind, Interrante et al. 2017).

In addition to the previously described risks, neonatal abstinence syndrome (NAS) due to opioid withdrawal in newborns may occur in the infant if the mother has been opioid-dependent. NAS may be characterized by poor feeding, failure to thrive, temperature dysregulation, and possibly seizures and may require prolonged neonatal intensive care hospitalization (Jansson and Patrick 2019).

The risks of using methadone, buprenorphine, or naltrexone, therefore, should be weighed against the pre- and postnatal risks of continued illicit opioid use. The goal of therapy during pregnancy is to lower the described risks by helping the mother maintain

abstinence from illicit opioids—and the use of either buprenorphine and methadone is preferable to the ongoing use of illicit
drugs (Mozurkewich and Rayburn 2014). An added goal is to avoid
opioid withdrawal (and likely hyperadrenergic state) during pregnancy given concerns about the potential for fetal distress, miscarriage, or preterm labor.

Historically, methadone had been favored for use in pregnant
patients; however, buprenorphine or buprenorphine/naloxone are
now frequently considered. Although buprenorphine without naloxone had been recommended initially for pregnant patients (due
to uncertainties regarding naloxone's risks to the fetus), the combination may be well-tolerated (Lund, Fischer et al. 2013; Wiegand,
Stringer et al. 2015; Debelak, Morrone et al. 2013).

There is mixed evidence suggesting that buprenorphine
may be associated with higher birth weights and lower preterm births than methadone, but overall outcomes including fetal death and congenital anomalies appear to be similar
(Wiegand, Stringer et al. 2015; Zedler, Mann et al. 2016). Still,
the risk of congenital abnormalities from both buprenorphine
and methadone exposure may be higher than in those who are
not exposed to opioids during pregnancy (Norgaard, Nielsson &
Heidi-Jorgensen 2015).

NAS is likely to be less severe and of shorter duration in newborns whose mothers were treated with buprenorphine than in
those who were treated with methadone (Norgaard, Nielsson et al.
2015; Grossman, Seashore & Holmes 2017; Tran, Griffin et al.
2017). Long-term developmental risks to the newborn from in
utero exposure to opioid agonists, or for those with severe NAS are
not known.

Injectable naltrexone is not preferred for initiation during pregnancy as it would require a period of withdrawal from existing opioids before starting treatment. Less is known about its potential
effects on the fetus (Tran, Griffin et al. 2017), although as expected

it should be associated with a much lower incidence of NAS (Kelty and Hulse 2017).

Irrespective of the previous comparisons between methadone and buprenorphine, whichever opioid agonist is used by the mother at conception is usually continued during pregnancy to avoid destabilization (Klaman, Isaacs et al. 2017), although dose adjustments may be needed later in pregnancy. Even for long-acting naltrexone for which there are less supporting data, one study showed that continuing it during pregnancy may have no greater risks than those of buprenorphine or methadone, and it may be associated with less congenital abnormalities than methadone (Kelty and Hulse 2017).

Alcohol Use Disorder

Alcohol use during pregnancy is associated with fetal alcohol syndrome and fetal alcohol spectrum disorders, which are characterized by growth retardation, facial dysmorphias, and neurological and neurobehavioral abnormalities (Denny, Coles et al. 2017). Increased maternal alcohol use is also associated with increases in preterm births and lower birth weights (Patra, Bakker et al. 2011), as well as increased incidence of stillbirths (Kesmodel, Wisborg et al. 2002). Despite the significant risks of alcohol use in pregnancy, there is insufficient evidence to recommend the use of available alcohol use disorder medications during pregnancy. It is not clear if experience from naltrexone use in opioid dependent mothers could be extrapolated to mothers with alcohol use disorders.

Tobacco Use Disorder

Smoking during pregnancy is associated with multiple complications such as an increased risk of miscarriage, preterm births, stillbirths, and low birth weights (Pineles, Park & Samet 2014;

Pineles, Hsu et al. 2016; Pereira, Da Mata et al. 2017; Soneji and Beltran-Sanchez 2019). Short- and long-term developmental effects on the fetus have also been suspected (Holbrook 2016). To decrease these risks, supportive counseling and psychoeducational interventions should be made available to pregnant women.

NRT in pregnancy does not seem to increase the risk of pregnancy related complications (Swamy, Roelands et al. 2009). However, recent results are mixed as to whether NRT is effective for smoking cessation during pregnancy (Coleman, Cooper et al. 2012; Berard, Zhao et al. 2016). Bupropion has been found to be beneficial for some patients (Berard, Zhao et al. 2016); however, an association with a small increased risked of congenital cardiac abnormalities is concerning (Louik, Kerr & Mitchell 2014; Hendrick, Suri et al. 2017). There are insufficient data to support the use of varenicline in pregnant women.

Breastfeeding

Opioid Use Disorder

Breastfeeding by mothers who are actively using illicit opioids is not recommended (D'Apolito 2013; Reece-Stremtan and Marinelli 2015). However, a very small study of seven infants who were breastfed while their mothers were treated with buprenorphine showed no adverse effects four weeks after birth (Gower, Bartu et al. 2014). Infant exposure to both methadone and buprenorphine in breast milk is considered to be low, and these are usually considered to be relatively safe for breastfeeding (despite potential risks of lethargy and respiratory depression; Sachs and Committee on Drugs 2013; Wachman, Saia et al. 2016). The Academy of Breastfeeding Medicine recommends that stable methadone- or buprenorphine-maintained mothers should be encouraged "to breastfeed regardless of dose" (Reece-Stremtan and Marinelli 2015). Breastfeeding may also decrease NAS symptoms (Holmes, Schmidlin & Kurzum 2017). If breastfeeding is to be discontinued, it may need to be gradually tapered off to decrease the risk of opioid withdrawal in the newborn. Limited information is available for breastfeeding while taking injectable naltrexone.

Alcohol Use Disorder

There are insufficient data to support the use of disulfiram, naltrexone (Sachs et al. 2013), or acamprosate while breastfeeding.

Tobacco Use Disorder

NRT can be used during breastfeeding as long as the daily doses are lower than the amount of nicotine that the mother would have otherwise received from smoking cigarettes. Short-acting gum and lozenges and low-dose patches may be preferred (Ilett, Hale et al. 2003; Sachs et al. 2013). There are insufficient data to establish the safety of breastfeeding while taking varenicline. The potential risk of seizures in breastfed infants whose mothers take bupropion is still of some concern (Chaudron and Schoenecker 2004).

Table of Medicines for Substance Use Disorders

Table 6.1 summarizes the characteristics of medications used for substance use disorders (Ansari and Osser 2015; World Health Organization 2019; PDR 2019; Lexicomp 2019).

TABLE 6.1 Medicines for Substance Use Disorders

Medication[a]	Adult Dosing[b]	Comments/FDA *Indication*
Methadone (Opioid agonist and analgesic) (Dolophine®, Methadose®)	Started at low doses and gradually increased over many months at specialized methadone maintenance centers only, to reach a target dose that would stop cravings for illicit opioids (e.g., 90–120 po mg daily)— see text; analgesic doses are much lower (e.g., 5 mg po tid prn pain). Start at lower doses, titrate more slowly, and monitor more carefully in patients with hepatic or renal impairments.	The use of prescribed opioids for patients with opioid use disorders is controversial, but effective; not curative; requires attendance at a methadone clinic for daily administration. Schedule II. May increase QTc; primarily a CYP3A4 substrate, however combination with CYP3A4 or CYP2B6, CYP2C19, CYP2C9, CYP2D6 inhibitors may increase risk of fatal respiratory depression. On WHO Essential Medicines List for psychoactive substance use. Black Box Warning: Addiction, abuse misuse; risk evaluation and mitigation strategy (REMS); life threatening respiratory depression; accidental ingestion/ overdose; QT prolongation/ serious arrhythmias; neonatal opioid withdrawal syndrome; dispense at certified program only; risks from concomitant use with benzodiazepines or other CNS depressants; risks of CYP450 interactions *Detoxification treatment of opioid addiction/ Maintenance treatment of opioid addiction in conjunction with appropriate social and medical services/ Management of moderate to severe pain (see package insert)*

TABLE 6.1 Continued

Medication[a]	Adult Dosing[b]	Comments/FDA *Indication*
Buprenorphine/ Naloxone (Partial opioid agonist with opioid antagonist) (Suboxone®, Suboxone Film®, Zubsolv®, Cassipa®);

Buprenorphine (Partial opioid agonist without opioid antagonist) (Subutex®)

Buprenorphine monthly injection (Sublocade®)

Buprenorphine 6-month subdermal implant (Probuphine®) | Do not start until patient is experiencing moderate opioid withdrawal. Then for Suboxone® start: buprenorphine/ naloxone 4 mg/1 mg sublingually bid-tid, usual maintenance dose is 16–20 mg/day or less, in divided doses. Max dose 24 mg/ day sublingually. (See package insert for other formulations).

For sublingual buprenorphine: Monitor more carefully in patients with moderate or severe hepatic impairments and reduce doses in the latter. Use with caution in patients with severe renal impairment. | May be given as take home prescription by trained physicians; less regulated than methadone, but considerable street usage is occurring. Schedule III. Suboxone® and Subutex® are available as generics; Suboxone Film® is available to decrease risk of diversion and to decrease risk of accidental ingestion by children; CYP3A4 substrate. On WHO Essential Medicines List for psychoactive substance use.

Black Box Warning: Accidental exposure; Addiction, abuse misuse; risk evaluation and mitigation strategy (REMS); life threatening respiratory depression; neonatal opioid withdrawal syndrome; risks from concomitant use with benzodiazepines or other CNS depressants; risks of harm or death from intravenous use; risks of insertion and removal of transdermal implant formulation.

Treatment of opioid dependence/ Maintenance treatment of opioid dependence and should be used as part of a complete treatment plan that includes counseling and psychosocial support |

(continued)

TABLE 6.1 Continued

Medication[a]	Adult Dosing[b]	Comments/FDA *Indication*
Naloxone (Opioid antagonist) (Narcan® Nasal Spray)	For nasal spray: Place unresponsive patient suspected of opioid overdose in supine position. Support the back of the neck and allow the head to tilt back. Insert device into one of patient's nostrils and administer contents (4 mg of naloxone). Repeated doses may be necessary every 2–3 minutes. Repeat dose if patient again has CNS or respiratory depression. After each dose turn patient on their side. Call EMS.	Also available in intramuscular, subcutaneous (absorption may be erratic), and intravenous formulations for use in medical and hospital settings. (Naloxone injection is on WHO Essential Medicines List). *For the emergency treatment of known or suspected opioid overdose, as manifested by respiratory and/or CNS depression*
Naltrexone (Opioid antagonist) (ReVia®) Naltrexone monthly injection (Vivitrol®)	Do not start until free from opioids for 7–10 days. For oral naltrexone, ReVia®: Start: 25 mg po q am after meal then increase to 50 mg po q am after 3 days. For Vivitrol® extended release: 380 mg IM gluteal injection every 4 weeks (alternating buttocks). Dose adjustments may be needed in patients with hepatic or renal impairment. Do not use in acute hepatitis or hepatic failure.	Check baseline LFTs. Do not use if LFTs are greater than 3 times the upper limit of normal. Monitor LFTs in one month, then every 6 months thereafter; available in long-acting IM form for every 4 weeks administration; Encourage patient medic-alert card or bracelet. Risk of hepatic injury. Black Box Warning (for Vivitrol®): Hepatic injury *Treatment of alcohol dependence and to block effects of exogenously administered opioids* For Vivitrol®: *Treatment of alcohol dependence in patients who are able to abstain from alcohol in an outpatient setting prior to initiation of therapy/ Prevention of relapse to opioid dependence following opioid detoxification*

TABLE 6.1 Continued

Medication[a]	Adult Dosing[b]	Comments/*FDA Indication*
Acamprosate (GABA analog) (Campral®)	Start: 333 mg po tid and increase to 666 mg po tid after 2–3 days. Do not use as first-line in patients with mild to moderate renal impairment—reduce doses if used; avoid in patients with severe renal impairment.	Renally cleared; check baseline kidney function and adjust dose with decreased function; can continue even with alcohol relapse; concurrent naltrexone may increase serum levels. *Maintenance of abstinence from alcohol in patients with alcohol dependence who are abstinent at treatment initiation*
Disulfiram (Aldehyde Dehydrogenase Inhibitor) (Antabuse®)	Start 24 hours or longer after last alcohol use. Start: 125 mg po q am and increase after 4 days to 250 mg po q am and continue; maximum 500 mg/day. Avoid, or use with extreme caution, in patients with hepatic cirrhosis or insufficiency and with extreme caution in patients with chronic or acute nephritis.	Check baseline LFTs before treatment and after 2 weeks and then every 3–6 months thereafter. Severe reactions, including death, have occurred. Not usual first-line. Black Box Warning: Never administer to patient with alcohol intoxication or without patient's knowledge. *Aid in the management of selected chronic alcoholics who want to remain sober in a state of enforced sobriety so that supportive and psychotherapeutic treatment may be applied to the best advantage*
Nicotine Replacement Therapy (NRT) (Nicoderm Patch®, Commit Lozenges®, Nicorette Lozenges®, Nicorette Gum®, Nicotrol Inhaler®, Nicotrol Nasal Spray®)	For Nicoderm Patch®: Stop smoking, then dosing depends on cigarette use: For example, if greater than 10 cigarettes/day then: 21 mg patch TD daily for 6 weeks, then 14 mg TD daily for 2 weeks, then 7 mg TD daily for 2 weeks then stop. Other dosing depends on formulation. Severe hepatic or renal impairments may reduce clearance of nicotine.	Nicotine replacement therapy also serves to eliminate hydrocarbon toxicity and carbon monoxide inhalation associated with cigarette use. Combination of nicotine patch with shorter acting formulation may be most beneficial. On WHO Essential Medicines List for psychoactive substance use. *To reduce withdrawal symptoms, including nicotine craving, associated with smoking cessation*

(continued)

TABLE 6.1 Continued

Medication[a]	Adult Dosing[b]	Comments/FDA *Indication*
Bupropion (Antidepressant) (Zyban®, Wellbutrin®, Aplenzin®, Buproban®, Wellbutrin SR®, Budeprion SR®, Wellbutrin XL®, Forfivo XL®)	For bupropion extended release, Zyban®, Wellbutrin SR®: Start while still smoking. Start: 150 mg sustained release po q am then 150 mg po bid (morning and afternoon) after 4–7 days, set cigarette cessation target date 2 weeks into treatment. (Different dosing for different bupropion formulations). Use 150 mg po q am in patients with schizophrenia. Reduce doses in patients with hepatic or renal impairments.	Contraindicated in patients with history of seizure, eating disorder or if otherwise at high seizure risk. May be combined with nicotine replacement therapy; risk of treatment-emergent suicidality in patients under 25 years old as with all antidepressants; CYP2D6 inhibitor. Black Box Warning: Suicidality *Aid to smoking cessation treatment/ MDD/Prevention of seasonal MDE in patients with seasonal affective disorder*
Varenicline (Nicotine Acetylcholine Receptor Agonist) (Chantix®)	Start: 0.5 mg po daily for 3 days, then 0.5 mg po bid for 4 days, then 1 mg po bid— which is the usual maximum dose. Set quit date one week after this dose. Continue for 12–52 weeks. Reduce doses in patients with renal impairment.	Treatment-emergent neuropsychiatric symptoms and suicidality initially reported but warning later removed by FDA. Patients with pre-existing psychiatric illness may still benefit from close monitoring when starting this medication. FDA warning regarding increased occurrence of cardiovascular events was later removed. Small risk of seizures. Minimal or no metabolism by liver. *Aid to smoking cessation treatment*

SEE PACKAGE INSERT FOR DOSING AND OTHER INFORMATION BEFORE PRESCRIBING MEDICATIONS. Dosing should be adjusted downwards ("start low, go slow" strategy) for the elderly and/or the medically compromised. Abbreviations: bid (bis in die), twice a day; CYP, cytochrome P450 enzyme; FDA, Food and Drug Administration; GABA, gamma aminobutyric acid; IM, intramuscular; LFT, liver function tests; MDD, major depressive disorder; MDE, major depressive episode; mg, milligram; po (per os), orally; q (quaque), every; TD, transdermally; tid (ter in die), three times a day; WHO, World Health Organization.

[a]Generic and U.S. brand name(s).

[b]Doses are provided for educational purposes only.

References

Addolorato G, Leggio L (2010). Safety and efficacy of baclofen in the treatment of alcohol-dependent patients. Curr Pharm Des 16(19): 2113–2117.

Agabio R, Trogu E, Pani PP (2018). Antidepressants for the treatment of people with co-occurring depression and alcohol dependence. Cochrane Database Syst Rev 4: CD008581.

Ahmed AI, Ali AN, et al. (2013). Neuropsychiatric adverse events of varenicline: a systematic review of published reports. J Clin Psychopharmacol 33(1): 55–62.

Ali B, Green KM, et al. (2017). Distress tolerance interacts with circumstances, motivation, and readiness to predict substance abuse treatment retention. Addict Behav 73: 99–104.

Ansari A, Osser DN (2015). *Psychopharmacology, A Concise Overview for Students and Clinicians, 2nd Edition*. North Charleston, SC: CreateSpace.

Anthenelli RM, Benowitz NL, et al. (2016). Neuropsychiatric safety and efficacy of varenicline, bupropion, and nicotine patch in smokers with and without psychiatric disorders (EAGLES): a double-blind, randomised, placebo-controlled clinical trial. Lancet 387(10037): 2507–2520.

Anton RF (2008). Naltrexone for the management of alcohol dependence. N Engl J Med 359: 715–721.

Anton RF, O'Malley SS, et al. (2006). Combined pharmacotherapies and behavioral interventions for alcohol dependence: the COMBINE study: a randomized controlled trial. JAMA 295: 2003–2017.

Anton RF, Oroszi G, et al. (2008). An evaluation of mu-opioid receptor (OPRM1) as a predictor of naltrexone response in the treatment of alcohol dependence: results from the Combined Pharmacotherapies and Behavioral Interventions for Alcohol Dependence study. Arch Gen Psychiatry 65: 135–144.

Arbaizar B, Diersen-Sotos T, et al. (2010). Topiramate in the treatment of alcohol dependence: a meta-analysis. Actas Esp Psiquiatr 38(1): 8–12.

Bachhuber MA, Saloner B, et al. (2014). Medical cannabis laws and opioid analgesic overdose mortality in the United States, 1999-2010. JAMA Intern Med 174(10): 1668–1673.

Baker TB, Piper ME, et al. (2016). Effects of nicotine patch vs varenicline vs combination nicotine replacement therapy on smoking cessation at 26 weeks: a randomized clinical trial. JAMA 315(4): 371–379.

Baldacara L, Cogo-Moreira H, et al. (2016). Efficacy of topiramate in the treatment of crack cocaine dependence: a double-blind, randomized, placebo-controlled trial. J Clin Psychiatry 77(3): 398–406.

Baltieri DA, Daro FR, et al. (2008). Comparing topiramate with naltrexone in the treatment of alcohol dependence. Addiction 103(12): 2035–2044.

Bao YP, Liu ZM, et al. (2009). A meta-analysis of retention in methadone maintenance by dose and dosing strategy. Am J Drug Alcohol Abuse 35(1): 28–33.

Bell J, Trinh L, et al. (2009). Comparing retention in treatment and mortality in people after initial entry to methadone and buprenorphine treatment. Addiction 104(7): 1193–1200.

Benowitz NL, Pipe A, et al. (2018). cardiovascular safety of varenicline, bupropion, and nicotine patch in smokers: a randomized clinical trial. JAMA Intern Med 178(5): 622–631.

Berard A, Zhao JP, Sheehy O (2016). Success of smoking cessation interventions during pregnancy. Am J Obstet Gynecol 215(5): e611–e618.

Bogenschutz MP, Forcehimes AA, et al. (2015). Psilocybin-assisted treatment for alcohol dependence: a proof-of-concept study. J Psychopharmacol 29(3): 289–299.

Bogenschutz MP, Podrebarac SK, et al. (2018). Clinical interpretations of patient experience in a trial of psilocybin-assisted psychotherapy for alcohol use disorder. Front Pharmacol 9: 100.

Bolliger CT, Issa JS, et al. (2011). Effects of varenicline in adult smokers: a multinational, 24-week, randomized, double-blind, placebo-controlled study. Clin Ther 33(4): 465–477.

Bonnet U, Scherbaum N (2017). How addictive are gabapentin and pregabalin? A systematic review. Eur Neuropsychopharmacol 27(12): 1185–1215.

Boothby LA, Doering PL (2005). Acamprosate for the treatment of alcohol dependence. Clin Ther 27: 695–714.

Bond C, LaForge KS, et al. (1998). Single-nucleotide polymorphism in the human mu opioid receptor gene alters beta-endorphin binding and activity: possible implications for opiate addiction. Proc Natl Acad Sci U S A 95: 9608–9613.

Breland AB, Spindle T, et al. (2014). Science and electronic cigarettes: current data, future needs. J Addict Med 8(4): 223–233.

Brensilver M, Heinzerling KG, Shoptaw S (2013). Pharmacotherapy of amphetamine-type stimulant dependence: an update. Drug Alcohol Rev 32(5): 449–460.

Brooks AC, Comer SD, et al. (2010). Long-acting injectable versus oral naltrexone maintenance therapy with psychosocial intervention for heroin dependence: a quasi-experiment. J Clin Psychiatry 71(10): 1371–1378.

Butler SF, Black RA, et al. (2018). Understanding abuse of buprenorphine/naloxone film versus tablet products using data from ASI-MV(R) substance use disorder treatment centers and RADARS(R) System Poison Centers. J Subst Abuse Treat 84: 42–49.

Cahill K, Stevens S, et al. (2013). Pharmacological interventions for smoking cessation: an overview and network meta-analysis. Cochrane Database Syst Rev 5: CD009329.

Caplehorn JR, Drummer OH (2002). Fatal methadone toxicity: signs and circumstances, and the role of benzodiazepines. Aust N Z J Public Health 26(4): 358–362; discussion 362–363.

Carroll KM, Fenton LR, et al. (2004). Efficacy of disulfiram and cognitive behavior therapy in cocaine-dependent outpatients: a randomized placebo-controlled trial. Arch Gen Psychiatry 61(3): 264–272.

Chaudron LH, Schoenecker CJ (2004). Bupropion and breastfeeding: a case of a possible infant seizure. J Clin Psychiatry 65(6): 881–882.

Chick J (1999). Safety issues concerning the use of disulfiram in treating alcohol dependence. Drug Saf 20(5): 427–435.

Coleman T, Cooper S, et al. (2012). A randomized trial of nicotine-replacement therapy patches in pregnancy. N Engl J Med 366(9): 808–818.

Cornelius JR, Chung T, et al. (2016a). Mirtazapine in comorbid major depression and an alcohol use disorder: A double-blind placebo-controlled pilot trial. Psychiatry Res 242: 326–330.

Cornelius JR, Chung TA, et al. (2016b). A review of the literature of mirtazapine in co-occurring depression and an alcohol use disorder. J Addict Behav Ther Rehabil 5(4).

Cornelius JR, Douaihy AB, et al. (2012). Mirtazapine in comorbid major depression and alcohol dependence: an open-label trial. J Dual Diagn 8(3): 200–204.

Correa Filho JM, Baltieri DA (2013). A pilot study of full-dose ondansetron to treat heavy-drinking men withdrawing from alcohol in Brazil. Addict Behav 38(4): 2044–2051.

Cullen KA, Ambrose BK, et al. (2018). Notes from the field: use of electronic cigarettes and any tobacco product among middle and high school students—United States, 2011–2018. MMWR Morb Mortal Wkly Rep 67: 1276–1277.

Dackis CA, Kampman KM, et al. (2005). A double-blind, placebo-controlled trial of modafinil for cocaine dependence. Neuropsychopharmacology 30(1): 205–211.

Daitch J, Frey ME, et al. (2012). Conversion of chronic pain patients from full-opioid agonists to sublingual buprenorphine. Pain Physician 15(3 Suppl): ES59–E66.

D'Apolito K (2013). Breastfeeding and substance abuse. Clin Obstet Gynecol 56(1): 202–211.

Debelak K, Morrone WR, et al. (2013). Buprenorphine + naloxone in the treatment of opioid dependence during pregnancy—initial patient care and outcome data. Am J Addict 22(3): 252–254.

Dell'Orto VG, Belotti EA, et al. (2014). Metabolic disturbances and renal stone promotion on treatment with topiramate: a systematic review. Br J Clin Pharmacol 77: 958–964.

De Sousa A (2010). The role of topiramate and other anticonvulsants in the treatment of alcohol dependence: a clinical review. CNS Neurol Disord Drug Targets 9(1): 45–49.

Denny L, Coles S, Blitz R (2017). Fetal alcohol syndrome and fetal alcohol spectrum disorders. Am Fam Physician 96(8): 515–522.

Diehl A, Ulmer L, et al. (2010). Why is disulfiram superior to acamprosate in the routine clinical setting? A retrospective long-term study in 353 alcohol-dependent patients. Alcohol 45(3): 271–277.

Dugosh K, Abraham A, et al. (2016). A systematic review on the use of psychosocial interventions in conjunction with medications for the treatment of opioid addiction. J Addict Med 10(2): 93–103.

Dundon W, Lynch KG, et al. (2004). Treatment outcomes in type A and B alcohol dependence 6 months after serotonergic pharmacotherapy. Alcohol Clin Exp Res 28(7): 1065–1073.

Dutra LM, Glantz SA (2014). Electronic cigarettes and conventional cigarette use among US adolescents: a cross-sectional study. JAMA Pediatr 168: 610–617.

Dutra L, Stathopoulou G, et al. (2008). A meta-analytic review of psychosocial interventions for substance use disorders. Am J Psychiatry 165: 179–187.

Ebbert JO, Elrashidi MU, Stead LF (2015). Interventions for smokeless tobacco use cessation. Cochrnae Database Syst Rev 10: CDC004306.

Ebbert JO, Hatsukami DK, et al. (2014). Combination varenicline and bupropion SR for tobacco-dependence treatment in cigarette smokers: a randomized trial. JAMA 311(2): 155–163.

Ehret GB, Voide C, et al. (2006). Drug-induced long QT syndrome in injection drug users receiving methadone: high frequency in hospitalized patients and risk factors. Arch Intern Med 166: 1280–1287.

Evans EA, Zhu Y, et al. (2019). Criminal justice outcomes over 5 years after randomization to buprenorphine-naloxone or methadone treatment for opioid use disorder. Addiction 114(8): 1396–1404.

Evins AE, Benowitz NL, et al. (2019). Neuropsychiatric safety and efficacy of varenicline, bupropion, and nicotine patch in smokers with psychotic, anxiety, and mood disorders in the EAGLES trial. J Clin Psychopharmacol 39(2): 108–116.

Evoy KE, Covvey JR, et al. (2019). Reports of gabapentin and pregabalin abuse, misuse, dependence, or overdose: an analysis of the Food and Drug Administration Adverse Events Reporting System (FAERS). Res Social Adm Pharm 15(8): 953–958.

Faggiano F, Vigna-Taglianti F, et al. (2003). Methadone maintenance at different dosages for opioid dependence. Cochrane Database Syst Rev 3: CD002208.

Fareed A, Casarella J, et al. (2010). Methadone maintenance dosing guideline for opioid dependence, a literature review. J Addict Dis 29(1): 1–14.

Fiellin DA, Pantalon MV, et al. (2006). Counseling plus buprenorphine-naloxone maintenance therapy for opioid dependence. N Engl J Med 355: 365–374.

Florez G, Saiz PA, et al. (2011). Topiramate for the treatment of alcohol dependence: comparison with naltrexone. Eur Addict Res 17(1): 29–36.

Follman S, Arora VM, et al. (2019). Naloxone prescriptions among commercially insured individuals at high risk of opioid overdose. JAMA Netw Open 2(5): e193209.

Food and Drug Administration (2016a). FDA Drug Safety Communication: FDA warns about serious risks and death when combining opioid pain or cough medicines with benzodiazepines; requires its strongest warning: https://www.fda.gov/drugs/drug-safety-and-availability/fda-drug-safety-communication-fda-warns-about-serious-risks-and-death-when-combining-opioid-pain-or

Food and Drug Administration (2016b). FDA Advisory Committee on the Most Appropriate Dose or Doses of Naloxone to Reverse the Effects of Life-threatening Opioid Overdose in the Community Settings: https://www.fda.gov/media/100409/download

Food and Drug Administration (2017). FDA Drug Safety Communication: FDA urges caution about withholding opioid addiction medications from patients taking benzodiazepines or CNS depressants: careful medication management can reduce risks: https://www.fda.gov/drugs/drug-safety-and-availability/fda-drug-safety-communication-fda-urges-caution-about-withholding-opioid-addiction-medications

Food and Drug Administration (2018). FDA Drug Safety Communication: FDA revises description of mental health side effects of the stop-smoking medicine Chantix (varenicline) and Zyban (bupriopion) to reflect clinical trial findings: https://www.fda.gov/drugs/drug-safety-and-availability/fda-drug-safety-communication-fda-revises-description-mental-health-side-effects-stop-smoking

Food and Drug Administration (2019a). FDA approves first generic naloxone nasal spray to treat opioid overdose: https://www.fda.gov/news-events/press-announcements/fda-approves-first-generic-naloxone-nasal-spray-treat-opioid-overdose

Food and Drug Administration (2019b). Statement from FDA Commissioner Scott Gottlieb, M.D., on unprecedented new efforts to support development of over-the-counter naloxone to help reduce opioid overdose deaths: https://www.fda.gov/news-events/press-announcements/statement-fda-commissioner-scott-gottlieb-md-unprecedented-new-efforts-support-development-over

Food and Drug Administration (2019c). Some e-cigarette users are having seizures, most reports involving youth and young adults: https://www.fda.gov/tobacco-products/ctp-newsroom/some-e-cigarette-users-are-having-seizures-most-reports-involving-youth-and-young-adults

Fox HC, Anderson GM, et al. (2012). Prazosin effects on stress- and cue-induced craving and stress response in alcohol-dependent individuals: preliminary findings. Alcohol Clin Exp Res 36(2): 351–360.

Freedman R (2007). Exacerbation of schizophrenia by varenicline. Am J Psychiatry 164: 1269.

Fucito LM, Park A, et al. (2012). Cigarette smoking predicts differential benefit from naltrexone for alcohol dependence. Biol Psychiatry 72(10): 832–838.

Fudala PJ, Bridge TP, et al. (2003). Office-based treatment of opiate addiction with a sublingual-tablet formulation of buprenorphine and naloxone. N Engl J Med 349: 949–958.

Garbutt JC, Kranzler HR, et al. (2005). Efficacy and tolerability of long-acting injectable naltrexone for alcohol dependence: a randomized controlled trial. JAMA 293: 1617–1625.

Gibbons RD, Mann JJ (2013). Varenicline, smoking cessation, and neuropsychiatric adverse events. Am J Psychiatry 170(12): 1460–1467.

Gibson A, Degenhardt L, et al. (2008). Exposure to opioid maintenance treatment reduces long-term mortality. Addiction 103(3): 462–468.

Goldenson NI, Leventhal AM, et al. (2017). Associations of electronic cigarette nicotine concentration with subsequent cigarette smoking and vaping levels in adolescents. JAMA Pediatr 171(12): 1192–1199.

Gonzales D, Rennard SI, et al. (2006). Varenicline, an alpha4beta2 nicotinic acetylcholine receptor partial agonist, vs. sustained-release bupropion and placebo for smoking cessation: a randomized controlled trial. JAMA 296: 47–55.

Gonzalez RA, Weiss F (1998). Suppression of ethanol-reinforced behavior by naltrexone is associated with attenuation of the ethanol-induced increase in dialysate dopamine levels in the nucleus accumbens. J Neurosci 18(24): 10663–10671.

Gower S, Bartu A, et al. (2014). The wellbeing of infants exposed to buprenorphine via breast milk at 4 weeks of age. J Hum Lact 30(2): 217–223.

Gowing LR, Farrell M, et al. (2006). Brief report: methadone treatment of injecting opioid users for prevention of HIV infection. J Gen Intern Med 21(2): 193–195.

Grossman M, Seashore C, Holmes AV (2017). Neonatal abstinence syndrome management: a review of recent evidence. Rev Recent Clin Trials 12(4): 226–232.

Guglielmo R, Martinotti G, et al. (2012). Pregabalin for alcohol dependence: a critical review of the literature. Adv Ther 29(11): 947–957.

Guglielmo R, Martinotti G, et al. (2015). Topiramate in alcohol use disorders: review and update. CNS Drugs 29(5): 383–395.

Haight BR, Learned SM, et al. (2019). Efficacy and safety of a monthly buprenorphine depot injection for opioid use disorder: a multicentre, randomised, double-blind, placebo-controlled, phase 3 trial. Lancet 393(10173): 778–790.

Haney M, Ramesh D, et al. (2015). Naltrexone maintenance decreases cannabis self-administration and subjective effects in daily cannabis smokers. Neuropsychopharmacology 40(11): 2489–2498.

Hartmann-Boyce J, Stead LF, et al. (2014). Efficacy of interventions to combat tobacco addiction: Cochrane update of 2013 reviews. Addiction 109(9): 1414–1425.

Helstrom AW, Blow FC, et al. (2016). Reductions in alcohol craving following naltrexone treatment for heavy drinking. Alcohol 51(5): 562–566.

Hendrick V, Suri R, et al. (2017). Bupropion Use during pregnancy: a systematic review. Prim Care Companion CNS Disord 19(5).

Heydari G, Marashian M, et al. (2012). Which form of nicotine replacement therapy is more effective for quitting smoking? A study in Tehran, Islamic Republic of Iran. East Mediterr Health J 18(10): 1005–1010.

Holbrook BD (2016). The effects of nicotine on human fetal development. Birth Defects Res C Embryo Today 108(2): 181–192.

Holmes AP, Schmidlin HN, Kurzum EN (2017). Breastfeeding considerations for mothers of infants with neonatal abstinence syndrome. Pharmacotherapy 37(7): 861–869.

Hser YI, Evans E, et al. (2016). Long-term outcomes after randomization to buprenorphine/naloxone versus methadone in a multi-site trial. Addiction 111(4): 695–705.

Hughes JC, Cook CC (1997). The efficacy of disulfiram: a review of outcome studies. Addiction 92: 381–395.

Hughes JR, Stead LF, et al. (2014). Antidepressants for smoking cessation. Cochrane Database Syst Rev 1: CD000031.

Hulse GK, Ngo HT, et al. (2010). Risk factors for craving and relapse in heroin users treated with oral or implant naltrexone. Biol Psychiatry 68(3): 296–302.

Hurd YL, Spriggs S, et al. (2019). Cannabidiol for the reduction of cue-induced craving and anxiety in drug-abstinent individuals with heroin use disorder: a double-blind randomized placebo-controlled trial. Am J Psychiatry 176: 911–922.

Ilett KF, Hale TW, et al. (2003). Use of nicotine patches in breast-feeding mothers: transfer of nicotine and cotinine into human milk. Clin Pharmacol Ther 74(6): 516–524.

Jansson LM, Patrick SW (2019). Neonatal abstinence syndrome. Pediatr Clin North Am 66(2): 353–367.

Johnson BA, Ait-Daoud N, et al. (2000). Combining ondansetron and naltrexone effectively treats biologically predisposed alcoholics: from hypothesis to preliminary clinical evidence. Alcohol Clin Exp Res 24: 737–742.

Johnson BA, Ait-Daoud N, et al. (2003). Oral topiramate for treatment of alcohol dependence: a randomized controlled trial. Lancet 361: 1677–1685.

Johnson BA, Ait-Daoud N, et al. (2013). Topiramate for the treatment of cocaine addiction: a randomized clinical trial. JAMA Psychiatry 70(12): 1338–1346.

Johnson BA, Roache JD, et al. (2000). Ondansetron for reduction of drinking among biologically predisposed alcoholic patients: a randomized controlled trial. JAMA 284: 963–971.

Johnson BA, Rosenthal N, et al. (2007). Topiramate for treating alcohol dependence: a randomized controlled trial. JAMA 298: 1641–1651.

Johnson MW, Garcia-Romeu A, et al. (2014). Pilot study of the 5-HT2AR agonist psilocybin in the treatment of tobacco addiction. J Psychopharmacol 28(11): 983–992.

Johnson TS (2010). A brief review of pharmacotherapeutic treatment options in smoking cessation: bupropion versus varenicline. J Am Acad Nurse Pract 22(10): 557–563.

Jonas DE, Amick HR, et al. (2014). Pharmacotherapy for adults with alcohol use disorders in outpatient settings: a systematic review and meta-analysis. JAMA 311(18): 1889–1900.

Jorenby DE, Hays JT, et al. (2006). Efficacy of varenicline, an alpha4beta2 nicotinic acetylcholine receptor partial agonist, vs. placebo or sustained-release bupropion for smoking cessation: a randomized controlled trial. JAMA 296: 56–63.

Jorenby DE, Leischow SJ, et al. (1999). A controlled trial of sustained-release bupropion, a nicotine patch, or both for smoking cessation. N Engl J Med 340: 685–691.

Jorgensen CH, Pedersen B, et al. (2011). The efficacy of disulfiram for the treatment of alcohol use disorder. Alcohol Clin Exp Res 35(10): 1749–1758.

Kalkhoran S, Glantz SA (2016). E-cigarettes and smoking cessation in real-world and clinical settings: a systematic review and meta-analysis. Lancet Respir Med 4(2): 116–128.

Kapur BM, Hutson JR, et al. (2011). Methadone: a review of drug-drug and pathophysiological interactions. Crit Rev Clin Lab Sci 48(4): 171–195.

Karam-Hage M, Kypriotakis G, et al. (2018). Improvement of smoking abstinence rates with increased varenicline dosage: a propensity score-matched analysis. J Clin Psychopharmacol 38(1): 34–41.

Kelty E, Hulse G (2017). A retrospective cohort study of birth outcomes in neonates exposed to naltrexone in utero: a comparison with methadone-, buprenorphine- and non-opioid-exposed neonates. Drugs 77(11): 1211–1219.

Kesmodel U, Wisborg K, et al. (2002). Moderate alcohol intake during pregnancy and the risk of stillbirth and death in the first year of life. Am J Epidemiol 155(4): 305–312.

Khan A, Tansel A, et al. (2016). Efficacy of psychosocial interventions in inducing and maintaining alcohol abstinence in patients with chronic liver disease: a systematic review. Clin Gastroenterol Hepatol 14(2): e191–e120; quiz e120.

Kintz P (2001). Deaths involving buprenorphine: a compendium of French cases. Forensic Sci Int 121: 65–69.

Kirchmayer U, Davoli M, et al. (2003). Naltrexone maintenance treatment for opioid dependence. Cochrane Database Syst Rev 4: CD001333.

Klaman SL, Isaacs K, et al. (2017). Treating women who are pregnant and parenting for opioid use disorder and the concurrent care of their infants and children: literature review to support national guidance. J Addict Med 11(3): 178–190.

Koegelenberg CF, Noor F, et al. (2014). Efficacy of varenicline combined with nicotine replacement therapy vs. varenicline alone for smoking cessation: a randomized clinical trial. JAMA 312(2): 155–161.

Kohen I, Kremen N (2007). Varenicline-induced manic episode in a patient with bipolar disorder. Am J Psychiatry 164: 1269–1270.

Kranzler HR, Armeli S, et al. (2011). A double-blind, randomized trial of sertraline for alcohol dependence: moderation by age of onset [corrected] and 5-hydroxytryptamine transporter-linked promoter region genotype. J Clin Psychopharmacol 31(1): 22–30.

Kranzler HR, Armeli S, et al. (2012). Post-treatment outcomes in a double-blind, randomized trial of sertraline for alcohol dependence. Alcohol Clin Exp Res 36(4): 739–744.

Kranzler HR, Burleson JA, et al. (1996). Fluoxetine treatment seems to reduce the beneficial effects of cognitive-behavioral therapy in type B alcoholics. Alcohol Clin Exp Res 20(9): 1534–1541.

Kranzler HR, Ciraulo DA, Zindel LH, Eds. (2014). Clinical Manual of Addiction Psychopharmacology, Second Edition. Washington, DC: American Psychiatric Publishing.

Kranzler HR, Van Kirk J (2001). Efficacy of naltrexone and acamprosate for alcoholism treatment: a meta-analysis. Alcohol Clin Exp Res 25: 1335–1341.

Krebs TS, Johansen PO (2012). Lysergic acid diethylamide (LSD) for alcoholism: meta-analysis of randomized controlled trials. J Psychopharmacol 26(7): 994–1002.

Krupitsky E, Nunes EV, et al. (2011). Injectable extended-release naltrexone for opioid dependence. Lancet 378(9792): 665; author reply 666.

Krupitsky E, Zvartau E, et al. (2012). Randomized trial of long-acting sustained-release naltrexone implant vs oral naltrexone or placebo for preventing relapse to opioid dependence. Arch Gen Psychiatry 69(9): 973–981.

Kunoe N, Lobmaier P, et al. (2009). Naltrexone implants after in-patient treatment for opioid dependence: randomised controlled trial. Br J Psychiatry 194(6): 541–546.

Kunoe N, Lobmaier P, et al. (2010). Retention in naltrexone implant treatment for opioid dependence. Drug Alcohol Depend 111(1–2): 166–169.

Kunoe N, Lobmaier P, et al. (2014). Injectable and implantable sustained release naltrexone in the treatment of opioid addiction. Br J Clin Pharmacol 77(2): 264–271.

Laaksonen E, Koski-Jannes A, et al. (2008). A randomized, multicentre, open-label, comparative trial of disulfiram, naltrexone and acamprosate in the treatment of alcohol dependence. Alcohol 43: 53–61.

Lee JD, Friedmann PD, et al. (2016). Extended-release naltrexone to prevent opioid relapse in criminal justice offenders. N Engl J Med 374(13): 1232–1242.

Lee JD, Nunes EV, et al. (2018). Comparative effectiveness of extended-release naltrexone versus buprenorphine-naloxone for opioid relapse prevention (X:BOT): a multicentre, open-label, randomised controlled trial. Lancet 391(10118): 309–318.

Lee SC, Klein-Schwartz W, et al. (2014). Comparison of toxicity associated with nonmedical use of benzodiazepines with buprenorphine or methadone. Drug Alcohol Depend 138: 118–123.

Levin FR, Mariani JJ, et al. (2011). Dronabinol for the treatment of cannabis dependence: a randomized, double-blind, placebo-controlled trial. Drug Alcohol Depend 116(1–3): 142–150.

Lexicomp (2019). https://www.wolterskluwercdi.com/lexicomp-online/

Lind JN, Interrante JD, et al. (2017). Maternal use of opioids during pregnancy and congenital malformations: a systematic review. Pediatrics 139(6).

Ling W, Wesson RD (1984). Naltrexone treatment for addicted health-care professionals: a collaborative private practice experience. J Clin Psychiatry 45: 46–48.

Ling W, Chang L, et al. (2014). Sustained-release methylphenidate in a randomized trial of treatment of methamphetamine use disorder. Addiction 109(9): 1489–500.

Lingford-Hughes AR, Welch S, et al. (2004). Evidence-based guidelines for the pharmacological management of substance misuse, addiction and comorbidity: recommendations from the British Association for Psychopharmacology. J Psychopharmacol 18: 293–335.

Littleton J, Zieglgansberger W (2003). Pharmacological mechanisms of naltrexone and acamprosate in the prevention of relapse in alcohol dependence. Am J Addict 12(Suppl 1): S3–S11.

Liu J, Wang LN (2013). Baclofen for alcohol withdrawal. Cochrane Database Syst Rev 2: CD008502.

Longo LP, Campbell T, et al. (2002). Divalproex sodium (Depakote) for alcohol withdrawal and relapse prevention. J Addict Dis 21(2): 55–64.

Louik C, Kerr S, Mitchell AA (2014). First-trimester exposure to bupropion and risk of cardiac malformations. Pharmacoepidemiol Drug Saf 23(10): 1066–1075.

Lund IO, Fischer G, et al. (2013). A comparison of buprenorphine + naloxone to buprenorphine and methadone in the treatment of opioid dependence during pregnancy: maternal and neonatal outcomes. Subst Abuse 7: 61–74.

Lyon JE, Khan RA, et al. (2011). Treating alcohol withdrawal with oral baclofen: a randomized, double-blind, placebo-controlled trial. J Hosp Med 6(8): 469–474.

Maisel NC, Blodgett JC, et al. (2013). Meta-analysis of naltrexone and acamprosate for treating alcohol use disorders: when are these medications most helpful? Addiction 108(2): 275–293.

Mann K, Lehert P, et al. (2004). The efficacy of acamprosate in the maintenance of abstinence in alcohol-dependent individuals: results of a meta-analysis. Alcohol Clin Exp Res 28: 51–63.

Maremmani I, Rolland B, et al. (2016). Buprenorphine dosing choices in specific populations: review of expert opinion. Expert Opin Pharmacother 17(13): 1727–1731.

Martinotti G, Di Nicola M, et al. (2007). High and low dosage oxcarbazepine versus naltrexone for the prevention of relapse in alcohol-dependent patients. Hum Psychopharmacol 22(3): 149–156.

Martinotti G, Di Nicola M, et al. (2010). Pregabalin versus naltrexone in alcohol dependence: a randomised, double-blind, comparison trial. J Psychopharmacol 24(9): 1367–1374.

Mason BJ, Quello S, et al. (2014). Gabapentin treatment for alcohol dependence: a randomized clinical trial. JAMA Intern Med 174(1): 70–77.

Mattick RP, Breen C, et al. (2009). Methadone maintenance therapy versus no opioid replacement therapy for opioid dependence. Cochrane Database Syst Rev 3: CD002209.

Mattick RP, Breen C, et al. (2014). Buprenorphine maintenance versus placebo or methadone maintenance for opioid dependence. Cochrane Database Syst Rev(2): CD002207.

Mattick RP, Kimber J, et al. (2008). Buprenorphine maintenance versus placebo or methadone maintenance for opioid dependence. Cochrane Database Syst Rev 2: CD002207.

McLellan AT, Arndt IO, et al. (1993). The effects of psychosocial services in substance abuse treatment. JAMA 269(15): 1953–1959.

Megarbane B, Hreiche R, et al. (2006). Does high-dose buprenorphine cause respiratory depression? Possible mechanisms and therapeutic consequences. Toxicol Rev 25: 79–85.

Medicines and Healthcare Products Regulatory Agency & Commission on Human Medicines (2006). Risk of QT interval prolongation with methadone. Report No. 31.

Miller SC, Fiellin DA, et al. (2019). *The ASAM Principles of Addiction Medicine, 6th Edition*. Philadelphia, PA: Wolters Kluwer.

Mills EJ, Wu P, et al. (2012). Comparisons of high-dose and combination nicotine replacement therapy, varenicline, and bupropion for smoking cessation: a systematic review and multiple treatment meta-analysis. Ann Med 44(6): 588–597.

Minozzi S, Amato L, et al. (2011). Oral naltrexone maintenance treatment for opioid dependence. Cochrane Database Syst Rev 4: CD001333.

Minozzi S, Saulle R, Rosner S (2018). Baclofen for alcohol use disorder. Cochrane Database Syst Rev 11: CD012557.

Mitchell JM, Grossman LE, et al. (2012). The anticonvulsant levetiracetam potentiates alcohol consumption in non-treatment seeking alcohol abusers. J Clin Psychopharmacol 32(2): 269–272.

Moore TJ, Furberg CD, et al. (2011). Suicidal behavior and depression in smoking cessation treatments. PLoS One 6(11): e27016.

Morley KC, Teesson M, et al. (2006). Naltrexone versus acamprosate in the treatment of alcohol dependence: a multi-centre, randomized, double-blind, placebo-controlled trial. Addiction 101: 1451–1462.

Mozurkewich EL, Rayburn WF (2014). Buprenorphine and methadone for opioid addiction during pregnancy. Obstet Gynecol Clin North Am 41(2): 241–253.

Mucke M, Phillips T, et al. (2018). Cannabis-based medicines for chronic neuropathic pain in adults. Cochrane Database Syst Rev 3: CD012182.

Mueller TI, Stout RL, et al. (1997). A double-blind, placebo-controlled pilot study of carbamazepine for the treatment of alcohol dependence. Alcohol Clin Exp Res 21(1): 86–92.

Mutschler J, Grosshans M, et al. (2016). Current findings and mechanisms of action of disulfiram in the treatment of alcohol dependence. Pharmacopsychiatry 49(4): 137–141.

Muzyk AJ, Rivelli SK, et al. (2012). Defining the role of baclofen for the treatment of alcohol dependence: a systematic review of the evidence. CNS Drugs 26(1): 69–78.

Norgaard M, Nielsson MS, Heide-Jorgensen U (2015). Birth and neonatal outcomes following opioid use in pregnancy: a Danish population-based study. Subst Abuse 9(Suppl 2): 5–11.

Olmsted CL, Kockler DR (2008). Topiramate for alcohol dependence. Ann Pharmacother 42(10): 1475–1480.

O'Malley SS, Garbutt JC, et al. (2007). Efficacy of extended-release naltrexone in alcohol-dependent patients who are abstinent before treatment. J Clin Psychopharmacol 27: 507–512.

O'Malley SS, Jaffe AJ, et al. (1996). Experience of a "slip" among alcoholics treated with naltrexone or placebo. Am J Psychiatry 153(2): 281–283.

Oslin DW, Leong SH, et al. (2015). Naltrexone vs placebo for the treatment of alcohol dependence: a randomized clinical trial. JAMA Psychiatry 72(5): 430–437.

Oulis P, Konstantakopoulos G (2012). Efficacy and safety of pregabalin in the treatment of alcohol and benzodiazepine dependence. Expert Opin Investig Drugs 21(7): 1019–1029.

Patra J, Bakker R, et al. (2011). Dose-response relationship between alcohol consumption before and during pregnancy and the risks of low birthweight, preterm birth and small for gestational age (SGA) —a systematic review and meta-analyses. BJOG 118(12): 1411–1421.

PDR (2019). Prescriber's digital reference. www.pdr.net

Pereira PP, Da Mata FA, et al. (2017). Maternal active smoking during pregnancy and low birth weight in the Americas: a systematic review and meta-analysis. Nicotine Tob Res 19(5): 497–505.

Petrov I, Krogh J, et al. (2011). Meta-analysis of pharmacological therapy with acamprosate, naltrexone, and disulfiram—a systematic review. Ugeskr Laeger 173(48): 3103–3109.

Pettinati HM, O'Brien CP, et al. (2006). The status of naltrexone in the treatment of alcohol dependence: specific effects on heavy drinking. J Clin Psychopharmacol 26: 610–625.

Pettinati HM, Oslin DW, et al. (2010). A double-blind, placebo-controlled trial combining sertraline and naltrexone for treating co-occurring depression and alcohol dependence. Am J Psychiatry 167(6): 668–675.

Pettinati HM, Silverman BL, et al. (2011). Efficacy of extended-release naltrexone in patients with relatively higher severity of alcohol dependence. Alcohol Clin Exp Res 35(10): 1804–1811.

Pettinati HM, Volpicelli JR, et al. (2000). Sertraline treatment for alcohol dependence: interactive effects of medication and alcoholic subtype. Alcohol Clin Exp Res 24(7): 1041–1049.

Pineles BL, Hsu S, et al. (2016). Systematic review and meta-analyses of perinatal death and maternal exposure to tobacco smoke during pregnancy. Am J Epidemiol 184(2): 87–97.

Pineles BL, Park E, Samet JM (2014). Systematic review and meta-analysis of miscarriage and maternal exposure to tobacco smoke during pregnancy. Am J Epidemiol 179(7): 807–823.

Piper ME, Smith SS, et al. (2009). A randomized placebo-controlled clinical trial of 5 smoking cessation pharmacotherapies. Arch Gen Psychiatry 66(11): 1253–1262.

Prochaska JJ, Hilton JF (2012). Risk of cardiovascular serious adverse events associated with varenicline use for tobacco cessation: systematic review and meta-analysis. BMJ 344: e2856.

Rasmussen DD, Kincaid CL, Froehlich JC (2017). Prazosin prevents increased anxiety behavior that occurs in response to stress during alcohol deprivations. Alcohol 52(1): 5–11.

Ray LA, Green R, et al. (2019). Naltrexone effects on subjective responses to alcohol in the human laboratory: a systematic review and meta-analysis. Addict Biol 24(6): 1138–1152.

Reece-Stremtan S, Marinelli KA (2015). ABM clinical protocol #21: guidelines for breastfeeding and substance use or substance use disorder, revised 2015. Breastfeed Med 10(3): 135–141.

Rezaei F, Emami M, et al. (2015). Sustained-release methylphenidate in methamphetamine dependence treatment: a double-blind and placebo-controlled study. Daru 23: 2.

Richter C, Effenberger S, et al. (2012). Efficacy and safety of levetiracetam for the prevention of alcohol relapse in recently detoxified alcohol-dependent patients: a randomized trial. J Clin Psychopharmacol 32(4): 558–562.

Rosenthal RN, Lofwall MR, et al. (2016). Effect of buprenorphine implants on illicit opioid use among abstinent adults with opioid dependence treated with sublingual buprenorphine: a randomized clinical trial. JAMA 316(3): 282–290.

Rosner S, Hackl-Herrwerth A, et al. (2010). Acamprosate for alcohol dependence. Cochrane Database Syst Rev 9: CD004332.

Rubio G, Jimenez-Arriero MA, et al. (2001). Naltrexone versus acamprosate: one year follow-up of alcohol dependence treatment. Alcohol 36: 419–425.

Rubio G, Martinez-Gras I, et al. (2009). Modulation of impulsivity by topiramate: implications for the treatment of alcohol dependence. J Clin Psychopharmacol 29(6): 584–589.

Saber-Tehrani AS, Bruce RD, Altice FL (2011). Pharmacokinetic drug interactions and adverse consequences between psychotropic medications and pharmacotherapy for the treatment of opioid dependence. Am J Drug Alcohol Abuse 37(1): 1–11.

Sachs HC; Committee on Drugs (2013). The transfer of drugs and therapeutics into human breast milk: an update on selected topics. Pediatrics 132(3): e796–e809.

Sass H, Soyka M, et al. (1996). Relapse prevention by acamprosate: results from a placebo-controlled study on alcohol dependence. Arch Gen Psychiatry 53: 673–680.

Savulich G, Riccelli R, et al. (2017). Effects of naltrexone are influenced by childhood adversity during negative emotional processing in addiction recovery. Transl Psychiatry 7(3): e1054.

Silagy C, Lancaster T, et al. (2004). Nicotine replacement therapy for smoking cessation. Cochrane Database Syst Rev 3: CD000146.

Silagy C, Mant D, et al. (2000). Nicotine replacement therapy for smoking cessation. Cochrane Database Syst Rev 3: CD000146.

Simpson TL, Malte CA, et al. (2015). A pilot trial of prazosin, an alpha-1 adrenergic antagonist, for comorbid alcohol dependence and posttraumatic stress disorder. Alcohol Clin Exp Res 39(5): 808–817.

Simpson TL, Saxon AJ, et al. (2009). A pilot trial of the alpha-1 adrenergic antagonist, prazosin, for alcohol dependence. Alcohol Clin Exp Res 33(2): 255–263.

Simpson TL, Saxon AJ, et al. (2018). Double-blind randomized clinical trial of prazosin for alcohol use disorder. Am J Psychiatry 175(12): 1216–1224.

Singh S, Loke YK, et al. (2011). Risk of serious adverse cardiovascular events associated with varenicline: a systematic review and meta-analysis. CMAJ 183(12): 1359–1366.

Smith RV, Havens JR, Walsh SL (2016). Gabapentin misuse, abuse and diversion: a systematic review. Addiction 111(7): 1160–1174.

Soneji S, Beltran-Sanchez H (2019). Association of maternal cigarette smoking and smoking cessation with preterm birth. JAMA Netw Open 2(4): e192514.

Sordo L, Barrio G, et al. (2017). Mortality risk during and after opioid substitution treatment: systematic review and meta-analysis of cohort studies. BMJ 357: j1550.

Soyka, M. (2017). Treatment of opioid dependence with buprenorphine: current update. Dialogues Clin Neurosci 19(3): 299–308.

Soyka M, Rosner S (2008). Opioid antagonists for pharmacological treatment of alcohol dependence—a critical review. Curr Drug Abuse Rev 1(3): 280–291.

Srisurapanont M, Jarusuraisin N (2005). Opioid antagonists for alcohol dependence. Cochrane Database Syst Rev 12: CD001867.

Stead LF, Koilpillai P, Lancaster T (2015). Additional behavioural support as an adjunct to pharmacotherapy for smoking cessation. Cochrane Database Syst Rev 10: CD009670.

Stead LF, Perera R, et al. (2012). Nicotine replacement therapy for smoking cessation. Cochrane Database Syst Rev 11: CD000146.

Suh JJ, Pettinati HM, et al. (2006). The status of disulfiram: a half of a century later. J Clin Psychopharmacol 26: 290–302.

Sullivan MA, Bisaga A, et al. (2019). A randomized trial comparing extended-release injectable suspension and oral naltrexone, both combined with behavioral therapy, for the treatment of opioid use disorder. Am J Psychiatry 176(2): 129–137.

Svanstrom H, Pasternak B, et al. (2012). Use of varenicline for smoking cessation and risk of serious cardiovascular events: nationwide cohort study. BMJ 345: e7176.

Swamy GK, Roelands JJ, et al. (2009). Predictors of adverse events among pregnant smokers exposed in a nicotine replacement therapy trial. Am J Obstet Gynecol 201(4): 354 e351–e357.

Tanum L, Solli KK, et al. (2017). Effectiveness of Injectable extended-release naltrexone vs daily buprenorphine-naloxone for opioid dependence: a randomized clinical noninferiority trial. JAMA Psychiatry 74(12): 1197–1205.

Taylor D, Paton C, Kapur S (2015). *The Maudsley Prescribing Guidelines in Psychiatry, 12th Edition*. London, England: John Wiley.

Tiihonen J, Krupitsky E, et al. (2012). Naltrexone implant for the treatment of polydrug dependence: a randomized controlled trial. Am J Psychiatry 169(5): 531–536.

Tonstad S, Tonnesen P, et al. (2006). Effect of maintenance therapy with varenicline on smoking cessation: a randomized controlled trial. JAMA 296: 64–71.

Tracqui A, Kintz P, Ludes B (1998). Buprenorphine-related deaths among drug addicts in France: a report on 20 fatalities. J Anal Toxicol 22(6): 430–434.

Tran TH, Griffin BL, Stone RH, et al. (2017). Methadone, buprenorphine, and naltrexone for the treatment of opioid use disorder in pregnant women. Pharmacotherapy 37(7): 824–839.

Wachman EM, Saia K, et al. (2016). Revision of breastfeeding guidelines in the setting of maternal opioid use disorder: one institution's experience. J Hum Lact 32(2): 382–387.

Walsh SL, Preston KL, et al. (1994). Clinical pharmacology of buprenorphine: ceiling effects at high doses. Clin Pharmacol Ther 55(5): 569–580.

Washton AM, Gold MS, et al. (1984). Successful use of naltrexone in addicted physicians and business executives. Adv Alcohol Subst Abuse 4: 89–96.

Whitworth AB, Fischer F, et al. (1996). Comparison of acamprosate and placebo in long-term treatment of alcohol dependence. Lancet 347: 1438–1442.

Wiegand SL, Stringer EM, et al. (2015). Buprenorphine and naloxone compared with methadone treatment in pregnancy. Obstet Gynecol 125(2): 363–368.

World Health Organization (2019). World Health Organization model list of essential medicines, 21st list. https://apps.who.int/iris/bitstream/handle/10665/325771/WHO-MVP-EMP-IAU-2019.06-eng.pdf?ua=1

Yoon SJ, Pae CU, et al. (2006). Mirtazapine for patients with alcohol dependence and comorbid depressive disorders: a multicentre, open label study. Prog Neuropsychopharmacol Biol Psychiatry 30(7): 1196–1201.

Zedler BK, Mann AL, et al. (2016). Buprenorphine compared with methadone to treat pregnant women with opioid use disorder: a systematic review and meta-analysis of safety in the mother, fetus and child. Addiction 111(12): 2115–2128.

Epilogue

Over the last five decades, multiple medications have become available for the treatment of patients with psychiatric disorders. Tricyclic antidepressants, monoamine oxidase inhibitors, selective serotonin reuptake inhibitors, serotonin-norepinephrine reuptake inhibitors, and other antidepressants have expanded current treatment options for depressive and anxiety disorders. Anxiolytics, including benzodiazepines and nondependence-producing alternatives, are available for the treatment of severe anxiety disorders. First- and second-generation antipsychotics with different receptor profiles and side effect profiles have expanded the choices for patients with psychotic disorders. Lithium and other medications with partial mood-stabilizing properties are available for use in patients with bipolar disorder. New formulations of stimulants and nonstimulant agents can be used in adults with attention-deficit/hyperactivity disorder. Finally, pharmacological therapies for the treatment of substance use disorders have been greatly expanded in recent years.

As noted earlier, students and clinicians should be aware that psychiatric medications are studied for the treatment of psychiatric disorders or syndromes and not for the alleviation of individual symptoms. But they are sometimes used for symptoms, although this is off-label and not evidence-supported. Furthermore, not all presenting symptoms and complaints should be seen as signs of medical illness or pathology.

The science and art of medicine comprise the ability to appropriately and carefully apply that which is learned in textbooks to a specific patient. In the clinical setting, pharmacotherapeutic treatments should be used judiciously. One should employ the least harmful strategies, for example, by using the lowest effective dose or using one medication at a time, so as to have the opportunity to know what is actually working or not working and to avoid subjecting a patient to unnecessary harm.

There is still much that is not known about available medications. We may have some understanding of the mechanisms of action of many medications at the level of the neuronal synapse and receptors, but we know far less about downstream effects that are actually responsible for the amelioration of clinical symptoms. We must not assume that we know all there is to know about every available medication. Every new drug presents promises for improved treatment—as well as potential adverse effects that temper those promises. There are times when potential adverse effects of current medications (especially those of the newest medications) cannot be fully appreciated or anticipated. Most initial studies are short-term studies; long-term risks become more clear only with long-term clinical experience. Even when short-term studies and long-term experiences inform us of the expected clinical effects of a medication, unexpected idiosyncratic reactions due to patient variability cannot be ruled out. Therefore, a degree of humility is necessary when considering pharmacotherapy for patients, both individually and on a large scale, and with older as well as the newest medicines.

As Hippocrates advised a long time ago, "to do nothing is sometimes a good remedy." William Osler added that it is sometimes more important to know when to "educate [patients] *not* to take medicine" (Garrison 1928; Bean 1961). Sometimes less is more—notwithstanding societal pressures to end every medical encounter with a prescription for a new medication.

In summary, as we anticipate future trends in psychophar-macology, we must maintain the cautious approach of our prede-cessors with a sober understanding of the risks and benefits of available treatments as they pertain to each individual patient. We need to remember, also, that the field of psychiatry is much larger than pharmacotherapy. The provision of psychosocial supports and psychotherapeutic treatments are likely to increase the chances that pharmacotherapeutic interventions and overall treatment will be successful. The ultimate goal is to provide relief and lessen suffering in the most cautious, humane, evidence-based, and cost-effective manner possible.

References

Bean RB, Ed. (1961). *Sir William Osler: Aphorisms From His Bedside Teachings and Writings.* Springfield, IL: Charles C. Thomas.

Garrison FH (1928). Medical proverbs, aphorisms and epigrams. Bull N Y Acad Med 4(10): 979–1005.

Index

Tables are indicated by *t* following the page number.

for bipolar disorder,
152–54, 195–97
and breastfeeding, 157
choice of, 141–44
complementary, alter-
native, and other
pharmacotherapies, 140–41
for depression, 152
drug interactions, 23, 193
for eating disorders, 154
emerging, 139–40, 166*t*
first-generation, 121–26, 325
long-acting injectable,
148–49, 197
for nonpsychiatric
disorders, 155
for personality
disorders, 154
in pregnancy, 155–57
second-generation, 124–39,
164*t*–65*t*, 165*t*–66*t*, 325
time to response, 144–45
treatment
continuation, 145–46
antiretroviral drugs, 269
anxiety, 85
anti-anxiety medicines, 85–119,
105*t*–10*t*, 325
anti-anxiety medicines without abuse potential, 90–95
antipsychotics for, 151–52
treatment-resistant, 102–3
anxiety disorders, 85–86,
99–101, 325
anxiolytics. *See* anti-anxiety
medicines
Aplenzin®. *See* bupropion
Aptensio XR®. *See*
methylphenidate

aripiprazole (Abilify®, Abilify
Discmelt®, Abilify
Maintena®, Abilify Mycite®,
Aristada®)
for bipolar disorder, 196–97
for depression, 42
effectiveness, 142
long-acting injectable, 148–49
for mania, 195
for psychotic disorders, 126,
131–33, 142, 148–49, 163*t*
for schizophrenia, 150
for tics, 155
armodafinil, 240–41
asenapine (Saphris®, Secuado®)
for bipolar disorder, 196–97
for mania, 195
for psychotic disorders, 126,
136–38, 165*t*
aspirin, 191
Atarax®. *See* hydroxyzine
Ativan®. *See* lorazepam
atomoxetine (Strattera®), 234,
238–39, 243, 248–49, 254*t*
attention-deficit/hyperactivity
disorder (ADHD)
diagnosis, 231, 241–42
prevalence, 245–46
and sleep, 244–45
treatment-resistant, 248–49
attention-deficit/hyperactivity
disorder (ADHD) medicines,
231–66, 253*t*–55*t*, 325
and breastfeeding, 252
clinical use, 241–42
for college students, 245–48
complementary, alternative,
and others, 241
drug holidays, 243–44

dyskinesia, tardive, 124–25
dyspepsia, functional, 49
dysthymic disorder, 41
dystonia, acute, 123–24

EAGLES (Evaluating Adverse
    Events in a Global Smoking
    Cessations Study), 285–86
eating disorders
    antidepressants for, 47–48
    antipsychotics for, 154
e-cigarettes (electronic
    cigarettes), 283–84
ECT. *See* electroconvulsive
    therapy
Edluar®. *See* zolpidem
effectiveness studies, 4–5
Effexor®. *See* venlafaxine
efficacy, 4
Elavil®. *See* amitriptyline
electroconvulsive
    therapy (ECT)
    for bipolar disorder, 205, 207
    for depression, 45
    for schizophrenia, 150–51
electronic cigarettes
    (e-cigarettes), 283–84
Emsam®. *See* transdermal
    selegiline
Equetro®. *See* carbamazepine
erythromycin, 269
escitalopram (Lexapro®)
    for depression, 40–41, 58t
    side effects, 22–23, 25–26
Eskalith®. *See* lithium carbonate
esketamine
    for bipolar disorder, 199
    for depression, 45, 63t
    nasal spray (Spravato®), 63t

eszopiclone (Lunesta®), 95,
    104, 110t
Evaluating Adverse Events in a
    Global Smoking Cessations
    Study (EAGLES), 285–86
evidence-based
    psychopharmacology, 4–7

Fanapt®. *See* iloperidone
fatigue
    mental, 251
    stimulants for, 251
FazaClo®. *See* clozapine
FD (functional dyspepsia), 49
fetal alcohol spectrum
    disorders, 299
fetal alcohol syndrome, 299
Fetzima®. *See*
    levomilnacipran ER
FGAs (first-generation
    antipsychotics), 121–26
first-generation antipsychotics
    (FGAs), 325
    for acute behavioral
        control, 146–48
    for bipolar disorder, 152–53
    and breastfeeding, 157
    choice of, 142–44
    dosing, 123
    for nonpsychiatric
        disorders, 155
    for psychotic disorders, 121–
        26, 142–43, 158t–59t
    side effects, 123–24
fluoxetine (Prozac®, Prozac
    Weekly®, Sarafem®)
    for alcohol use
        disorder, 281–82
    for bipolar depression, 196

hydroxyzine (Atarax®,
  Vistaril®)
  for anxiety, 93, 102–4, 108t
  for insomnia, 102, 104, 108t
  in pregnancy, 104
hyperparathyroidism,
  lithium-induced, 189
hypertensive crisis, 20
hypnotics, 95–99, 109t–10t
  clinical use of, 99–103
  side effects, 96–97
hypothyroidism, 189

IBS (irritable bowel
  syndrome), 49
iloperidone (Fanapt®), 126,
  136–37, 164t
imipramine (Tofranil®), 17, 53t
impulsivity, 208
Inderal®. See propranolol
injectable antipsychotics,
  long-acting, 148–49
Innopran XL® (propranolol). See
  propranolol
inositol, 200
insomnia
  anxiolytics and hypnotics
    for, 101–2
  complementary, alternative,
    and other pharmacothera-
    pies for, 98
  non-antidepressant medicines
    for, 104, 105t–10t
Intermezzo®. See zolpidem
international guidelines, 5
Intuniv®. See guanfacine
  extended release
Invega®. See paliperidone
iproniazid, 20

irritable bowel syndrome
  (IBS), 49
isocarboxazid (Marplan®),
  20, 62t

JORNAY PM®. See
  methylphenidate

Kapvay®. See clonidine
kava (Piper methysticum), 98
ketamine
  for bipolar disorder, 198–99
  for depression, 34–35, 45
ketoconazole, 269
Khedezla®. See desvenlafaxine
Klonopin®. See clonazepam

lactation. See breastfeeding
LactMed database (TOXNET), 8
lamotrigine (Lamictal®,
  Lamictal XR®)
  for bipolar depression, 201–2
  for bipolar disorder, 190, 193–
    94, 200–203, 211, 214t
  and breastfeeding, 211–12
  drug interactions, 194
  for maintenance
    therapy, 202–3
  in pregnancy, 211
  side effects, 192
Latuda®. See lurasidone
lavender, 98
lemborexant, 97
levetiracetam
  for alcohol use disorder, 280
  for bipolar disorder, 197–98
levomilnacipran ER (Fetzima®),
  28, 30, 62t
levothyroxine, 199